THE
ESSENTIAL GUIDE
TO VITAMINS
AND MINERALS

THE ESSENTIAL GUIDE TO VITAMINS AND MINERALS

Health Media of America

AND

Elizabeth Somer, M.A., R.D.

HarperPerennial
A Division of HarperCollinsPublishers

HarperCollins books may be purchased for educational, business, or sales promotional use. For information, please call or write: Special Markets Department, HarperCollins Publishers, Inc., 10 East 53rd Street, New York, NY 10022. Telephone: (212) 207–7528; Fax: (212) 207–7222.

Library of Congress Cataloging-in-Publication Data

Somer, Elizabeth.
    The essential guide to vitamins and minerals / Health Media of America and Elizabeth Somer.
      p. cm.
    Includes bibliographical references and index.
    ISBN 0-06-271516-X — ISBN 0-06-273045-2 (pbk.)
    1. Vitamins in human nutrition. 2. Minerals in human nutrition.
I. Health Media of America (Firm) II. Title.
    [DNLM: 1. Minerals. 2. Nutrition Disorders—diagnosis.
3. Nutrition Disorders—therapy. 4. Vitamins. QU 160 S694e]
QP771.S66   1992
612.3'99—dc20
DNLM/DLC for Library of Congress   91-55390

93 94 95 PS/HC 10 9 8 7 6 5 4 3

Health Media of America Editorial Board

Contents

SECTION 2
VITAMINS AND MINERALS IN THE PREVENTION
AND TREATMENT OF DISEASE

SECTION 3
THE VITAMIN/MINERAL-RICH DIET

CHAPTER 1

Nutrition as a Way of Life

People want to feel and look their best no matter what their ages. Most people want the energy, enthusiasm, and good health to enjoy life and they want freedom from crippling disorders that interfere with that enjoyment. Although a person's level of health throughout life will vary based on hereditary uniqueness, achieving optimal health depends in large part on what and how much a person eats.

The phrase "you are what you eat" is now supported by scientific research. A balanced diet of wholesome, nutritious, low-fat foods reduces a person's risk for developing many of the common degenerative diseases, such as heart disease, stroke, high blood pressure, cancer, diabetes, osteoporosis, and obesity. A diet that supplies optimal amounts of vitamins and minerals helps a person not only avoid disease, but also feel his or her best, with the emotional and physical health necessary to enjoy life to its fullest.

The opposite is also true. A diet unbalanced in favor of high-fat, high-sugar, low-fiber, or salty foods is associated with low vitamin and mineral intake and a higher risk for developing disease, or at best not feeling "up to par." Since people do not possess a natural instinct for choosing nutritious, wholesome foods, it is important to learn which nutrients the body needs and what to eat to meet these nutrient needs. "You are what you eat" is a promise of better health if a person takes the time to choose nutritious foods and to practice good eating habits.

1

THE CHANGING AMERICAN DIET

The typical American diet today is much different than the diet chosen at the beginning of the century. Many traditional foods, such as milk, broccoli, bread, and meat, still grace American dining tables, but they are now outnumbered by thousands of new processed, refined, or convenience foods, such as French fries, soda pop, frozen dinners, and ready-to-eat cereals. In some ways the changes in the way individuals in America eat are an improvement; in other ways good eating habits in this country are on the decline.

Advertising has proven "you are what you are told to eat." Millions of dollars are spent each year by large food and restaurant corporations to convince people they should eat one processed food or another. Food selection has changed dramatically as a result. The marketing of food, however, is motivated by sales, not nutrition, and can cause a person to make food choices based on generalities, misconceptions, half-truths, and superstitions. For example, a person concerned about nutrition might choose a commercial granola cereal because it is "natural" and contains no "additives" or white sugar. The cereal, however, might provide more than 30% of its calories from a highly saturated fat called coconut oil. One person might swallow a half dozen vitamin and mineral supplements instead of taking the time to make good food choices while another person grabs a "breakfast bar," containing more sugar than is found in a candy bar, in an effort to lose weight. In most cases, these unhealthful food choices are based on misconceptions and marketing strategies.

Food selections have never been greater. Approximately 500 new foods enter the marketplace each year. However, more than one-half of all foods are processed or refined and their nutrient quality never equals their natural, unprocessed counterparts. Most advertisements are for convenience foods high in fat, salt, sugar, air, or water. Seldom are fresh fruits and vegetables, whole grain breads, non-fat dairy products, or extra lean beef advertised.

Changes in the family structure also have influenced eating patterns. Dual-career and single-parent families have increased the demand for time-saving, highly processed convenience foods. In addition, people today as compared to people in 1910 are more likely to skip meals, snack, diet, and eat away from home.

Today, people consume fewer calories than did their ancestors. The reduced food intake means these diets cannot always guarantee daily recommended amounts of vitamins and minerals, especially for those people who diet, have irregular eating habits, skip meals, or choose poorly from the wealth of food selections available. Consequently, the nutritional changes in the American diet since 1910 include a 31% increase in fat consumption; a 43% reduction in complex carbohydrate (starch) consumption; and a 50% increase in sugar consumption. The influences of these dietary changes are reflected in the disease statistics in the United States since 1910. The incidence of cardiovascular disease, including heart disease, high blood pressure, and stroke; cancer; diabetes; and obesity has increased.

Major national surveys repeatedly show that diets consumed by many Americans are not well-balanced. Inadequate intake of vitamins and minerals are frequently reported, including vitamin A, vitamin C, vitamin B_1, vitamin B_2, folic acid, vitamin B_6, calcium, copper, iron, manganese, and zinc. In addition, 9 in 10 diets are estimated to be low in chromium, and magnesium intake is approximately half the amount recommended in the RDAs.

Although more than 80% of adult consumers think ". . . it is alright to eat what you want when you want it," good eating habits are not instinctive. The body and mind do not automatically choose nutritious foods, especially in light of modern distractions and highly sophisticated marketing and advertising techniques. Even the well-planned diet can be lacking in vitamins and minerals when processed foods are overused or foods are not stored or prepared properly. If an individual chooses a diet that contains less than 2,000 calories, he or she cannot be guaranteed an optimal supply of all vitamins and minerals.

The best way to guarantee optimal intake of all vitamins and minerals is to understand which of the nutrients in the diet are most likely to be low and to learn how to design and consume a nutritious diet based on individual needs. At no other time in history has nutritious and safe food been more accessible. The challenge is learning how to wisely select the most healthful food while planning a diet that tastes good, looks good, and fits into your lifestyle.

SECTION 1

VITAMIN AND MINERAL BASICS

CHAPTER 2

Vitamins, Minerals, and the Body

The body requires more than 45 nutrients from the diet to maintain health. Those 45-plus nutrients can be obtained from a variety of foods and diet patterns within a wide range of calorie intakes. Although in theory it is a simple task to meet the body's daily nutritional needs, in practice many people make the wrong food choices, consume too many calories or too few vitamins or minerals, or choose foods that promote rather than prevent the development of degenerative diseases. In addition, undetected marginal deficiencies of vitamins and minerals can interfere with the quality and length of life. The epidemic of cancer, cardiovascular disease, adult-onset diabetes, osteoporosis, iron deficiency anemia, and obesity in the United States will attest to the difficulty some people have in designing an optimal diet for life (Table 1).

The first step in providing the best nutrition for the body is to understand the basics about nutrients, how information about individual nutrients can be organized into simple guidelines for dietary intake, and the importance of designing a diet that provides optimal, not minimal, amounts of all vitamins and minerals.

7

Table 1.
THE ESSENTIAL NUTRIENTS

CARBOHYDRATE
Glucose

AMINO ACIDS

Arginine	Methionine
Histidine	Phenylalanine
Isoleucine	Threonine
Leucine	Tryptophan
Lysine	Valine

FATS
Linoleic Acid

VITAMINS

Biotin	Vitamin B_6
Folic Acid	Vitamin B_{12}
Niacin	Vitamin C
Pantothenic Acid	Vitamin D
Vitamin A	Vitamin E
Vitamin B_1	Vitamin K
Vitamin B_2	

MINERALS

Calcium	Molybdenum
Chloride	Nickel
Chromium	Phosphorus
Cobalt	Potassium
Copper	Selenium
Fluorine	Silicon
Iodine	Sodium
Iron	Sulfur
Magnesium	Vanadium
Manganese	Zinc

WATER

THE NUTRIENT CATEGORIES

A nutrient is a substance obtained from food and used by the body for growth, maintenance, or repair of tissues. Nutrients are divided into six categories: protein, carbohydrate, fat, vitamins, minerals, and water. Water is the most abundant nutrient in the body, followed by protein, fat, and carbohydrate. Vitamins and minerals constitute the smallest percentage of body weight, but are just as important as the other four nutrient categories.

Three categories of nutrients—protein, carbohydrate, and fat—provide calories. They are called the *energy nutrients*. The energy they provide is used by the body to fuel the billions of chemical reactions that sustain life each day, heat the body and maintain body temperature, move muscles, build structures such as bones, or is stored as fat for later use. (See Appendix page 327 for more information on calories.) The primary role of protein is to build tissues and other essential compounds, such as hormones. Vitamins and minerals are important in the regulation of all body processes and also act as structural components, such as calcium and magnesium in bone, but they do not provide calories or energy.

Alcohol also supplies calories, but is not a nutrient because it does not contribute to the maintenance, repair, and growth of body tissues. In contrast, it is damaging to tissues when consumed in even moderate amounts or over long periods of time. Calories from alcohol can be converted to fat when total calorie consumption exceeds the daily requirement.

Most foods provide a combination of the six categories of nutrients. For example, chicken is a protein-rich food that contains a generous supply of niacin, iron, and other trace minerals. Whole wheat bread is called a carbohydrate-rich food, but also supplies protein, vitamins, minerals, and small amounts of fat and water. Milk is more than a source of calcium; it also contains vitamin B_2, protein, carbohydrate, vitamin D, water, magnesium, and other nutrients. The exceptions to this rule are sugar, which is pure carbohydrate, and oils or other fats, which are pure fat.

Essential nutrients are substances the body is unable to make in adequate amounts to sustain life and therefore must be obtained from the diet. Up to 8 or 10 amino acids (the building blocks of protein), most of the 13 vitamins, 15 to 20 minerals, and 1 oil, called linoleic acid, are essential nutrients. Carbohydrates can be made from amino acids, but this is an inefficient use of protein; therefore, dietary sources of carbohydrate, such as starchy foods, are also important in the daily diet. Most fats, including cholesterol, are manufactured from other substances in the diet and body and are nonessential nutrients. Vitamin D must be obtained from dietary sources and is considered an essential nutrient if a person is not exposed to sunlight. Niacin becomes an essential nutrient when the diet supplies insufficient amounts of the amino acid tryptophan, which the body can convert to niacin. Essential does not only mean necessary, as nonessential nutrients are also necessary, but refers to the body's *dependency* on the diet for a source of the nutrient.

Nutrients always work as teams; no vitamin or mineral works alone in the body. For example, the B vitamins are essential for extracting energy from the calorie-containing nutrients. Calcium, phosphorus, and magnesium are essential components of bones. Nerve impulses require adequate amounts of sodium, potassium, and chloride, as well as calcium and vitamin B_{12}. The digestion of food requires a healthy digestive tract dependent on a constant supply of all vitamins and minerals. Healthy skin requires a frequent supply of most nutrients, including vitamin B_2, niacin, folic acid, iron, vitamin E, and the essential fat linoleic acid. Red blood cell formation and the maintenance of a constant oxygen supply to the brain and body tissues are dependent on a constant supply of iron, vitamin C, copper, vitamin B_6, vitamin B_{12}, folic acid, and protein.

A person eats only two to six times a day, but the tissues require a constant supply of nutrients. The body is efficient in regulating the storage and release of nutrients entering from the digestive tract so that constant blood levels of vitamins, minerals, and other substances are maintained if the diet is adequate. The liver is a primary organ in the control of many nutrients. For example, vitamin A entering from the digestive tract is transported in the blood to the liver where small amounts are released gradually to maintain blood levels while the rest is stored for later use. Calcium is stored in bones and constantly released in small amounts to maintain blood calcium levels. Excess calories are stored in fat tissue and released when extra energy is needed.

Optimal and regular intake of all vitamins and minerals is necessary to maintain storage levels and readily available supplies of nutrients for all body functions. The Recommended Dietary Allowances (RDAs) are the most commonly used guidelines for determining how much of each vitamin and mineral people need to maintain health.

THE RECOMMENDED DIETARY ALLOWANCES

The Recommended Dietary Allowances (RDAs) are suggested levels of intake for several essential nutrients. They are established by the Food and Nutrition Board, National Research Council of the National Academy of Sciences—a group composed of scientists and other nutrition experts. The RDAs have become the primary nutrient standards used in the United States and throughout the world. Since 1943 they have evolved and are updated from current research approximately every 5 years. The RDAs are based on a person's age, weight, height, and gender. The RDAs provide dietary intake guidelines for:

Calories	Folic acid	Phosphorus
Protein	Niacin	Iodine
Vitamin A	Vitamin B_2	Iron
Vitamin D	Vitamin B_1	Magnesium
Vitamin E	Vitamin B_6	Selenium
Vitamin K	Vitamin B_{12}	Zinc
Vitamin C	Calcium	

An additional table of "safe and adequate daily dietary intakes" provides ranges of intakes for biotin, pantothenic acid, copper, manganese, fluoride, chromium, molybdenum, sodium, potassium, and chloride.

The RDAs replaced the now outdated "Minimum Daily Requirements" or MDRs. The RDA for each nutrient is designed to meet or exceed most people's requirement for that nutrient and, in most cases, the RDA contains a wide margin of safety. What does this margin of safety mean? It means that the "R" in RDA stands for recommendation, not requirement, and that the RDAs are not minimum requirements, but meet the nutrient requirements and contain an extra allowance for most people.

The RDAs are the "best game in town" when it comes to deciding the nutritional adequacy of a person's diet. However, they are not without limitations. The RDAs are designed for the "reference" person, the average woman or man with an average weight, body fat percentage, nutrient absorption and excretion rate, stress level, and heredity pattern. The RDA for many nutrients would require adjustment if one falls outside these descriptions.

The RDAs are only estimates of nutrient needs. In many cases the available research on a nutrient is scarce and a recommendation is based on the amount of a nutrient found in the "normal" diet. In addition, the following considerations influence the usefulness of the RDAs:

1. The RDAs are expressed as daily amounts, but actually are averages for each nutrient to be consumed over a week's time.
2. The RDAs are based on nutrient requirements for healthy persons and might not be adequate during illness or chronic use of medications, for the elderly, or when other factors alter nutrient requirements. They are recommendations for maintenance of nutrient status and might be inadequate if a person needs to restore depleted vitamin and mineral stores because of long-term illness or poor dietary habits.

3. Recommendations for some nutrients, especially the nutrients included in the Safe and Adequate Ranges are based on limited information and can be considered, at best, estimates of nutrient needs.
4. Interactions between nutrients or between nutrients and other substances in the diet were not considered in the development of the RDAs but could affect absorption, utilization, and excretion of vitamins and minerals. For example, excessive intake of calcium or protein might interfere with absorption and use of magnesium. Large doses of iron upset the absorption of zinc and copper.
5. The RDAs are based on the assumption that people will store and prepare foods with reasonable care to ensure retention of vitamins and minerals. Improper storage or preparation techniques could result in excessive loss of nutrients from food and potential vitamin or mineral deficiencies.
6. The RDAs are recommendations to prevent classical nutrient deficiency diseases and to maintain growth, maintenance, and repair of tissues. They do not consider the relationship between nutrients and the prevention of disease. For example, the RDA for vitamin A is based on maintenance of normal blood levels of the fat-soluble vitamin and the prevention of vitamin A deficiency symptoms. The dietary advice from the Institute of Medicine of the National Academy of Sciences (a different branch of the same umbrella organization that oversees the development of the RDAs) and the Cancer Institute of the National Institutes of Health includes a recommendation to increase dietary intake of vitamin A to reduce the risk of developing cancer. This recommendation and the research on which it is based are not considered in the RDA for vitamin A.

Until more precise recommendations are developed, or the RDAs are revised to include recommendations for optimal health and the prevention of degenerative diseases, it is wise for a person to consider the following when designing an individualized nutritious diet:

1. The RDAs are the best guidelines available for vitamin, mineral, protein, and energy intakes; however, they are not perfect. They are based on the most reliable information available, but still remain only estimates of nutrient needs. Although the RDAs are generous in their recommendations, it is wise to strive for an average dietary intake that meets 100% of the RDAs.
2. When some is good, more is not necessarily better. Excessive intake of one or more nutrients can be dangerous, can upset the

delicate balance between nutrients and result in secondary deficiencies of other vitamins or minerals, and can result in temporary or permanent damage to the body. Vitamins in large doses can act more like drugs than nutrients, and megadoses should be taken only with the supervision of a physician.

MARGINAL DEFICIENCIES

Classical nutrient deficiency symptoms are described in detail in all nutrition textbooks and are memorized by all conscientious nutrition authorities. However, scurvy (the classic disease of vitamin C deficiency), beriberi (an extreme deficiency of vitamin B_1), and xerophthalmia (the final stage of vitamin A deficiency) are unusual in the United States. These symptom-diseases are characteristic of long-term and severe vitamin or mineral deficiencies. Long before the gums recede in scurvy or dermatitis develops in beriberi, a series of harmful, yet subtle, changes have taken place in the body. These subclinical changes are characteristic of marginal nutrient deficiencies.

A marginal nutrient deficiency is a condition where the body's vitamin or mineral stores are gradually drained, resulting in loss of optimal health and impairment of body processes that depend on that nutrient. Marginal nutrient deficiencies can develop from long-term poor dietary intake; altered absorption, use, or excretion of a nutrient; or chronic use of medications or alcohol, which interfere with the absorption or use of a nutrient.

Nutrient deficiencies develop in stages. During the initial stage, marginal deficiencies develop over time as body stores are gradually emptied. The second stage of deficiency is characterized by impairment of body processes dependent on the nutrient. No signs of a deficiency are visually detected during these two stages of nutrient loss. During the third stage of nutrient deficiency the loss becomes so great that personality and emotions are affected. A person might feel depressed, irritable, or anxious. The loss of health is not severe and the person does not usually seek medical care. However, some quality of life is lost. The initial stages in nutrient deficiency are actually a gradual continuum with no clearly defined separation between stages. Classical deficiency symptoms develop if the nutrient deficiency continues to the fourth stage. The fifth and final stage is when death is likely if immediate action is not taken to restore the lacking nutrient (Table 2).

Table 2.
Sequence Of Events In The Development Of A Vitamin Deficiency

Deficiency Stage	Symptoms
1. Preliminary	1. Depletion of tissue stores (caused by diet, poor absorption, abnormal metabolism, etc.). Urinary excretion of the nutrient is decreased.
2. Biochemical	2. Enzyme activity is reduced because of nutrient lack. Urinary excretion of nutrient is negligible.
3. Physiological/Behavioral	3. Loss of appetite, reduced body weight, insomnia or excessive sleepiness, irritability, personality changes.
4. Clinical	4. Nonspecific symptoms worsen. Specific deficiency syndrome appears.
5. Anatomical	5. Clear specific syndromes with tissue damage. Death ensues unless treated.

A marginal nutrient deficiency occurs somewhere between optimal nutritional status and a classical nutrient deficiency disease. The symptoms of a marginal deficiency are vague and poorly defined and often are described as "feeling under the weather" or "not at one's best." General feelings of tiredness, irritability, insomnia, poor concentration, or depression are common symptoms of marginal nutrient deficiency. These emotional or behavioral changes also result from numerous other factors such as lack of sleep, stress, or the presence of disease, which makes it difficult to establish the primary cause of the mood or behavior change. Marginal nutrient deficiencies consequently often progress undetected, undermining the quality of life and health.

The subject of marginal deficiencies is controversial. Many nutrition experts presume a person is adequately nourished if he or she shows no clinical signs of classical deficiency disease, such as scurvy, beriberi, or anemia. These deficiency diseases are diagnosed by simple physical or blood examinations. Other nutrition experts support the presence and importance of marginal deficiencies.

Treating a disease in its early stages is more advantageous than waiting until the disease has progressed to final and severe stages. For example, the identification and treatment of cell changes on the cervix found during an annual Pap smear has an almost 100% cure rate as compared to the poor prognosis if cervical cancer is allowed to progress. If other diseases develop in a progressive fashion from early to advanced stages, it is only reasonable to suspect nutritional deficiencies proceed through similar stages.

More advanced tests for nutritional status have proven this theory correct. As researchers learned more about vitamins and minerals and their chemical pathways and storage in the body, they recognized classical deficiency diseases to be one of the final stages in long-term depletion of vitamin or mineral status. Current laboratory tests can assess the vitamin or mineral concentrations in blood, urine, and more specifically in the cells or tissues. Marginal nutrient status is detected at this level long before overt symptoms are recognized. For example, iron deficiency anemia is the fourth or clinical stage of iron deficiency. Iron levels in the tissues slowly have been drained prior to the loss of red blood cells in anemia. Poor concentration and changes in personality or mood are likely to develop during the stages of marginal iron deficiency, although no signs of iron loss, indicative of the clinical stage of deficiency, are detected in routine blood tests.

There is evidence that marginal nutrient deficiencies exist in the United States. Marginal nutrient deficiencies are found in all segments of the population, but especially in pregnant women, alcoholics and drug abusers, children, and the elderly. School children who consume diets low in zinc develop a marginal zinc deficiency and as a result are shorter in stature than children who consume optimal amounts of zinc. Marginal nutrient deficiencies are common in hospitalized patients who consume inadequate diets during illness and stress, when nutrient needs are highest. Poor nutrition during times of illness can weaken the body's natural defense against disease and infection and can hamper the healing process. Vague discomfort and muscle weakness in the elderly has been attributed to marginal intake and status of vitamin C. The body is more susceptible to colds and infections when dietary intake of vitamins and minerals, especially iron, zinc, vitamin A, vitamin B_{12}, vitamin B_6, and folic acid, is marginal. Depression, anxiety, and nausea are reported long before the appearance of clinical signs of nutrient deficiency when people consume a diet marginal in vitamin B_1.

Long-term marginal intake of nutrients might be associated with the development of the degenerative diseases. Low intake of chromium is associated with high blood sugar levels and adult-onset diabetes, which in some cases is corrected or improved when intake of chromium is increased. Suboptimal consumption of magnesium is linked to an increased risk for sudden death from heart attack, and the risk for experiencing a heart attack or irregular heartbeat associated with heart disease declines when adequate amounts of magnesium are consumed. Low dietary intake or blood levels at the low end of the normal range for vitamin A are associated with an increased risk for developing several forms of cancer. Low blood or tissue levels of calcium or long-term poor dietary intake of the mineral are associated with an increased risk for developing high blood pressure. In all cases, the diet contains some of the nutrient but not enough to either maintain adequate tissue stores or prevent disease. Many degenerative diseases, such as osteoporosis and heart disease, once thought to be the natural result of aging, are now recognized as preventable, in many cases, with a lifetime of healthy habits.

Many questions remain to be answered about marginal nutrient deficiencies.

- What are the long-term effects of suboptimal nutrient intakes?
- Do marginal nutrient deficiencies produce subtle changes in mood and personality that current tests are unable to detect?
- How do marginal vitamin or mineral deficiencies affect the body's immune system and ability to ward off disease and infection?
- Are there additional signs of malnutrition as yet not identified?

It is hoped that future well-designed research studies might provide more information and answers to these questions. In the meantime, it is important to consume a diet optimal in all vitamins and minerals to avoid the potential effects of even marginal intake of nutrients.

CHAPTER 3

The Vitamins

Vitamins are essential, noncaloric substances—needed in very small amounts from the diet—that promote growth, health, and life. They are produced by living material, such as plants and animals, as compared to minerals that originate from the soil. The 13 recognized vitamins cannot be made by the body in sufficient amounts to maintain life, so they must be obtained from the diet.

Vitamins participate in a variety of life-building processes, including the formation and maintenance of blood cells, hormones, nervous system chemicals, genetic material, and all the cells and tissues of the body. Characteristic deficiency symptoms develop if the diet does not supply optimal amounts of a vitamin. For example, poor dietary intake of folic acid or vitamin B_{12} results in anemia, inadequate intake of vitamin A affects vision, and a vitamin B_6 deficiency is characterized by mood disorders and nausea. If a substance does not produce a deficiency symptom when it is removed from the diet, it is not considered a vitamin. Each vitamin functions in many diverse roles and always with other essential nutrients. A deficiency interferes with many different body processes, including how the body uses other nutrients.

Unlike carbohydrates, protein, and fat, vitamins do not supply energy. Only calories provide energy, and vitamins do not contain calories. Several vitamins, however, do help convert the calories in carbohydrates, protein, and fat into usable energy for the body. They are like the ignition switch that sparks the fuel and keeps the engine running.

17

Vitamins are grouped into two categories: fat-soluble and water-soluble. The fat-soluble vitamins A, D, E, and K are found in the fat or oil of food and require some dietary fat to be absorbed. The water-soluble vitamins C and the B vitamins—B_1, B_2, niacin, B_6, folic acid, B_{12}, pantothenic acid, and biotin are found in the watery portion of foods, are easily lost when foods are overcooked, and do not require fat for their absorption. Fat-soluble vitamins generally are stored in the body, while water-soluble vitamins mix easily in the blood, are excreted in the urine, and only small amounts are stored in the tissues.

The vitamin content of food varies depending on how and where the food is grown, when it is harvested, and how it is stored and processed. In general, the fresher the food, the colder the storage temperature (below 40° F for refrigeration), and the shorter the cooking and holding time, the higher the vitamin content.

VITAMIN A (RETINOL, RETINAL, BETA CAROTENE)

Overview

Vitamin A was the first vitamin to be discovered. The substance was termed vitamin A in 1913 after studies found that the eyes of animals became inflamed and infected when the diet lacked sufficient amounts of foods now recognized as rich sources of vitamin A. In 1932 researchers discovered that a substance in plants, called *beta carotene*, could be converted in the body to vitamin A and was as useful as cod liver oil in preventing eye disorders.

Vitamin A is a family of compounds that includes retinol, retinal, and the carotenoids. Retinol and retinal are found in foods of animal origin, such as liver and eggs. These forms of vitamin A are ready to be used by the body directly from the food source and are called *preformed* vitamin A. The carotenoids are a group of fat-soluble pigments found in orange, dark yellow, and dark green vegetables and fruits. Some carotenoids, such as beta carotene, can be converted to vitamin A once ingested and are called a *building block* or *provitamin* form of vitamin A. A provitamin is any compound in the diet that can be converted to an active vitamin. The vitamin A content of the diet is a combination of the preformed vitamin A and the provitamin beta carotene.

The factors that affect fat absorption also influence the absorption of dietary vitamin A and beta carotene. A small amount of fat is needed in the diet to stimulate the secretion of digestive juices that aid in fat digestion. In contrast, absorption of vitamin A and beta carotene decreases if a person has an intestinal disorder that alters or reduces the absorption of dietary fat. One form of vitamin A found in some supplements, retinyl palmitate, can be absorbed even in the absence of dietary fat and is useful for people with long-term intestinal disorders.

Functions

VISION. Vitamin A is essential for normal eyesight. The vitamin combines with a specialized protein in the retina of the eye that is necessary for night vision.

EPITHELIAL TISSUE. Vitamin A helps develop and maintain moist, healthy epithelial tissue, the tissue that lines the body's external and internal surfaces. In this capacity, vitamin A is necessary in the maintenance of the cornea in the eye, all mucous membranes, the digestive tract, the urinary tract, the reproductive tract, the skin, and the lungs. Adequate vitamin A intake also maintains the lining of the stomach and might aid in the prevention and treatment of gastric ulcer.

GROWTH AND BONE FORMATION. Vitamin A is important in normal body growth and the formation of bones and soft tissue. The formation of tooth enamel and the proper spacing of teeth are also dependent on adequate amounts of vitamin A in the body.

RESISTANCE TO INFECTION. Vitamin A is called the "anti-infective vitamin" because it functions in the development and maintenance of the body's "barriers" to infection, such as the skin, lungs, and linings of the mouth and throat. This vitamin also enhances the activity of the immune system, the body's natural defense system against infection and disease. Vitamin A or beta carotene, when given before or shortly after exposure to a bacteria, reduces infection. Vitamin A's influence on immunity might be one of the reasons for the vitamin's beneficial effect in the prevention and treatment of cancer.

REPRODUCTION. Vitamin A might assist normal pregnancy and lactation (breastfeeding). How vitamin A functions in the reproductive system is unclear, but it might encourage the activity of certain hormones or aid in the normal changes in cells characteristic of early growth in the developing baby.

ANTI-CANCER AGENT. Ample intake of vitamin A and normal to high levels of vitamin A or beta carotene in the blood are associated with a reduced risk for developing certain forms of cancer, such as breast, stomach, cervical, and lung cancer. Vitamin A might prevent cancer by maintaining healthy epithelial tissues or by discouraging the formation of abnormal cells. Beta carotene might aid in the prevention of certain cancers by acting as an antioxidant to maintain healthy cell membranes. (See pages 126–128 for more information on antioxidants and disease.) Beta carotene and other carotenoids found in dark green, orange, and dark yellow vegetables and fruits might protect the skin from damage and cancer caused by overexposure to sunlight and its harmful ultraviolet (UV) light. (See pages 150–159 for more information on vitamin A, beta carotene, and cancer.)

LIVER DISORDERS. Adequate intake of vitamin A might prevent liver damage caused by exposure to toxic chemicals.

Deficiency

Prolonged deficiency of vitamin A results in changes in the skin, eyes and eyesight, and teeth.

CANCER. A low intake of vitamin A, either retinol or beta carotene, has been linked to cancer. People who smoke cigarettes, cigars, or pipes, or chew tobacco show low levels of vitamin A and an increase in the amount of precancerous cells in the tissues of the mouth, throat, and lungs.

SKIN. Long-term poor intake of vitamin A results in skin problems called "goose flesh" or "toad skin." The skin develops small hard bumps because the hair follicles are plugged with a hardened protein called *keratin*. The skin becomes dry, scaly, and rough. The condition is called *xeroderma* or *follicular keratinosis*. The most common locations are the shoulders, neck, back, forearms, thighs, and abdomen.

EYE. Chronic, severe vitamin A deficiency results in ulceration and distortion of the cornea of the eye and blindness. This vitamin deficiency disease, called *xerophthalmia*, begins as dryness, thickening, and wrinkling of the conjunctiva, the membrane that covers the eye. If poor dietary intake of vitamin A continues, the condition worsens, hardened patches (Bitot's spots) appear on the eye, and a milky appearance to the eye develops that eventually results in infection of the iris, the formation of scar tissue, and blindness. Xerophthalmia is common in third world countries, especially in infants and children, but is seldom found in the United States.

VISION. A specialized protein in the eye cannot be formed without adequate supplies of vitamin A. As a result, night vision is diminished or lost. Night blindness is a primary symptom of vitamin A deficiency.

TOOTH FORMATION. Inadequate intake of vitamin A during the formative years can result in improper tooth formation, crooked teeth, and poor spacing between teeth.

GROWTH. Poor intake of vitamin A results in growth retardation, loss of appetite, weight loss, and bone deformities. Because the tongue is lined with epithelial tissue, a vitamin A deficiency results in keratinosis (hardening) of the taste buds and loss of appetite.

Groups at high risk for developing vitamin A deficiency are alcohol abusers; adolescents; people with celiac disease and other intestinal malabsorption disorders; people with liver disease; people who use tobacco; and people who consume few or irregular amounts of dark green, dark yellow, or orange fruits and vegetables. Low-income groups, cancer patients, and people at risk for developing cancer might have low blood levels of the vitamin, which indicates inadequate dietary intake or poor absorption of the vitamin.

Daily Recommended Intake

The need for vitamin A increases with increasing body size and weight. The Recommended Dietary Allowances (RDAs) for vitamin A are expressed in either RE (retinol equivalents) or IU (international units). (1 RE = 3.33 IU of vitamin A or 10 IU of beta carotene.) The RDAs assume more than half of the vitamin A intake will come from beta carotene, so the guidelines are based on 1 RE = 5 IU. The 1989 RDAs for vitamin A are:

	Retinol Equivalents (RE)	International Units (IU)
INFANTS		
0–1 year	375	1875
CHILDREN		
1–3 years	200	2000
4–6 years	500	2500
7–10 years	700	3300
YOUNG ADULTS AND ADULTS		
Males 11+ years	1000	5000
Females 11+ years	800	4000
Pregnant	800	4000
Lactating, 1st 6 mo	+500	+2500
Lactating, 2nd 6 mo	+400	+2000

The RDAs for infants are based on the normal vitamin A content in breastmilk. The RDA for women is based on 80% of the RDA for men because women generally weigh less and therefore probably need a smaller intake of the vitamin. Exact daily requirements have not been determined for any age or sex group. Some researchers suggest that doses larger than the RDAs, between 10,000 IU and 25,000 IU for adults, might be necessary to decrease the risk for developing cancer. However, more evidence is necessary before higher recommendations can be made.

Sources in the Diet

The dietary sources of preformed vitamin A are liver, kidney, egg yolk, butter, fortified margarine, cheese made with whole milk or cream, fortified non-fat milk, whole milk, and cream. However, with the exception of non-fat milk, these dietary sources also are high in saturated fat and cholesterol. Cod liver oil is a low-cholesterol, low-saturated fat source of vitamin A.

The dietary sources of beta carotene are dark green, dark yellow, and orange vegetables, such as spinach, collard greens, broccoli, carrots, and sweet potatoes, and yellow fruits, such as apricots and peaches. These foods supply significant amounts of vitamin A and are low in fat and calories. The deeper the green, yellow, or orange color, the higher the content of beta carotene. At least one serving of a dark green or orange vegetable and three additional servings of other vegetables and fruits should be included in the diet daily (Table 3).

Dietary sources of vitamin A are preferable to supplements. Preliminary research shows that other carotenoids in dark green vegetables, such as canthaxanthin and lycopene, may reduce a person's risk for developing cancer. Canthaxanthin is related to beta carotene, but cannot be converted to vitamin A. These findings suggest that there are other substances in vitamin A-rich foods not found in supplements that are beneficial to health.

Toxicity

The preformed vitamin A is not excreted and can accumulate in the body to toxic levels if large amounts are consumed over long periods of time. In some adults, prolonged daily intake of 50,000 IU to 100,000 IU can cause vomiting, nausea, loss of appetite and weight, joint pain, abdominal discomfort, irritability, bone deformities, itching, hair loss, liver enlargement, or dry and cracked lips. Headaches are reported in adults who daily consume between 60,000 IU and 341,000 IU or more of vitamin A. Children develop toxicity symptoms more readily than adults and can experience the above symptoms as well as slowed growth when much smaller doses, such as 25,000 IU, are

Table 3.
THE VITAMIN A CONTENT OF SELECTED FOODS*

Food	Amount	Vitamin A (IU)
Liver, beef	3 ½ ounces	43,900
Carrot, raw	1	11,000
Sweet potato, baked	1 small	8,100
Spinach, cooked	½ cup	7,300
Apricots, dried	8 large halves	5,500
Beet greens, cooked	½ cup	5,100
Squash, winter	½ cup	4,200
Cantaloupe	¼ melon	3,400
Broccoli	1 stalk	2,500
Peach	1 medium	2,170
Lettuce, romaine	3½ ounces	1,900
Egg yolk	1	850
Peas, cooked	⅔ cup	540
Milk, non-fat	1 cup	500
Milk, whole	1 cup	370
Cheese, cheddar	1 ounce	370
Orange	1 medium	300
Butter	1 tsp	165
Margarine, fortified	1 tsp	165
Apple	1 medium	140
Celery, raw	1 stalk	48

*Preformed vitamin A and beta carotene.

consumed. Birth defects have occurred in animals who received overdoses of vitamin A. Symptoms disappear quickly when vitamin A toxicity is detected and the vitamin therapy is discontinued. Individual tolerance to vitamin A varies widely among people. Vitamin A toxicity from dietary sources is rare and is associated primarily with arctic explorers who consumed excessive amounts of polar bear liver.

Beta carotene is not toxic. Large amounts of dark green, yellow, or orange fruits and vegetables can be consumed over long periods of time with no ill effects other than a harmless yellowing of the skin, which disappears when fruit and vegetable intake is reduced.

Nutrient-Nutrient Interactions

• Vitamin A's function is enhanced by the amount of vitamin E in the body.
• Adequate intake of zinc is necessary for the proper use and transportation of vitamin A within the body. Deficiency symptoms of

vitamin A can occur when intake is adequate, but the diet is low in zinc.
- Vitamin A is important for calcium metabolism in the formation of healthy bones and teeth.

VITAMIN D (CALCIFEROL, CHOLECALCIFEROL, ERGOCALCIFEROL)

Overview

Vitamin D was recognized as an essential substance in cod liver oil almost a decade after the discovery of vitamin A. Vitamin D is a family of compounds labeled vitamins D_1, D_2, and D_3.

Vitamin D is unique from other essential nutrients because it can be produced in the body after exposure to sunlight or obtained from the diet. The production of vitamin D in the body is blocked by several factors such as skin pigment (the darker the skin, the less readily vitamin D is formed) or substances that screen the sun's ultraviolet rays (smog, fog, smoke, clothing, screens and windows, or hats). In addition, as a person ages, his or her ability to manufacture vitamin D decreases and longer exposure to sunlight or a greater dependency on dietary sources is required to meet daily needs. A healthy, young, fair-skinned person can theoretically produce up to 10,000 IU of vitamin D in one day. Adequate annual stores of vitamin D probably are obtained with 10 minutes of sunbathing daily during the summer months.

The second source of vitamin D is the diet. As with other fat-soluble vitamins, vitamin D requires at least a small amount of fat in the diet for absorption and any intestinal disorder that alters absorption of fat could affect dietary vitamin D absorption. Vitamin D from both the diet and internal production is not readily excreted and is stored in the liver, skin, brain, bones, and other tissues.

Functions

FORMATION AND MAINTENANCE OF BONES AND TEETH. The primary function of vitamin D is to regulate the absorption and use of calcium and phosphorus and to aid in the formation of normal bones and teeth. Vitamin D also stimulates the specialized cells in the small intestine to absorb calcium and phosphorus, prevents excessive urinary loss of calcium and phosphorus, maintains normal blood levels of calcium and phosphorus to support normal mineralization of bones and teeth, and aids in the deposition of calcium into bones and teeth.

MAINTENANCE OF NORMAL NERVES AND MUSCLES. Vitamin D aids in the maintenance of a healthy nerve and muscle system by regulating the level of calcium in the blood. Calcium is necessary for normal nerve transmission and muscle contraction (including the heartbeat), and the nerves and muscles depend on a constant supply of this mineral from the blood.

HEARING. Vitamin D aids in the maintenance of all bones, including the small bones of the ear.

INSULIN SECRETION. Vitamin D might function in the normal production or secretion of the hormone insulin from the pancreas. In this capacity, the vitamin might aid in the regulation of normal blood sugar.

CANCER. Vitamin D might aid in the prevention or treatment of cancer. The vitamin might alter the growth of several different types of cancer, including colon cancer and non-Hodgkin's lymphoma. Further information is needed, however, before the link between vitamin D and cancer can be confirmed.

IMMUNE SYSTEM. Vitamin D might assist the regulation of normal immune function and, therefore, would function to defend the body against infection and disease.

Deficiency

Prolonged deficiency of vitamin D results in changes in the bones of children and adults, and possible hearing loss with aging.

RICKETS AND OSTEOMALACIA. Rickets is a childhood nutrient-deficiency disease caused by a lack of vitamin D in the diet or inadequate exposure to sunlight. As a result of this disease, the bones are malformed and weak from poor calcium and phosphorus deposition. The weight-bearing bones buckle under the strain of supporting the body, the chest bone bows to resemble a pigeon breast, the head is malformed, and the wrists and ankles are enlarged. Less severe symptoms occur when the deficiency is mild.

Often rickets is not detected in infants until they begin to walk. Prior to this time, the infant is restless, may sweat profusely, and repeatedly turns his or her head from side to side. Delayed development of teeth could be a sign of mild vitamin D deficiency. Death can result when internal organs are impaired by the weakened surrounding bone structure. Rickets is treated by adding vitamin D to the diet.

Rickets was more common in the past, prior to vitamin D fortification of milk. It is still seen in some parts of the world, especially in northern climates where sunlight is limited and the intake of vitamin D fortified foods is inadequate. Prolonged breastfeeding of infants without supplementation with vitamin D or inadequate consumption of vitamin D-fortified milk by children can result in rickets. Black children in the United States are more prone to rickets than are white children because dark skin pigment limits the amount of vitamin D produced during exposure to sunlight. Children on long-term anticonvulsant therapy for epilepsy or who have a fat-malabsorption disorder such as celiac disease are at risk for vitamin D deficiency and rickets.

Osteomalacia is the adult form of rickets and results from long-term poor dietary intake of vitamin D or exposure to sunlight. (See pages 211–213 for more information on vitamin D and osteomalacia.)

Rickets and osteomalacia respond well to vitamin D supplementation and there is improvement in symptoms within 2 months of initiating vitamin D therapy. Most bone loss can be corrected, but some damage might be irreversible. However, supplementation will prevent further deformities.

OSTEOPOROSIS. Osteomalacia should not be confused with osteoporosis (see page 212), although the two bone disorders often occur together. Although controversial, vitamin D, in conjunction with calcium supplementation, might be useful in the prevention and treatment of osteoporosis.

HEARING LOSS. Slow, progressive hearing loss might be caused by an inadequate intake of vitamin D. A lack of vitamin D causes a small, snail-shaped bone in the inner ear, called the *cochlea*, to become porous. The cochlea is then unable to transmit messages to the nerves that lead to the brain and hearing loss can result. In some cases, the loss will respond to vitamin D supplementation. Supplementation is not effective when hearing loss is a result of causes other than vitamin deficiency (Figure 1).

Daily Recommended Intake

There is no established requirement for vitamin D. The main function of the RDAs is to emphasize that the vitamin is needed throughout life. However, if an individual is healthy and frequently exposed to unfiltered sunlight no dietary intake is necessary. Dietary sources are necessary if a person lives in a smoggy, foggy, or overcast environment; wears heavy clothing; is indoors or exposed to sunlight only through windows or screens; or is housebound. Dark-skinned people are most dependent on dietary sources of vitamin D as their skin can screen out as much as 95% of the vitamin D-producing ultraviolet rays.

Figure 1

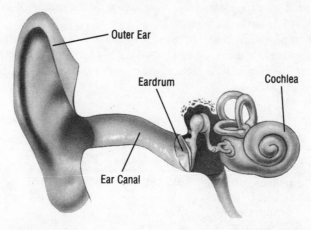

Vitamin D might improve hearing by strengthening the inner bones of the ear, including the cochlea.

The 1989 RDAs for vitamin D are:

	Micrograms (mcg)	*International Units (IU)*
INFANTS		
0–0.5 year	7.5	300
INFANTS, CHILDREN, AND YOUNG		
ADULTS		
0.5–24 years	10	400
ADULTS		
25+	5	200
Pregnant and Lactating	10	400

Sources in the Diet

The most reliable dietary source of vitamin D is vitamin D-fortified milk. One quart of whole, low-fat, or non-fat milk supplies 400 IU of vitamin D, or the RDA for infants, children, adults up to 24 years old, and pregnant and lactating women. Some dried or evaporated milks contain vitamin D. Other dairy products, such as cheese, yogurt, cottage cheese, cream cheese, raw milk, and goat's milk do not contain vitamin D, as fortified milk seldom is used in the production of these products. Liver, egg yolk, butter, and cream contain varying amounts of the vitamin and are not reliable sources. Some ready-to-eat processed breakfast cereals are fortified with vitamin D. Vitamin D supplementation is recommended for breastfed infants. Cod liver oil and other fish oils are excellent sources of vitamin D. Salmon, herring, mackerel, and sardines contribute substantial amounts of vitamin D to the body if consumed frequently.

Foods from plant sources are poor sources of the vitamin and people on strict vegetarian diets have few dietary choices in meeting their requirement of vitamin D other than processed, fortified foods or supplements (Table 4).

Table 4.
THE VITAMIN D CONTENT OF SELECTED FOODS

Food	Amount	Vitamin D (IU)
Sardines, canned	3½ ounces	1150–1570
Mackerel, fresh	3½ ounces	1100
Herring, fresh	3½ ounces	315
Salmon, fresh	3½ ounces	154–550
Shrimp	3½ ounces	150
Milk, fortified	1 cup	100
Egg yolk	1 average	25
Liver, beef	3½ ounces	9–42
Cheese	1 ounce	3–4
Butter	1 pat	1.8

Toxicity

Vitamin D can be toxic if taken in doses more than four times the RDA. The symptoms of vitamin D overdose include diarrhea, dermatitis, headache, nausea, weakness, loss of appetite, calcium deposits in soft tissues (kidney, arteries, heart, ear, and lungs), irreversible kidney or heart damage, retarded growth, and mental retardation. Large doses of vitamin D used in the treatment of some kidney disorders might increase urinary calcium loss and increase the risk for developing osteoporosis. Large doses of vitamin D also are linked to increased risk for premature heart attack and atherosclerosis. Vitamin D overdose develops over time and there is wide variation among individuals in their tolerance to toxicity.

Children and infants are more susceptible than adults to vitamin D toxicity. A parent should monitor vitamin D intake as toxic levels could accumulate in the child's small body from regular combined ingestion of fortified milk or formula, children's vitamin supplements, and fortified cereals. Pregnant women also should avoid large doses of vitamin D. Toxicity can be reversed by removal of excess vitamin D from the daily diet; however, the deposition of calcium into soft tissues could cause irreversible organ damage.

Prolonged exposure to sunlight does not cause vitamin D toxicity. The body has an efficient feedback system and reduces the production of vitamin D with increased exposure to sunlight.

Nutrient-Nutrient Interactions

- Vitamin D is important for the absorption of calcium and phosphorus and for the normal depositing of these minerals into bone.
- Cadmium can block the production of vitamin D.
- Fat must provide at least 10% of the total dietary calories for adequate absorption of vitamin D.
- Pantothenic acid is necessary for the synthesis of vitamin D.
- Vitamin D might improve zinc status in kidney disease patients on dialysis.

VITAMIN E (TOCOPHEROL)

Overview

Vitamin E was discovered in the 1920s and is a family of fat-soluble compounds, including the tocopherols. Alpha tocopherol is the most common and most potent form of the vitamin and requires a small amount of dietary fat for absorption.

Functions

ANTIOXIDANT. The main function of vitamin E is as an antioxidant. In this capacity, vitamin E protects fats and vitamin A in the body from destruction by oxygen fragments called *free radicals*. In the absence of antioxidants, free radicals damage the fats in cell membranes and other important components of the body's cells and tissues. As an antioxidant, vitamin E stabilizes cell membranes and protects the cells and tissues from damage, protects the tissues of the lungs and mouth from damage by air pollutants, and might aid in the prevention of tumor growth. Vitamin E protects tissues of the eyes, skin, liver, breast, and calf muscles; helps regulate the use and storage of vitamin A; and protects red blood cells from damage, thus preventing a special form of anemia called *hemolytic anemia*.

Vitamin E also might affect the production of hormone-like substances in the body called *prostaglandins* that regulate a variety of body processes including blood pressure, reproduction, and muscle contraction.

AGING. Vitamin E might aid in the prevention of premature aging because of its role as an antioxidant. Free radicals destroy connective tissues that provide firmness to tissues such as the skin, might contribute to the development of atherosclerosis, and accumulate during the aging process. The combination of vitamin E and vitamin C reduces free radical levels by 26% in older adults. Whether or not this reduction slows the aging process is unclear.

Preliminary reports show that vitamin E might aid in the maintenance of normal, active brain function. Accumulation of free radicals in brain tissue has been associated with age-related memory loss, and antioxidants might prevent this sign of premature aging.

CANCER. The evidence linking vitamin E with cancer is incomplete. Vitamin E might protect against the development of cancer because of its role as an antioxidant. Antioxidants, such as vitamin E, selenium, and vitamin C, protect tissues from hazardous oxygen fragments. The oxidative damage is possibly linked to cancer as tissues that are cancerous are low in antioxidants. Antioxidants such as vitamin E might stabilize cell membranes, scavenge free radicals, and reduce risk for developing cancer (Graph 1). (See pages 126–128 and 154–155 for more information on vitamin E, antioxidants, and cancer.)

Graph 1
**THE EFFECT OF VITAMIN E AND SELENIUM
ON THE PROTECTION OF CELL MEMBRANES**

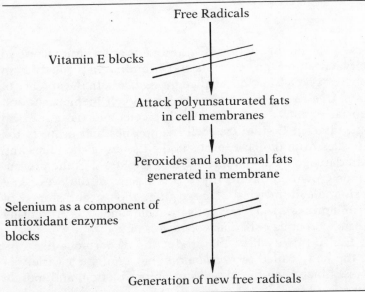

Free Radicals

Vitamin E blocks

Attack polyunsaturated fats
in cell membranes

Peroxides and abnormal fats
generated in membrane

Selenium as a component of
antioxidant enzymes
blocks

Generation of new free radicals

DIABETES. A few reports show that vitamin E might reduce blood sugar levels in some diabetics. In one study, blood sugar levels decreased 20% when patients increased vitamin E intake to 2,000 IU a day.

HEART DISEASE. A few studies have found a possible link between vitamin E and heart disease. The vitamin might aid in the prevention of premature heart disease by inhibiting the clumping of blood cell fragments called *platelets* that are associated with atherosclerosis. When taken in doses exceeding 600 IU a day, vitamin E also might improve blood cholesterol levels. However, the effects of vitamin E on the prevention or treatment of heart disease are not confirmed, nor are they as strong as the effects of reducing dietary fat and cholesterol and increasing the intake of fiber. Vitamin E also is used to treat intermittent claudication (pain and tension in the legs when walking) that occurs in some heart disease patients.

LUPUS ERYTHEMATOSUS. Recent evidence shows that vitamin E might be effective in the treatment of lupus erythematosus. The skin disorder associated with lupus usually appears on the face and might be a result of alteration of cell membranes in skin tissue. Doses between 800 IU and 2,000 IU of vitamin E relieve symptoms in some individuals with no apparent side effects. Sensitivity to sunlight in some patients with lupus is also reduced or eliminated with use of vitamin E.

RHEUMATOID ARTHRITIS. Limited evidence exists that vitamin E in conjunction with selenium might help alleviate some of the pain and morning stiffness of rheumatoid arthritis.

There is no scientific evidence that vitamin E is effective in the following disorders:

Menstrual disorders
Muscular dystrophy
Poor athletic performance
Rheumatic fever
Sterility and impotence
Toxemias of pregnancy

Deficiency

A deficiency of vitamin E is difficult to diagnose as low intakes of the vitamin develop in a variety of ways in different animals. Symptoms of vitamin E deficiency in animals include nervous system disorders, infant malformations, muscular dystrophy, anemia, degeneration of heart tissue, damage to liver tissue, and destruction of tissues in the testes. Anemia in infants and nerve damage in adults are the only known disorders that occur as a result of vitamin E deficiency. Premature infants have not accumulated ample amounts of the fat-soluble vitamin in their tissues and are susceptible to a type of anemia where the red blood cells break easily. Breastmilk contains enough vitamin E to prevent this "hemolytic" anemia in normal term infants. Infant anemia in formula-fed infants is rarely seen as most formulas now contain vitamin E.

People with rare fat malabsorption syndromes, such as celiac disease, cystic fibrosis, and sprue, are susceptible to nerve damage, muscle weakness, poor coordination, involuntary movement of the eyes, damage to the eyes, and anemia probably caused by vitamin E deficiency. Symptoms are improved or alleviated with vitamin E supplementation. Low tissue levels are also found in people who abuse alcohol.

Daily Recommended Intake

The need for vitamin E increases with increasing body size and dietary intake of polyunsaturated fats, including fish oil. Vitamin E protects these fats from rancidity caused by oxygen fragments and other free radicals. Vigorous exercise also might increase the need for vitamin E.

The RDAs are only estimates based on the assumption that the average person consumes a diet that provides a 2:5 ratio of vitamin E (as a mix of different tocopherols) to polyunsaturated fat. More information is needed about the dietary factors that influence vitamin E requirements.

The 1989 RDAs for vitamin E are:

	Milligrams (mg)	International Units (of alpha tocopherol)
INFANTS	3–4	4.5–6.0
CHILDREN 1–10 years	6–7	9.0–10.5
YOUNG ADULTS AND ADULTS		
Males 11+ years	10	15
Females 11+ years	8	12
Pregnant	10	15
Lactating, 1st 6 mo	12	18
Lactating, 2nd 6 mo	11	16.5

Sources in the Diet

The primary dietary sources of vitamin E are vegetable oils, seeds, wheatgerm, and nuts. Varying amounts of different tocopherols are found in different vegetable oils. For example, 90% of the vitamin E in safflower oil is alpha tocopherol, the most potent or "biologically active" form of the vitamin. Corn oil is only 10% alpha tocopherol and soybean oil is primarily gamma tocopherol, a form of vitamin E with little potency. The diet is likely to be deficient in vitamin E if soybean oil, the major oil used in salad dressings, mayonnaise, and other commercial oils, constitutes the major source of polyunsaturated fat. Other plant sources of the vitamin include avocados, peaches, whole grain breads and cereals, spinach, broccoli, asparagus, and dried prunes. Foods of animal origin are usually poor sources of vitamin E. Wide variations exist, however, and depend on the vitamin E content of the animal's diet (Table 5).

Table 5.
THE VITAMIN E CONTENT OF SELECTED FOODS

Food	Amount	Vitamin E (IU)
Wheatgerm oil	¼ cup	63.6
Safflower oil	¼ cup	19.5
Sunflower oil	¼ cup	18.3
French Dressing (cottonseed oil)	¼ cup	13
Spinach	½ cup	2.2–3.3
Peaches, canned	½ peach	2.1–2.4
Dried Prunes	10 prunes	1.61–1.85
Asparagus	5 spears	1.1–1.6
Avocados	½ avocado	0.95–2.0
Broccoli	3 stalks	0.8–3.4
Whole Wheat Cereal, shredded	1 cup	0.4–0.6
Beef	3½ ounces	0.33–1.0
Turkey	3½ ounces	0.09
Milk, whole	1 cup	0.02

Cooking and processing of foods reduce their vitamin E content. Vitamin E is lost when flours and oils are processed and bleached. So much vitamin E is lost from bleaching vegetable oils that the by-product is used for vitamin E supplements. The vitamin E content of a vegetable oil, such as soybean oil, is not always adequate to maintain an optimal ratio of vitamin E to polyunsaturated fat. Cold-pressed, unbleached vegetable oils, especially safflower oil, are the best sources of vitamin E.

Toxicity

Unlike the other fat-soluble vitamins, few toxicity symptoms have been identified for vitamin E. Large doses of the vitamin might interfere with vitamin K activity and result in prolonged bleeding time. This effect is most likely to occur in people who take anticoagulant medications for heart disease or in people with low amounts of vitamin K in the body because of liver disease. The recorded history of vitamin E is short and much remains to be learned. Because of potential toxicity in animals, it is recommended that people avoid chronic large doses of any fat-soluble vitamin.

Nutrient-Nutrient Interactions

- Vitamin E protects vitamin A, beta carotene, and vitamin C in foods from destruction by oxygen.
- Vitamin E improves the use of vitamin A in the body.
- Selenium enhances the antioxidant capabilities of vitamin E.
- Vitamin C might work with vitamin E to prevent premature aging.
- Vitamin E might be necessary for the conversion of vitamin B_{12} to its biologically active form.
- Vitamin E might reduce some of the symptoms of a zinc deficiency and a zinc deficiency might increase dietary requirements for vitamin E.
- Vitamin E provides protection from the toxic effects of silver, mercury, and lead.
- Large doses of vitamin E can interfere with the coagulant functions of vitamin K.

VITAMIN K

Overview

There are two naturally-occurring forms of vitamin K and one synthetic form. All forms of the vitamin require the presence of a small amount of dietary fat in the small intestine for absorption.

Functions

BLOOD CLOTTING. The primary function of vitamin K is to regulate normal blood clotting. The vitamin is important for the production of *prothrombin*, a protein essential for blood coagulation.

CANCER. Experiments on tumor cells removed from the body show that vitamin K might inhibit the growth of several forms of cancer, including cancer of the breast, ovary, colon, stomach, bladder, liver, and kidney. The effectiveness is enhanced when vitamin K is used in conjunction with the medication warfarin. However, the research on vitamin K is limited and more conclusive information is needed before recommendations can be made.

Deficiency

A deficiency of vitamin K is rare, except in newborn infants. The vitamin is synthesized by microorganisms in the mature intestinal tract, but the establishment of bacteria takes days to weeks to develop in the newborn. The mother is often given vitamin K supplements prior to delivery to increase the amount of vitamin K that crosses the placenta and is available in breastmilk. Additionally, vitamin K injections are often given to the baby at delivery.

A deficiency in the adult is likely only if the diet is low in dark green leafy vegetables or the growth of intestinal bacteria is inhibited by chronic use of antibiotic medications. Other medications that affect vitamin K absorption or use include coumarin, warfarin, heparin, and salicylates. In addition, any malabsorption syndrome that affects fat digestion would inhibit vitamin K absorption. Severe liver disease would hinder the utilization of the vitamin in the formation of prothrombin. These conditions require the attention of a physician and therapeutic doses of the vitamin to maintain normal blood clotting.

Daily Recommended Intake

It is assumed that half of the daily intake comes from bacterial synthesis in the intestines. A normal, mixed diet contains between 300 mcg and 500 mcg. The 1989 RDAs for vitamin K are:

	Vitamin K (mcg)
INFANTS	
0–0.5 year	5
0.5–1 year	10
CHILDREN	
1–3 years	15
4–6 years	20
7–10 years	30
YOUNG ADULTS AND ADULTS	
Males 11–14 years	45
Males 15–18 years	65

	Vitamin K (mcg)
Males 19–24 years	70
Males 25+ years	80
Females 11–14 years	45
Females 15–18 years	55
Females 19–24 years	60
Females 25+ years	65
Pregnant	65
Lactating	65

Sources in the Diet

Vitamin K is found in green or leafy vegetables, such as broccoli, turnip greens, romaine lettuce, and cabbage. Cheese, egg yolk, and liver contain small amounts of the vitamin (Table 6).

Table 6.
THE VITAMIN K CONTENT OF SELECTED FOODS

Food	Amount	Vitamin K (mcg)
Turnip greens	²/₃ cup	650
Broccoli	²/₃ cup	200
Lettuce	2 cups	129
Cabbage	²/₃ cup	125
Spinach	²/₃ cup	89
Liver, beef	3½ ounces	92
Cheese	3½ ounces	35
Egg, yolk	1 medium	11
Peach	½ medium	8
Liver, pork	3½ ounces	7
Potato, baked	1 medium	6

Toxicity

Large doses of synthetic vitamin K can cause anemia in animals and a severe form of jaundice in infants that results in degeneration of the brain. The less potent forms of vitamin K found in alfalfa leaves have a wider range of safety. Vitamin K supplements are available only through prescription as the vitamin can be toxic.

Nutrient-Nutrient Interactions

- Large doses of vitamin E might interfere with the blood clotting functions of vitamin K.

VITAMIN B₁ (THIAMIN)

Overview

Vitamin B_1 was called "water-soluble B" until 1926 when it was found that the vitamin consisted of two substances. The first compound, vitamin B_1, cured beriberi and was easily deactivated by heat. The second compound, niacin, cured another disease called pellagra and was not affected by heat.

Functions

Vitamin B_1 is required for normal functioning of all body cells, especially nerves. Vitamin B_1 is involved in numerous body processes that break down carbohydrates, protein, and fat for energy and convert excess carbohydrate to fat for storage.

Deficiency

Symptoms of vitamin B_1 deficiency occur primarily in the nervous, gastrointestinal, and cardiovascular systems. Early symptoms include fatigue, loss of appetite, weight loss, gastrointestinal upsets, nausea, and weakness. Caution must be exercised in self-diagnosing the problem at this stage as these symptoms are vague and can be an indication of numerous other health or lifestyle problems unrelated to vitamin B_1 intake. The following symptoms are signs of a clinical deficiency:

Mental confusion	Muscular weakness
Paralysis of the extremities	Calf muscle tenderness
Muscle fatigue	Abnormal heart action
Emaciation	Slowing of the heart rate
Enlargement of the heart	Tingling in the extremities
Numbness	Loss of reflexes

Personality changes also can develop and include memory loss, emotional instability, reduced attention span, irritability, confusion, and depression. Permanent damage to the nervous system can occur if a severe deficiency is not corrected in time.

Beriberi, the classic vitamin B_1 deficiency disease, is classified into two main types: wet beriberi and dry beriberi. Wet beriberi is characterized by the accumulation of fluids in the tissues (edema), especially in the ankles, feet, and legs. This excess of fluid affects heart function and can be fatal. There is no accumulation of fluid in dry beriberi; instead there is severe muscle wasting, emaciation, and paralysis of the legs.

Although the causes of some symptoms of vitamin B_1 deficiency are not fully understood, many deficiency symptoms are probably a result of accumulation of substances that cannot be completely broken apart for energy without vitamin B_1. The effects of this accumulation are felt in every cell in the body, especially those cells that depend primarily on carbohydrate for energy, such as the brain and nervous system, or tissues that have immediate contact with nerves, such as the muscles. Anything that increases the demand for the conversion of carbohydrate to energy (ie, exercise, alcohol, and carbohydrate foods, especially sugary foods) will increase the likelihood of deficiency symptoms if the diet is low in vitamin B_1.

Vitamin B_1 deficiency occurs primarily in people who either consume a diet comprised mainly of polished rice or who abuse alcohol. Alcohol is associated with poor dietary intake, reduced absorption, increased requirements, and increased urinary loss of vitamin B_1. Alcohol's effect on vitamin B_1 status results in Wernicke-Korsakoff syndrome with loss of immediate memory, disorientation, jerky movements of the eyes, and a staggering gait. Many symptoms of this form of alcohol-induced nerve damage are reversible if the individual stops drinking alcohol and starts eating a nutrient-rich diet. However, if the problem is not treated, the person's brain can be permanently damaged leading to psychosis and death. Enrichment of white rice and white bread with vitamin B_1 has reduced the incidence of overt vitamin B_1 deficiency, so beriberi is rare in the United States. However, subclinical or mild deficiencies might be more common.

A diet high in fats, sugar, or other nutrient-poor foods is likely to be low in vitamin B_1. Mild forms of mental illness have been reported with the consumption of such diets and the neuroses are eliminated when dietary intake of vitamin B_1 is increased. Vitamin B_1 deficiency can develop during fasting, chronic dieting, or when a person consumes a limited variety or amount of food. The diet should be adequate in vitamin B_1 if a person consumes at least 10 servings a day of nutrient-rich foods, such as fresh vegetables, whole grain breads and cereals, lean meats or cooked dried beans and peas, and low-fat or nonfat dairy foods. The tannins in tea can inhibit vitamin B_1 absorption and prolonged, excessive intake might result in vitamin B_1 deficiency.

Daily Recommended Intake

Because vitamin B_1 is water-soluble, excesses are excreted in the urine rather than stored, and a daily supply of the vitamin is necessary to maintain normal body processes. The daily need for vitamin B_1 is based on the amount of calories consumed, especially calories from carbohydrates as the vitamin will be needed to convert those calories to energy. Other factors that affect vitamin B_1 requirements are body weight, growth, and the small amount of vitamin B_1 that is absorbed from bacterial synthesis in the intestines.

Deficiency symptoms have been noted when vitamin B_1 intake drops below 0.2 mg to 0.3 mg for every 1,000 calories. The RDAs are based on 0.5 mg/1,000 calories. Daily intake of vitamin B_1 on diets less than 2,000 calories should not drop below 1.0 mg/day. Vitamin B_1 needs increase during pregnancy and breastfeeding, and during physical or emotional stress.

The 1989 RDAs for vitamin B_1 are:

	Vitamin B_1 (mg)
INFANTS	
0–0.5 year	0.3
0.5–1 year	0.4
CHILDREN	
1–3 years	0.7
4–6 years	0.9
7–10 years	1.0
YOUNG ADULTS AND ADULTS	
Males 11–14 years	1.3
Males 15–50 years	1.5
Males 51+ years	1.2
Females 11–50 years	1.1
Females 50+ years	1.0
Pregnant	1.5
Lactating	1.6

Sources in the Diet

Pork, organ meats, oysters, green peas, collard greens, oranges, dried beans and peas, and wheatgerm are the richest sources of vitamin B_1. Other good sources of the vitamin include brewer's or nutritional yeast, fish, peanuts and peanut butter, whole grain breads and cereals, nuts, and cooked dried beans and peas. Moderate dietary sources include avocados, lean meat, milk, spinach, cauliflower, and dried fruit (Table 7).

Vitamin B_1 is lost when the cooking water is discarded or when baking soda is added to cooked vegetables to maintain their green color. Vitamin B_1 is lost when sulfur dioxide is used in the drying of fruits.

Table 7.
THE VITAMIN B₁ CONTENT OF SELECTED FOODS

Food	Amount	Vitamin B_1 (mg)
Wheatgerm	¼ cup	0.44
Ham	3 ounces	0.40
Brewer's (nutritional) Yeast	1 Tbsp	0.34
Oysters	¾ cup	0.25
Liver, beef	3 ounces	0.23
Peanuts	½ cup	0.22
Green peas	½ cup	0.22
Raisins	1 cup	0.21
Collard greens	½ cup	0.14
Orange	1	0.13
Dried beans and peas (cooked)	½ cup	0.13
Asparagus	1 cup	0.12
Cauliflower	1 cup	0.11
Milk, non-fat	1 cup	0.09
Potato, small	1	0.08
Bread, whole wheat	1 slice	0.06
Brussels sprouts	½ cup	0.06
Beef, lean	3 ounces	0.05
Chicken, meat only	3 ounces	0.05

Toxicity

There are no known toxic levels of vitamin B_1 when the vitamin is taken orally. As the vitamin is not stored well in the body it is unlikely vitamin B_1 could accumulate to toxic levels. Repeated intravenous injections of vitamin B_1 might cause anaphylactic shock in some people. The safety levels for vitamin B_1 appear to be at least 300 mg/day, possibly higher. However, there is no known reason to consume this quantity and the consumption of a nutritious diet should supply a safe and ample intake of this B vitamin.

Nutrient-Nutrient Interactions

The B vitamins, especially vitamin B_1, vitamin B_2, niacin, biotin, pantothenic acid, and vitamin B_6 are generally found in the same foods and they work together in converting dietary protein, carbohydrates, and fat to energy or storage fat. In humans, a deficiency of one B vitamin is usually associated with poor intake of several B vitamins.

VITAMIN B₂ (RIBOFLAVIN)

Overview

Vitamin B_2 is one of a number of compounds that have similar chemical structures. Vitamin B_2 is easily absorbed from food, but only approximately 15% of the vitamin is absorbed when taken alone in supplemental form on an empty stomach. The vitamin is not well stored and excesses are excreted in the urine, giving the urine a fluorescent yellow color.

Functions

Vitamin B_2, as with vitamin B_1, is essential for the normal release of energy from carbohydrate, protein, and fat in food. Vitamin B_2 is important for normal growth and development, the production of and regulation of certain hormones, and the formation of red blood cells. Vitamin B_2 might be a necessary adjunct to iron supplementation in the treatment of anemia and it might aid in the prevention of prostate cancer.

Deficiency

Clinical symptoms of vitamin B_2 deficiency are rare, except in alcohol abusers, and are usually accompanied by vitamin B_1 or niacin deficiencies. Subclinical or mild deficiencies are more common.

Early symptoms include soreness and burning of the lips, mouth, and tongue; burning and itching of the eyes; loss of vision; sensitivity to light; and cracks in the corners of the mouth. As the deficiency progresses, the mucous membranes of the mouth become inflamed, the eyes redden, dermatitis with simultaneous dryness and greasy scaling develops, and/or depression or hysteria develop. Infants born to malnourished mothers are malformed or have retarded growth. Symptoms are difficult to detect as other nutrient deficiencies are most likely occurring simultaneously. Similar deficiency symptoms also occur as a result of niacin, iron, or vitamin B_6 deficiencies. Supplementation usually reverses symptoms within a few days to weeks.

Daily Recommended Intake

The daily need for vitamin B_2 increases as calorie intake increases, and the RDA is based on 0.6 mg/1,000 calories. Vitamin B_2 intake should not drop below 1.2 mg/day regardless of calorie intake, as tissue reserves cannot be maintained on low intakes. Daily needs increase during pregnancy, lactation, and possibly during strenuous exercise or use of oral contraceptives.

The 1989 RDAs for vitamin B_2 are:

	Vitamin B_2 (mg)
INFANTS	
0–0.5 year	0.4
0.5–1 year	0.5
CHILDREN	
1–3 years	0.8
4–6 years	1.1
7–10 years	1.2
YOUNG ADULTS AND ADULTS	
Males 11–14 years	1.5
Males 15–18 years	1.8
Males 19–50 years	1.7
Males 51+ years	1.4
Females 11–50 years	1.3
Females 51+ years	1.2
Pregnant	1.6
Lactating, 1st 6 mo	1.8
Lactating, 2nd 6 mo	1.7

Sources in the Diet

Small amounts of vitamin B_2 are distributed in a variety of foods; however, the most concentrated sources of the vitamin include milk and milk products and liver. Children, adolescents, and adults who avoid dairy products are likely to consume inadequate amounts of vitamin B_2 as dairy products supply half of the daily vitamin B_2 most people consume in the United States. Other dietary sources of the vitamin include oysters, lean meat, green leafy vegetables, mushrooms, asparagus, broccoli, avocados, Brussels sprouts, and salmon (Table 8).

Vitamin B_2 is stable to heat so little is lost in cooking, unless baking soda is added during the cooking of vegetables. The vitamin is easily destroyed in the presence of light. Foods stored in clear containers, such as milk in glass bottles, sun drying of fruits and vegetables, noodles and other grains in glass or clear plastic jars, or mushrooms and other vegetables left uncovered, will lose large portions of their vitamin B_2 content in a short period of time.

Table 8.
THE VITAMIN B₂ CONTENT OF SELECTED FOODS

Food	Amount	Vitamin B_2 (mg)
Liver, beef	3 ounces	0.63
Milk, low-fat	1 cup	0.52
Yogurt, low-fat	1 cup	0.39
Oysters	¾ cup	0.30
Avocado	½	0.22
Collard greens	½ cup	0.19
Chicken, meat only	3 ounces	0.16
Salmon, canned	3 ounces	0.16
Asparagus	½ cup	0.13
Broccoli	½ cup	0.12
Brussels sprouts	½ cup	0.11
Spinach	½ cup	0.11
Whole wheat bread	1 slice	0.05

Toxicity

No known toxicity levels are identified for vitamin B_2. The vitamin is excreted in the urine in proportion to intake when intake is greater than 1.3 mg/day.

Nutrient-Nutrient Interactions

- Vitamin B_2 works with other B vitamins, such as vitamin B_1, niacin, biotin, pantothenic acid, and vitamin B_6 in the breakdown of the calorie nutrients (carbohydrate, protein, and fat) for energy. A deficiency of any of these nutrients will compromise the other vitamins' ability to function.
- Vitamin B_2 might enhance the effectiveness of iron supplementation in the treatment of anemia.
- Vitamin B_2 is necessary for the activation of vitamin B_6.

Vitamin B_2 is needed to convert tryptophan to niacin. Although pellagra is the nutrient deficiency disease associated with niacin, it is actually a multiple deficiency of niacin, vitamin B_6, tryptophan, and vitamin B_2.

NIACIN (NICOTINIC ACID, NIACINAMIDE)

Overview

Niacin is the common name for two compounds: nicotinic acid and niacinamide (also called nicotinamide). The name niacin was chosen to avoid confusion with the toxic drug nicotine found in tobacco. Niacin is absorbed in the small intestine and, as it is a water-soluble vitamin, it is not stored in the body. Excess intakes of niacin are excreted in the urine.

Functions

CELL FUNCTION. Niacin functions in more than 50 body processes and is primarily important in the release of energy from carbohydrates. Niacin aids in the breakdown of protein and fats, in the synthesis of fats and certain hormones, in the formation of red blood cells, and in the detoxification of several drugs and chemicals. The diversity of niacin's roles makes it essential for the supply of energy to and the maintenance of all body cells.

BLOOD CHOLESTEROL. Large daily doses of niacin, as nicotinic acid, decrease blood cholesterol, LDL-cholesterol, and triglyceride levels; increase HDL-cholesterol levels; and reduce the risk for developing cardiovascular disease in people with elevated blood fat levels. Smaller doses of nicotinic acid can be used with similar effectiveness when this B vitamin is combined with vitamin A and vitamin E. The cholesterol-lowering effect of many medications is even more pronounced when nicotinic acid is included in the therapy. Nicotinic acid as a treatment for elevated blood cholesterol should be supervised by a physician as there are side effects. (See page 162 for more information on nicotinic acid and heart disease.)

DRUG TOXICITY. Adriamycin is a medication used in the treatment of cancer. One of the adverse side effects of adriamycin is possible damage to heart tissue. Niacin might reduce the toxic effects of this medication on heart tissue without reducing its effectiveness in the treatment of cancer.

EPILEPSY. Niacinamide might enhance the effectiveness of anti-epileptic medications such as phenobarbital or primidone.

PSYCHIATRIC DISORDERS. Large doses of niacin have been used with varying success in the treatment of schizophrenia. The vitamin was first investigated because the psychiatric symptoms of pellagra resemble schizophrenia.

Some psychiatric disorders might be caused by a genetic defect in the absorption of substances necessary for normal brain function. Psychological symptoms, such as aggressive behavior, temper tantrums, restlessness, depression, hyperactivity, and sleep disturbances, are sometimes a result of impaired absorption of the amino acid tryptophan, but symptoms improve with increased daily intake of niacinamide. Treatment for psychological problems with niacin only should be used with the supervision of a physician.

Deficiency

In 1945 it was found that either an amino acid called *tryptophan* found in protein or niacin could cure pellagra, and later it was recognized that tryptophan could be converted to niacin in the body. In more recent years, pellagra has been suspected to be a more complex nutrient deficiency disorder that also involves vitamin B_1, vitamin B_2, and other nutrients.

Pellagra is the classic deficiency disease associated with niacin. All tissues are affected by inadequate intake of niacin, but those tissues where the cells are replaced more frequently, such as the skin and the digestive tract, show symptoms first. The nervous system is also a prime target for deficiency symptoms. The classic description of pellagra is the four "Ds": dermatitis, diarrhea, dementia, and death.

Early symptoms of niacin deficiency include weakness, loss of appetite, indigestion, skin eruptions, and lethargy. The 4 "Ds" of pellagra develop as the deficiency worsens. The dermatitis of pellagra is a scaly, dark pigmentation that develops on areas of the skin exposed to sunlight, heat, or mild irritation or trauma. The tongue is swollen, the person may experience tremors, and damage to the central nervous system can result in disorientation, irritability, headaches, insomnia, loss of memory, delirium, and emotional instability. These symptoms are often accompanied by other deficiency symptoms from poor intake of protein, vitamin B_2, iron, vitamin B_1, or vitamin B_6.

Niacin deficiency is rare unless a person consumes a diet composed primarily of corn or cornmeal with little protein, or the diet is so poor that numerous vitamin, mineral, protein, and calorie deficits are present. The niacin and tryptophan content of corn is low and poorly absorbed. In Mexico, where corn is treated with lye before use, the alkali increases the absorption of the amino acid tryptophan in the corn. Once in the body, tryptophan is converted to niacin, which lowers the risk for deficiency. In fact, pellagra and niacin deficiency can be cured by increasing the dietary intake of tryptophan with no increased intake of niacin. Wheat and other grains contain a poorly absorbed form of niacin, but provide adequate amounts of tryptophan so their use is not associated with pellagra.

Daily Recommended Intake

Either adequate amounts of niacin or high-quality protein are needed to cure the symptoms of pellagra. Niacin is a vitamin, but it also can be produced in the body from the amino acid tryptophan. More than half of the daily requirement for niacin is obtained by the conversion of tryptophan to niacin with the help of vitamin B_6.

The total daily niacin intake is expressed as niacin equivalents and includes both the dietary intake of the vitamin and the amount of niacin formed as a result of tryptophan intake. Food composition tables provide information on the amount of niacin in a food but do not include the niacin from the tryptophan-to-niacin conversion. To estimate total niacin equivalents:

1. Estimate total grams of protein consumed in a day.
2. Multiply by 0.01 to determine total tryptophan intake (tryptophan constitutes 1% of total protein intake).
3. Convert grams to milligrams (1 gram = 1,000 mg).
4. Divide by 60 mg to determine niacin equivalents from tryptophan conversion (it takes 60 mg of tryptophan to produce 1 mg of niacin).
5. Add the niacin equivalents to the dietary intake of preformed niacin to determine total niacin available in the diet.

It can be assumed that niacin intake is adequate if the daily diet contains more than three servings of protein-rich foods, such as low-fat milk and cheese, lean meat, chicken, fish, or cooked dried beans and peas. Most diets in the United States contain about 500 mg to 1,000 mg or more of tryptophan and about 8 mg to 17 mg of preformed niacin, for a total daily intake of 34 mg of niacin equivalents (Table 9).

Table 9.
THE NIACIN EQUIVALENT CONTENT OF SELECTED FOODS

Food	Amount	Niacin (mg)	Tryptophan (mg/100gr)	Niacin Equivalent (mg/serving)
Chicken	½ breast	15.5	205	21.5
Salmon	3 ounces	6.8	200	9.6
Beef	2.9 ounces	4.4	198	7.1
Peanut butter	2 Tbsp	4.8	305	6.2
Peas, green	1 cup	2.7	66	4.5

Table 9. (*continued*)
THE NIACIN EQUIVALENT CONTENT OF SELECTED FOODS

Food	Amount	Niacin (mg)	Tryptophan (mg/100gr)	Niacin Equivalent (mg/serving)
Potato	1 medium	2.7	33	3.6
Brewer's (nutritional) yeast	1 Tbsp	3.0	429	3.6
Milk	1 cup	0.2	50	2.2

The RDAs for niacin are based on calorie intake, 6.6 mg of niacin/1,000 calories. No less than 13 mg of niacin should be consumed each day to maintain tissue stores in adults.

The 1989 RDAs for niacin are:

	Niacin (mg)
INFANTS	
0–0.5 years	5
0.5–1 years	6
CHILDREN	
1–3 years	9
4–6 years	12
7–10 years	13
ADOLESCENTS AND YOUNG ADULTS	
Males 11–14 years	17
Males 15–18 years	20
Females 11–18 years	15
ADULTS	
Males 19–50 years	19
Males 50+	15
Females 19–50 years	15
Females 50+	13
Pregnant	17
Lactating	20

Sources in the Diet

The best sources of niacin and tryptophan are protein-rich foods such as lean meat, chicken, fish, cooked dried beans and peas, brewer's (nutritional) yeast, peanut butter, non-fat or low-fat milk and cheese, soybeans, and nuts. Milk contains little preformed niacin, but is a good selection because of its high tryptophan content. Fruit, except for orange juice, is a poor source of niacin.

The vitamin is relatively stable to heat and light and little is lost during cooking and preparation of food unless cooking water is discarded.

Toxicity

Daily doses of niacin up to 1,000 mg appear to be safe. A single 1,000 mg dose of nicotinic acid can cause dilation of the blood vessels and skin flushing, headaches, tingling, and burning within 15 minutes of ingestion. In the past, snake oils and medicinal elixirs often contained nicotinic acid. The characteristic flushing that occurred when the product was used was mistakenly attributed to the healing effects of the potion.

The flushing effect is caused by a sudden release of histamine and for this reason people with asthma or peptic ulcer disease are cautioned against taking large dose of nicotinic acid. Niacinamide does not produce these effects, regardless of the dose.

Niacin is likely to be toxic for some people who consume several gram doses of the vitamin. Large doses of niacin (more than 3 grams) also might increase the risk for liver damage and might increase uric acid levels.

Nutrient-Nutrient Interactions

- Niacin deficiency alone is rare. The vitamin works closely with vitamin B_1, vitamin B_2, pantothenic acid, biotin, and vitamin B_6 in energy metabolism and is found in similar foods. A deficiency of one of these nutrients usually means that other B vitamins are deficient, too.
- Protein, specifically the amino acid tryptophan, can partially or totally substitute for niacin in the prevention and treatment of pellagra.
- The addition of vitamin A and vitamin E to nicotinic acid therapy in the treatment of heart disease might allow a lower, less toxic dose of niacin to be used.
- Vitamin B_6 is needed to convert tryptophan to niacin in the body.
- Tryptophan competes with another amino acid, leucine, for absorption and use in the body. Chronic, excess intake of leucine can cause a secondary tryptophan and niacin deficiency.

VITAMIN B₆ (PYRIDOXINE, PYRIDOXAMINE, PYRIDOXAL)

Overview

Vitamin B_6 is a family of water-soluble compounds that includes pyridoxine, pyridoxamine, and pyridoxal. Excess intake is excreted in the urine.

Functions

Vitamin B_6 is involved in the building and breakdown of carbohydrates, fats, and proteins; however, its primary role involves protein and its building blocks, the amino acids. Vitamin B_6 aids in the conversion of one amino acid to another, the synthesis of new amino acids from carbohydrate, the conversion of amino acids to carbohydrate or fat for storage or energy, and the conversion of the amino acid tryptophan to niacin. Thus, vitamin B_6 is involved in the manufacture of most protein-related compounds, such as hormones, the protein hemoglobin in red blood cells, protein-derived neurotransmitters that regulate nerve function, and many enzymes (the catalysts for all body processes), such as those responsible for the release of sugar from storage in the liver. In addition, vitamin B_6 is necessary for the conversion of one type of essential fat to another and in the formation of fat-derived hormone-like substances called *prostaglandins* that regulate a variety of body processes including blood pressure, muscle contraction, and heart function. Vitamin B_6 also aids in the formation and maintenance of the nervous system.

ASTHMA. Supplementation with vitamin B_6 might be an effective aid in the treatment of asthma. Some people who consume additional vitamin B_6 daily report a reduction in severity and frequency of wheezing and asthmatic attacks. Asthmatics might have an altered ability to use vitamin B_6 and might require increased intake to maintain normal body functions.

BEHAVIOR. Mood and sleep disorders might improve if the vitamin B_6 content of the diet is increased. Billions of nerve cells transmit signals throughout the body to regulate behavior and body functions. These signals are conducted from one nerve cell to another by chemicals called *neurotransmitters*. Vitamin B_6 aids in the production of the neurotransmitter serotonin that regulates sleep, pain, mood, and eating habits. When the diet is low in vitamin B_6, the nerve cells cannot produce adequate amounts of serotonin and the result is insomnia, depression, irritability, and nervousness. Low levels of serotonin are found in suicidal patients, in people with low thresholds to pain, and in those suffering from depression. Mood stabilizes and depression is improved when vitamin B_6 intake is increased.

CARPAL TUNNEL SYNDROME. Carpal tunnel syndrome is a neurological disorder of the wrists and hands that often requires surgery. Supplementation with vitamin B_6 might alleviate pain and stiffness and prevent the need for surgery.

DRUG TOXICITY. Vitamin B_6 might reduce the harmful effects of some medications used in the treatment of cancer. The toxic effects of vincristine on the nervous system are reduced without affecting the medication's effectiveness in treating cancer when the intake of vitamin B_6 is increased. Azauridine triacetate is another medication used in the treatment of cancer. Adverse side effects of this medication are alleviated when vitamin B_6 intake is increased.

HEART DISEASE. Low levels of vitamin B_6 are found in patients who have suffered a heart attack; however, it is unknown whether a marginal deficiency of vitamin B_6 is a cause or a result of the disease. In addition, limited information shows that inadequate intake of vitamin B_6 might encourage the formation of atherosclerosis and increase the risk for developing premature heart disease.

IMMUNE SYSTEM. Adequate intake of vitamin B_6 aids in the regulation and maintenance of a healthy immune system; however, large doses do not provide additional benefits. Older adults who consume a diet inadequate in vitamin B_6 might be especially susceptible to infection and disease.

KIDNEY DISORDERS. Vitamin B_6 might be beneficial in the treatment of certain kidney disorders, such as hyperoxaluria—an excess amount of oxalates in the urine that can lead to kidney stones—and kidney damage or failure. Vitamin B_6 supplementation might lower the amount of oxalic acid in the urine and reduce the risk for kidney stone formation.

PREMENSTRUAL SYNDROME. Supplementation with vitamin B_6 might relieve the symptoms of premenstrual syndrome (PMS) in some women. Reduction in depression, irritability, tension, breast tenderness, edema (fluid retention), headaches, and acne has been reported by some women who take vitamin B_6 supplements (25 mg to 200 mg/day). However, symptoms also improve in many cases when women take placebos, which are sugar tablets with no nutritional or medicinal value. More research is necessary before recommendations can be made about the effectiveness of vitamin B_6 as a treatment for PMS.

Deficiency

Deficiency symptoms of vitamin B_6 are widespread and vague because of the vitamin's variety of functions. Symptoms include depression, vomiting, increased susceptibility to disease and infection, dermatitis, anemia, inflammation of the nerves, oxalate kidney stones, nausea, and lethargy. Infants fed formulas lacking in vitamin B_6 become irritable and develop convulsions. Deficiency symptoms can result from either inadequate intake of the vitamin or the use of antagonistic medications such as isoniazid, a medication used in the treatment of tuberculosis. A deficiency of vitamin B_6 also might be associated with an increased risk for developing cancer.

Pregnant women show low blood levels of vitamin B_6, possibly because of the developing infant's increased need for the vitamin. Vitamin B_6 has been used as a treatment for the nausea and vomiting of pregnancy and for the depression experienced by some women on oral contraceptives. The below-normal blood levels of vitamin B_6 found in these women result in lethargy, fatigue, and depression. Symptoms improve with increased intake of the vitamin.

Vitamin B_6 deficiency can accompany alcohol abuse, as alcohol reduces liver function and interferes with normal vitamin B_6 metabolism.

Infants born with a defect in how their body uses vitamin B_6 can develop mental retardation and uncontrollable convulsions. Treatment for the disorder requires physician supervision and large daily doses of vitamin B_6 initiated in the early days of life.

A low intake of vitamin B_6 might be associated with reduced bone width, malformation of bones, and epileptic seizures.

Daily Recommended Intake

The daily need for vitamin B_6 is based on protein intake. Measurements for the adult RDA are based on the assumption that the average daily protein intake is 100 grams; more of the vitamin would be needed if the protein intake was greater than this. Women on oral contraceptives, people exposed to radiation, patients with heart disease, and people on certain medications, such as amphetamines, chlorpromazine, and reserpine, need to increase the vitamin B_6 content of their diets above the adult RDAs. Inadequate intake of vitamin B_6 is common in adolescents, women, older adults, people on restricted diets, alcoholics, and people who consume diets high in sugar and fat.

The 1989 RDAs for vitamin B_6 are:

	Vitamin B_6 (mg)
INFANTS	
0–0.5 year	0.3
0.5–1 year	0.6
CHILDREN	
1–3 years	1.0
4–6 years	1.1
7–10 years	1.4
Males 11–14 years	1.7
Females 11–14 years	1.4
YOUNG ADULTS AND ADULTS	
Males 15+ years	2.0
Females 15–18 years	1.5
Females 19+ years	1.6
Pregnant	2.2
Lactating	2.1

Sources in the Diet

The best dietary sources of vitamin B_6 are protein-rich foods, such as lean meat, wheatgerm, brewer's (nutritional) yeast, poultry, fish, soybeans, cooked dried beans and peas, and peanuts. Moderate sources include bananas, avocados, cabbage, cauliflower, potatoes, whole grain breads and cereals, and dried fruit. Significant amounts of vitamin B_6 are lost during the processing and refining of flours. As much as 70% of the vitamin is lost when foods are frozen or when cooking water is discarded (Table 10).

Table 10.
THE VITAMIN B_6 CONTENT OF SELECTED FOODS

Food	Amount	Vitamin B_6 (mg)
Banana	1 medium	0.480
Avocado	½ medium	0.420
Hamburger	3 ounces	0.391
Chicken	3 ounces	0.340
Fish	3 ounces	0.289
Potato	1 medium	0.200
Collard greens	½ cup	0.170
Spinach, cooked	½ cup	0.161
Rice, brown	½ cup	0.127
Peas, green	½ cup	0.110

Table 10. (*continued*)
THE VITAMIN B_6 CONTENT OF SELECTED FOODS

Food	Amount	Vitamin B_6 (mg)
Walnuts	8 to 10 halves	0.109
Peanut butter	2 Tbsp	0.096
Wheatgerm	1 Tbsp	0.055

Toxicity

Vitamin B_6 is one of the few water-soluble vitamins that can be toxic to the nervous system when taken in large doses. Doses greater than 2,000 mg/day can produce tingling sensations in the neck and feet, lack of muscle coordination, a stumbling gait, and degeneration of nerve tissue. Lower doses of 200 mg might be toxic if taken daily for months or years. Most symptoms improve when supplementation is discontinued; however, some nerve damage might be permanent. Vitamin B_6 in doses exceeding 100 times the RDA or 200 mg should be taken only with the supervision of a physician.

Nutrient-Nutrient Interactions

- Vitamin B_6 requires vitamin B_2 for its normal function in the body.
- Vitamin B_6, in conjunction with vitamin B_2, is necessary for the conversion of tryptophan to niacin.
- Vitamin B_6 deficiency results in reduced absorption and low blood and liver levels of vitamin B_{12}.
  Vitamin C deficiency causes increased urinary excretion of vitamin B_6 and vitamin B_6 deficiency results in low blood levels of vitamin C.

VITAMIN B_{12} (COBALAMIN, CYANOCOBALAMIN)

Overview

Cobalamin is the general name for vitamin B_{12} and reflects the inclusion of cobalt in the vitamin's structure. Cyanocobalamin, the most stable form of vitamin B_{12} and the main form of synthetic vitamin B_{12}, has a cyanide group attached to the vitamin. The cyanide group is not found on the vitamin naturally, but is a consequence of processing.

The amount of cyanide derived from this form of vitamin B_{12} is minimal and well below toxic levels.

A form of anemia that affected older adults and usually resulted in death within 2 to 5 years was identified in the 1800s and named pernicious anemia (meaning deadly or fatal). More than 70 years later researchers found that a daily intake of 1 pound of raw liver cured pernicious anemia, and investigators theorized that "intrinsic" and "extrinsic" factors were responsible for the disease. The extrinsic factor in liver was identified as vitamin B_{12} in the late 1940s.

Intrinsic factor is a substance in digestive juices that binds to vitamin B_{12} and assists in the absorption of the vitamin in the lower small intestine. Absorption decreases with age or with a deficiency of iron and vitamin B_6, and increases during pregnancy. Unlike other water-soluble nutrients, vitamin B_{12} is stored in the liver, kidney, and other tissues, and symptoms of deficiency do not develop for 5 to 6 years despite poor dietary intake or inadequate secretion of intrinsic factor. Excess intake of the vitamin is excreted in the urine.

Functions

Vitamin B_{12} is necessary for normal processing of carbohydrate, protein, and fat in the body. It is important for the normal production of certain amino acids and fats and in the formation and maintenance of the nervous system. The formation of the insulation sheath around nerve cells, called the *myelin sheath*, requires vitamin B_{12}. This sheath speeds the conduction of signals along nerve cells. The vitamin functions in the replication of the genetic code within each cell, and in this capacity vitamin B_{12} is essential for the replacement and maintenance of all cells in the body.

Deficiency

A deficiency of vitamin B_{12} can result from poor dietary intake of the vitamin or inadequate secretion of intrinsic factor. In either case, anemia is the first clinical symptom. Vitamin B_6 deficiency also can be caused by intestinal disorders that impair vitamin B_{12} absorption, such as intestinal infections, or surgical removal of the portion of the small intestine where vitamin B_{12}-intrinsic factor is absorbed or the portion of the stomach that secretes intrinsic factor.

Vitamin B_{12} deficiency affects the growth and repair of all body cells. Poor vitamin B_{12} intake or absorption results in faulty formation of nerve cells. Irreversible nerve damage results, including disorientation, numbness, tingling, moodiness, confusion, agitation, dimmed vision, delusions, hallucinations, or dizziness. The improper replication of the genetic code that results from vitamin B_{12} deficiency causes poor formation of blood cells. Reduced numbers of red blood cells cause anemia and fatigue, and reduced numbers of white blood cells cause increased susceptibility to colds and disease. Reduced formation of blood cell fragments called *platelets* causes poor blood clotting and bruising. Poor cell formation in the digestive tract causes nausea, vomiting, loss of appetite, poor absorption of food, diarrhea, and increased likelihood of malnutrition. Faulty cell production in the skin causes dermatitis and changes in the lips and tongue.

The classic deficiency symptom of vitamin B_{12} is either pernicious anemia or megaloblastic (macrocytic) anemia. As with iron deficiency anemia, both of these forms of anemia start with fatigue and poor concentration; however, under the microscope the red blood cells are larger, more fragile, and fewer in number than the small, pale red blood cells seen in iron deficiency samples. Macrocytic means "large cell." The condition is called pernicious anemia when the cause is a lack of intrinsic factor; it is called megaloblastic or macrocytic anemia when poor dietary intake of vitamin B_{12} is the cause.

The symptoms of vitamin B_{12} deficiency and the nerve disorders associated with diabetes are similar. Possible disturbances in vitamin B_{12} metabolism might be associated with diabetic neuropathy.

Patients with Alzheimer's disease, a chronic and progressive brain disorder associated with memory loss, confusion, and nerve damage, also have low blood levels of vitamin B_{12}. Whether the low vitamin levels are a cause or a result of the disease is unclear.

The body's ability to conserve and store the vitamin combined with minimal daily needs means that a deficiency takes years to develop. Deficiency more often results from poor absorption than from dietary lack. Vitamin B_{12} deficiency is usually found in mid to later life when the production of intrinsic factor declines, and injections or large oral doses of vitamin B_{12} are often necessary to correct the problem. Strict vegetarians—people who do not consume any foods of animal origin—and their children whose diet is composed entirely of breastmilk are at risk for vitamin B_{12} deficiency. Other vegetarian diets that contain milk, yogurt, cheese, or eggs supply adequate amounts of the vitamin.

Daily Recommended Intake

The daily need for vitamin B_{12} is minimal, but essential. A diet that contains 4 or more servings a day of foods from animal origin contains between 7 mcg and 30 mcg of vitamin B_{12}, or 3 to 10 times the adult RDA.

The 1989 RDAs for vitamin B_{12} are:

	Vitamin B_{12} (mcg)
INFANTS	
0–0.5 year	0.3
0.5–1 year	0.5
CHILDREN	
1–3 years	0.7
4–6 years	1.0
7–10 years	1.4
YOUNG ADULTS AND ADULTS	
11+ years	2.0
Pregnant	2.2
Lactating	2.1

Sources in the Diet

Foods of animal origin or fermented foods are the only sources of vitamin B_{12}. The vitamin is produced only by bacteria and is not a natural component of plants unless they are fermented by bacteria, as is the case with fermented soybean products such as miso. Vitamin B_{12} produced by bacteria in the intestines of animals is also absorbed. Lean meats, poultry, fish, shellfish, milk, organ meats, cheese, and eggs are excellent dietary sources of the vitamin. Some of the vitamin is lost when food is cooked to temperatures above 100° C (Table 11).

Table 11.
THE VITAMIN B_{12} CONTENT OF SELECTED FOODS

Food	Amount	Vitamin B_{12} (mcg)
Liver, beef	3 ounces	68.0
Clams, canned	½ cup	19.1
Oysters, canned	3½ ounces	18.0
Tuna	2 ounces	1.32
Yogurt	1 cup	1.06
Milk, non-fat	1 cup	0.95
Halibut	3 ounces	0.85
Egg	1 large	0.77
Chicken	3 ounces	0.36
Cheese, cheddar	1 ounce	0.23

Toxicity

There are no known toxic effects in adults when the vitamin is consumed in amounts several times the RDA.

Nutrient-Nutrient Interactions

- Calcium is necessary for normal absorption of vitamin B_{12}.
- A deficiency of either iron or vitamin B_6 decreases the absorption of vitamin B_{12}.
- A high intake of folic acid can mask the anemia caused by vitamin B_{12} deficiency.
- Vitamin E deficiency might impair the conversion of vitamin B_{12} to its active form.
- A deficiency of vitamin B_6 results in reduced absorption and low blood and liver concentrations of vitamin B_{12}.

FOLIC ACID (FOLACIN)

Overview

In 1941, a substance extracted from spinach leaves and named folic acid from the Latin word "folium" for leaf was found to be effective in the treatment of anemia. Folic acid, also called folacin, is a family of water-soluble compounds. The folic acid in the diet is converted to its biologically active form in the body with the help of vitamin B_{12}, niacin, and vitamin C. The vitamin is absorbed from the small intestine and small amounts are stored in the liver and other tissues. Excess is excreted in the urine.

Functions

The main function of folic acid is to maintain the cells' genetic code and regulate cell division and the transfer of inherited traits from one cell to another. It is essential for the normal growth and maintenance of all cells.

Deficiency

A deficiency of folic acid limits cell function and affects the growth and repair of all cells and tissues in the body. The tissues that have the fastest rate of cell replacement are affected first, including red blood cells, the digestive tract, the cervix and vagina, and the skin. Symptoms of folic acid deficiency are macrocytic (megaloblastic) anemia, poor growth, digestive disorders, impaired nutrient absorption and malnutrition, diarrhea, loss of appetite, weight loss, weakness, apathy, sore tongue, headaches, heart palpitations, irritability, and behavioral disorders.

CANCER. A folic acid deficiency causes damage to cells that resembles the initial stage of cancer, and preliminary research shows low intake of folic acid might increase a woman's risk for developing cervical cancer. Women who take folic acid supplements show less precancerous cervical tissue as compared to women who consume a diet low in the vitamin. Folic acid might prevent the transformation of abnormal cells to cancer cells and might return damaged tissue to a healthy condition.

Folic acid is one of the most common vitamin deficiencies. Surveys show that the folic acid content of the American diet is half the recommended dietary intake. Stressful situations, including disease, alcohol consumption, and chronic use of medication add to the risk of developing a deficiency by increasing daily needs for the vitamin or reducing the absorption of the vitamin. Many major categories of drugs, including oral contraceptives, aspirin, and anticonvulsants, can produce a folic acid deficiency. A deficiency can develop within a few weeks to months of low dietary intake.

Daily Recommended Intake

Information on folic acid needs is limited and the latest RDAs are only estimates based on assumptions that the adult requires about 100 mcg to 200 mcg to maintain normal body functions and that approximately 25% to 50% of dietary intake is absorbed. RDAs for infants and children are based on body weight and the folic acid content of breastmilk. The small amount of folic acid stored in the liver is not adequate to meet the additional needs imposed by pregnancy, stress, lactation, ingestion of certain medications, or alcohol abuse. More information is necessary to determine more precise amounts of folic acid required for different age and sex groups.

The folic acid allowances in the 1989 edition of the RDAs are much lower than previous recommendations. Studies repeatedly showed that diets did not meet the previous allowances of 400 mcg for adults to 800 mcg for pregnant women, so the 1989 allowances were reduced based on the amount typically consumed by adults who show no clinical signs of deficiency. However, the new RDAs remain controversial as they do not consider marginal or subclinical status or the association between folic acid and the possible development of cancer. References in this book to the RDAs refer to previous recommendations for higher intakes than the latest 1989 allowances.

The 1989 RDAs compared to previous RDAs for folic acid:

	Folic Acid (mcg)	
	Previous RDAs	*1989 RDAs*
INFANTS		
0–0.5 year	30	25
0.5–1 year	34	35
CHILDREN		
1–3 years	100	50
4–6 years	200	75
7–10 years	300	100
11–14 years	400	150
ADULTS		
Males 15+ years	400	200
Females 15+ years	400	180
Pregnant	800	400
Lactating	500	260–280

Sources in the Diet

The best dietary sources of folic acid are brewer's (nutritional) yeast, dark green leafy vegetables, and liver. Orange juice, avocado, beets, and broccoli are also good sources. Whereas romaine lettuce and other leaf lettuce are good sources, iceberg or head lettuce contains minimal amounts of folic acid.

The vitamin is easily lost when foods are improperly stored for too long or at too warm a temperature or are overcooked or reheated. The vitamin is also lost when the cooking water is discarded. Salads that contain dark green or leaf lettuce should be consumed daily to ensure adequate folic acid intake (Table 12).

Table 12.
THE FOLIC ACID CONTENT OF SELECTED FOODS

Food	Amount	Folic Acid (mcg)
Brewer's (nutritional) yeast	1 Tbsp	313
Liver, beef	3 ounces	123
Spinach, raw	1 cup	106
Spinach, cooked	½ cup	82
Orange juice	6 ounces	102
Lettuce, romaine	1 cup	98
Lettuce, iceberg	1 cup	0–20
Beets, cooked	½ cup	66
Avocado	½ medium	59
Broccoli, cooked	½ cup	44

Table 12. (*continued*)
THE FOLIC ACID CONTENT OF SELECTED FOODS

Food	Amount	Folic Acid (mcg)
Wheatgerm	2 Tbsp	40
Beans, red, cooked	1/2 cup	34
Banana	1 medium	33
Brussels sprout, cooked	1/2 cup	28
Bread, whole wheat	1 slice	16
Bread, white	1 slice	10

Toxicity

Folic acid works closely with vitamin B_{12} in the maintenance and replication of the genetic code within each cell and the two vitamins share similar symptoms of deficiency. A diet high in folic acid or supplementation with the vitamin can cure the symptoms of anemia that result from a vitamin B_{12} deficiency, but folic acid is ineffective against the more serious nerve damage. Thus, folic acid could mask a vitamin B_{12} deficiency and nerve problems could progress undetected to irreversible stages. For this reason, the amount of folic acid in vitamin preparations is limited by law to 400 mcg for adults and 800 mcg for pregnant women.

Large doses of folic acid should not be taken unless the possibility of vitamin B_{12} deficiency has been first ruled out. A simple blood test would not be sufficient as the red blood cells will appear normal if folic acid intake is adequate. Strict vegetarians who consume large amounts of folic acid-rich foods and little or no vitamin B_{12} are at particular risk.

No toxic effects are known for folic acid even when doses 1,000 times the RDA are consumed; however, the vitamin might interfere with the effectiveness of anticonvulsant medications.

Nutrient-Nutrient Interactions

- Folic acid requires vitamin B_{12}, niacin, and vitamin C to be converted to its biologically active form.
- Folic acid can mask an underlying vitamin B_{12} deficiency.

BIOTIN (VITAMIN B₇)

Overview

The history of biotin is unique because this B vitamin was "discovered" several times and acquired several names prior to its final identification. It was originally discovered in 1901 and named "bios." Another group of researchers isolated a substance many years later that they called coenzyme R, and yet another group of investigators discovered "protective factor X" and "vitamin H." Eventually bios, biotin, coenzyme R, protective factor X, and vitamin H were identified as the same substance.

Biotin is water-soluble, absorbed in the small intestine, and excesses are excreted in the urine. Significant amounts are produced by bacteria in the intestines and are probably available for absorption as more biotin is excreted in the urine than is consumed in the diet.

Functions

Biotin is essential for numerous body processes that manufacture and break down fats, amino acids, and carbohydrates. The vitamin works closely with folic acid, pantothenic acid, and vitamin B_{12}, and also might minimize the symptoms of a zinc deficiency.

Deficiency

A biotin deficiency is rare, even when a person consumes a diet low in the B vitamin. However, long-term consumption of large doses of raw egg whites, more than 15 to 20 raw eggs a day, can result in biotin deficiency. A protein in raw egg white called *avidin* binds to biotin in the intestine and prevents its absorption. Avidin is deactivated by cooking. An occasional raw egg in the diet will not produce a biotin deficiency.

Infants might develop deficiency symptoms from poor absorption of the vitamin. Some hospitalized patients on formulated tube or intravenous feedings also have developed a biotin deficiency. Symptoms include dermatitis, depression, conjunctivitis, progressive hair loss and color, elevated blood levels of cholesterol, anemia, loss of appetite, tingling and numbness in the hands and feet, nausea, lethargy, muscle pain, and enlargement of the liver.

Long-term use of antibiotics interferes with the production of biotin in the intestine and might increase the risk for deficiency. Oxytetracycline and sulfonamides are two antibiotics that specifically reduce the growth of intestinal bacteria that produce biotin.

Daily Recommended Intake

The biotin content of the average American diet is estimated to be between 150 to 300 mcg each day. Dietary intake combined with bacterial production in the intestine apparently is adequate to prevent deficiency symptoms.

The 1989 Safe and Adequate Intakes for biotin are:

	Biotin (mcg)
INFANTS	
0–0.5 year	10
0.5–1 year	15
CHILDREN AND ADULTS	
1–3 years	20
4–6 years	25
7–10 years	30
11+ years	30-100

Sources in the Diet

Good sources of biotin are organ meats such as kidney and liver, oatmeal, egg yolk, soybeans, clams, mushrooms, bananas, peanuts, and brewer's (nutritional) yeast (Table 13).

Table 13.
THE BIOTIN CONTENT OF SELECTED FOODS

Food	Amount	Biotin (mcg)
Liver, beef	3 ounces	82
Oatmeal, cooked	1 cup	58
Soybeans, cooked	½ cup	22
Clams, canned	½ cup	20
Egg, cooked	1 medium	13
Peanut butter	2 Tbsp	12
Salmon	3 ounces	10
Milk	1 cup	10
Rice, brown, cooked	½ cup	9
Chicken	3 ounces	9
Mushrooms, canned	½ cup	7
Banana	1 medium	6
Rice, white, cooked	½ cup	4

Toxicity

Biotin has no known toxic effects.

Nutrient-Nutrient Interactions

- Biotin works closely with folic acid, pantothenic acid, and vitamin B_{12}.
- Biotin lessens the symptoms of a pantothenic acid and a zinc deficiency.

PANTOTHENIC ACID (CALCIUM PANTOTHENATE, VITAMIN B_3)

Overview

Pantothenic acid is a B vitamin named after the Greek word *pantos*, meaning "everywhere." The name reflects the vitamin's widespread appearance in plants and animals. Pantothenic acid is available commercially as calcium pantothenate. The B vitamin is water-soluble, absorbed from the intestine, and excesses are excreted in the urine. The body has a limited ability to store the vitamin.

Functions

Pantothenic acid is said to function at the "crossroads of metabolism." The vitamin is converted to a substance called *coenzyme A*, an important catalyst in the breakdown of fats, carbohydrates, and protein for energy. Pantothenic acid also functions in the production of fats, cholesterol, bile, vitamin D, red blood cells, and some hormones and neurotransmitters. The vitamin prevents graying of hair in some animals and stimulates wound healing.

Deficiency

A deficiency of pantothenic acid has not been reported in humans. A deficiency can be induced in laboratory animals and in volunteer subjects fed a highly refined synthetic diet complete in all nutrients except pantothenic acid and also given a medication that depletes the tissues of the vitamin. Under these severe conditions animals and humans show a variety of symptoms including fatigue, cardiovascular and digestive problems, upper respiratory infections, dermatitis, burning sensations, lack of coordination, staggering gait, restlessness, and muscle cramps. Additional symptoms include irritability, poor wound healing, loss of appetite, indigestion, fainting, rapid pulse, increased susceptibility to infection, depression, and numbness and tingling in the hands and feet.

Daily Recommended Intake

The pantothenic acid content of the average American diet is between 5 mg and 20 mg a day. This amount is assumed to be sufficient as no deficiency has been reported. Bacterial synthesis of the vitamin in the intestine that is available for absorption might be another source. Stressful situations, such as pregnancy and lactation, increase daily needs. However, there is not enough information to establish a specific recommended allowance for this B vitamin.

The 1989 Safe and Adequate Intakes for pantothenic acid are:

	Pantothenic Acid (mg)
INFANTS	
0–0.5 year	2
0.5–1 year	3
CHILDREN AND ADULTS	
4–6 years	3–4
7–10 years	4–5
11+ years	4–7

Sources in the Diet

Pantothenic acid is found in a wide variety of foods including liver, fish, chicken, cheese, whole grain breads and cereals, avocados, cauliflower, green peas, cooked dried beans and peas, nuts, dates, and potatoes. Significant amounts of pantothenic acid are lost in the milling and refining of grains. As this vitamin is not added in the "enrichment" process, refined flour, breads, rice, and noodles are a poor source of pantothenic acid. As much as 50% of the pantothenic acid is lost in the thawing and cooking of meat (Table 14).

Table 14.
THE PANTOTHENIC ACID CONTENT OF SELECTED FOODS

Food	Amount	Pantothenic Acid (mg)
Liver, beef	3 ounces	6.035
Egg	1 medium	1.100
Avocado	½ medium	1.100
Mushrooms, canned	½ cup	1.000
Milk	1 cup	0.984
Chicken	3 ounces	0.765
Soybeans, cooked	½ cup	0.525
Peanut butter	2 Tbsp	0.476
Banana	1 medium	0.450

Table 14. (*continued*)
THE PANTOTHENIC ACID CONTENT OF SELECTED FOODS

Food	Amount	Pantothenic Acid (mg)
Orange	1 medium	0.450
Collard greens, cooked	½ cup	0.425
Potato	1 medium	0.400
Broccoli, cooked	½ cup	0.315
Rice, brown, cooked	½ cup	0.300
Rice, white, cooked	½ cup	0.150
Cantaloupe	¼ melon	0.300
Bread, whole wheat	1 slice	0.184
Bread, white	1 slice	0.092
Wheatgerm	1 Tbsp	0.132

Toxicity

Large doses of pantothenic acid can be consumed with no serious toxic effects other than diarrhea. There is no known benefit to taking large doses of the vitamin other than a possible improvement in athletic performance.

Nutrient-Nutrient Interaction

- Pantothenic acid works with vitamin B_1, vitamin B_2, niacin, vitamin B_6, and biotin in the breakdown of carbohydrates, protein, and fats for energy.
- Pantothenic acid is necessary for the production of vitamin D.
- Biotin lessens the symptoms of a pantothenic acid deficiency.

VITAMIN C (L-ASCORBIC ACID, L-DEHYDROASCORBIC ACID)

Overview

Vitamin C cures the oldest known nutrient-deficiency disease: scurvy. In fact, ascorbic is the Latin word for "without scurvy." Prior to the discovery of vitamin C, scurvy was responsible for the death of one-half to two-thirds of the crew on prolonged ocean voyages where the diet consisted solely of cereals and meat. James Lind's recommendation to include limes or lemons (rich sources of vitamin C) in the daily menu was ignored at first by the British Navy, but eventually became the source of the nickname for British sailors—"limeys."

Vitamin C is a water-soluble vitamin that is easily absorbed in the intestine. Excesses of vitamin C are excreted in the urine. Humans are one of the few species that cannot manufacture vitamin C and must depend on the diet as their only source of the vitamin.

Functions

Vitamin C functions in the formation and maintenance of collagen, a protein that forms the basis for the most abundant tissue in the body: connective tissue. The shape and function of all tissues depend on collagen, which acts as a cementing substance between cells. Collagen is found in bones, the cornea of the eye, teeth, tendons, skin, and other tissues; is the supporting material in blood vessel walls; maintains the shape of the discs of the backbone; allows joints to move; and binds muscle cells together. Collagen, and therefore vitamin C, promotes the healing of wounds, bone fractures, bruises, hemorrhages, and bleeding gums; and forms a protective barrier between infections or disease and the surrounding healthy tissues.

ALLERGY. Vitamin C might reduce the bronchial constriction and impaired breathing that results from allergic reactions.

ANTIOXIDANT. Vitamin C is an antioxidant and might reduce tissue damage associated with premature aging, cancer, and rheumatoid arthritis.

CANCER. Nitrites, added to processed meats and found naturally in some foods, combine with other compounds in the stomach to form potent cancer-causing substances called *nitrosamines*. Vitamin C inhibits the conversion of nitrites to nitrosamines and apparently reduces the risk for developing cancer of the stomach, bladder, and colon. Vitamin C also might inhibit the growth of cancer cells. (See pages 153–154 for more information on vitamin C and cancer.)

CATARACTS. Vitamin C might inhibit the progression and encourage the regression of some types of cataracts in the eyes.

DIABETES. Adequate intake and maintenance of high blood levels of vitamin C might help regulate blood sugar, and low vitamin C levels in white blood cells are found in diabetics.

HEART AND ARTERY DISEASE. Vitamin C helps regulate cholesterol production in the liver and conversion of cholesterol to bile for excretion. The vitamin also might aid in the removal of cholesterol from artery walls and sometimes is used in the treatment of atherosclerosis. Vitamin C might lower total blood cholesterol and LDL-cholesterol, increase HDL-cholesterol, and reduce risk for developing heart disease, atherosclerosis, and stroke. (See page 162 for more information on vitamin C and heart disease.)

IMMUNE RESPONSE. Adequate intake of vitamin C might increase resistance to colds and infection. Vitamin C does not prevent infection, but, in some studies, adequate intake is associated with fewer colds of shorter duration and less severity. (See page 129 for more information on vitamin C and immunity.)

STRESS. Vitamin C is important in the formation of the stress hormones produced in the adrenal glands. Vitamin C is depleted from these tissues and urinary excretion of the vitamin increases during times of stress.

Vitamin C is necessary for the conversion of folic acid to its potent or biologically active form. The vitamin also enhances the absorption and use of iron; is important in the conversion of tryptophan to the hormone-like substance serotonin, which regulates sleep, pain, depression, and other behaviors; and is necessary for the formation of a hormone related to adrenaline.

Deficiency

The major symptoms of scurvy result from vitamin C's role in the formation of collagen. Poorly formed collagen results in small, pinpoint hemorrhages under the skin; poor wound healing or breakdown of old scars; spongy, bleeding gums; dry, scaly skin; damage to blood vessels; swollen, tender joints and aching bones; gangrene; muscle cramps; and loosened teeth. General weakness and lethargy, loss of appetite, depression, swollen legs and arms, and shortness of breath also are symptoms of scurvy.

Stomach disorders, such as gastritis and skin problems associated with rheumatoid arthritis, might result from poor vitamin C intake. Low intake of vitamin C can result in delayed healing, reduced resistance to colds and infections, and increased susceptibility to disease.

Severe vitamin C deficiency and scurvy are rare in the United States; however, marginal deficiencies and poor dietary intake of vitamin C are common. Most large-scale national nutrition surveys in the United States report inadequate intake of vitamin C. Alcohol and tobacco, stress, limited food intake and poor intake of fruits and vegetables, chronic illness, and long-term use of some medications contribute to vitamin C deficiency. Bottle-fed infants should be given a vitamin C supplement or given vitamin C-rich fruit juice within the first 6 months; breastmilk contains adequate amounts of the vitamin if the mother's diet is adequate.

Daily Recommended Intake

Scurvy is prevented when the dietary intake of vitamin C is approximately 10 mg a day. Tissues stores are saturated at 100 mg to 120 mg a day and the antioxidant functions of vitamin C are enhanced at intakes of 150 mg or more. Daily needs increase above the adult RDA during physical and emotional stress such as fever, infection, elevated environmental temperatures, or burns; illness such as congestive heart failure, kidney and liver disease, gastrointestinal disturbances, and cancer; alcohol and tobacco abuse; or use of medications such as oral contraceptives. The 1989 RDAs acknowledge the negative effect tobacco use has on vitamin C status and recommend that people who use tobacco consume at least 100 mg of vitamin C each day. One study found that 1,000 mg of vitamin C were required to counteract some of the harmful effects of cigarette smoking.

The 1989 RDAs for vitamin C are:

	Vitamin C (mg)
INFANTS	
0.0–0.5 years	30
0.5–1.0 years	35
CHILDREN	
1–3 years	40
4–10 years	45
11–14 years	50
YOUNG ADULTS AND ADULTS	
15+ years	60
Pregnant	70
Lactating, 1st 6 mo	95
Lactating, 2nd 6 mo	90

Sources in the Diet

The best sources of vitamin C are fresh fruits and vegetables. Poor sources of vitamin C include milk, meat, eggs, poultry, fish, cereals and bread, and nuts. Freezing has little effect on vitamin C content, so frozen vegetables are an excellent source of the vitamin. Some vitamin C is lost when fruits and vegetables are heated during the canning process and more vitamin C is lost if canning water is discarded.

The vitamin is easily lost when foods are handled or prepared improperly. Aging, bruising, storing at temperatures above 40° F, overwashing, cooking too long, discarding cooking water, and reheating or holding foods at room temperature or higher destroys the vitamin. Baking soda added to vegetables to retain their color destroys vitamin C. Slicing or chopping vegetables exposes a greater surface area to air and light and more of the vitamin is lost. For example, French fries contain less vitamin C than a baked potato, and vegetables cut and exposed to air at a salad bar lose substantial amounts of vitamin C.

To maximize vitamin C intake, purchase only the amount of food that can be used within a few days. Fruits and vegetables should be sun-ripened, chilled and used immediately after picking, eaten raw or cooked for a short time in a minimum amount of water, and only enough should be cooked for immediate consumption (Table 15).

Table 15.
THE VITAMIN C CONTENT OF SELECTED FOODS

Food	Amount	Vitamin C (mg)
Orange juice	6 ounces	90
Brussels sprouts	½ cup	68
Strawberries	½ cup	66
Orange	1 medium	66
Broccoli	½ cup	52
Collard greens	½ cup	44
Cantaloupe	¼	32
Tomato juice	6 ounces	30
Cabbage	½ cup	24
Asparagus	½ cup	19
Green peas	½ cup	17
Potato	1 small	15
Lima beans	½ cup	15
Pineapple	½ cup	15
French fried potaotes	8	10
Mashed potatoes	½ cup	10
Corn on the cob	1 small	7
Banana	1 medium	6
Carrots	½ cup	5

Toxicity

Vitamin C is water-soluble, and as excesses are excreted in the urine, large amounts of the vitamin can be consumed without risk for toxicity. However, some toxic effects might be experienced when doses greater than 1 gram are consumed regularly. Megadoses of vitamin C might reduce the absorption or utilization of selenium and copper and might produce a conditioning effect that results in scurvy when supplementation is stopped, especially in infants born to mothers who consumed large doses of this vitamin during pregnancy. Vitamin C might aggravate kidney stone formation in patients with kidney disease. Excess intake of vitamin C gives a false positive test for diabetes and interferes with test results for hemoglobin. Large doses of vitamin C can cause nausea, stomach cramping, diarrhea, vomiting, and increased susceptibility to colds and infections, especially in children.

Nutrient-Nutrient Interactions

- Deficiency of vitamin C is associated with increased urinary excretion of vitamin B_6 and a vitamin B_6 deficiency results in low blood levels of vitamin C.
- Vitamin C enhances the absorption of iron when both are consumed in the same meal.
- Vitamin C has a protective function against the toxic effects of cadmium.
- Toxic symptoms caused by high doses of copper, vanadium, cobalt, mercury, and selenium are reduced by vitamin C.
- Large doses of vitamin C might lower blood levels of copper and selenium.
- Calcium or manganese supplementation might decrease urinary excretion of vitamin C.
- Vitamin C supplementation might increase absorption of manganese.

VITAMIN-LIKE FACTORS (BIOFLAVONOIDS, CHOLINE, INOSITOL, LIPOIC ACID, UBIQUINONE)

Several naturally-occurring substances in foods have been investigated for their use in the body. Some have no known functions. Others are essential to animals but do not appear to be necessary for humans. Still others are necessary for health but are manufactured in the body and dietary requirements, if any, are unknown.

Bioflavonoids

Initial research in the 1930s indicated that flavonoids might be a useful treatment for patients with fragile, easily torn blood vessels, and these substances were given the name vitamin P. Over four decades of research have not supported this initial claim and the substances have been renamed bioflavonoids.

There are over 200 substances grouped under the name of bioflavonoids, or flavonoids; rutin, hesperidin, and quercetin are examples. Limited evidence exists to support the claim that bioflavonoids are essential to humans or that they serve a purpose in health or the prevention of disease. There are no accepted uses for these substances in the treatment of damaged blood vessels, hypertension, rheumatic fever, arthritis, or cancer, although a few studies show the bioflavonoids might function as antioxidants. Claims are unsubstantiated that bioflavonoids improve the effects of vitamin C, although limited evidence suggests the bioflavonoids in citrus fruits might increase the absorption and retention of vitamin C. Bioflavonoids are broken down in the intestine and little, if any, intact bioflavonoids are absorbed from the diet.

The average diet contains approximately 1,000 mg of bioflavonoids. The best dietary sources are the skin, peel, and outer layer of fruits and vegetables such as citrus fruits; leafy vegetables; tea, coffee, and wine; and red onions.

Choline

Choline is an essential nutrient for some animals. The human body can make choline with the help of vitamin B_{12}, folic acid, and an amino acid called *methionine*, although not always in sufficient amounts to meet daily needs. Choline is not considered a vitamin, however, as no deficiency symptoms have been identified and limited evidence exists that the human body requires choline from the diet, unless the amino acid methionine and the B vitamin folic acid are low in the diet.

Choline functions in the production and transportation of fats from the liver and thus aids in the prevention of fat accumulation in this organ. Choline is also used in the formation of lecithin and in the structure of cell membranes. As a component of acetylcholine, choline is necessary for normal nerve and brain function. Levels of this nerve regulator increase in proportion to dietary intake of choline. Pharmacological doses of choline have been experimentally used with varying success in the treatment of Huntington's disease and tardive dyskinesia, disorders of the nervous system related to low levels of acetylcholine in brain or nerve tissue.

No recommended daily intakes or toxicity levels have been established for choline. The average daily diet supplies between 400 mg and 900 mg of choline. This amount is apparently adequate to maintain health, but should not be considered a dietary requirement.

The best dietary sources of choline are eggs, liver and other organ meats, lean meat, brewer's (nutritional) yeast, wheatgerm, soybeans, peanuts, and green peas.

Inositol

Inositol was a recognized component of food for years before it was accepted as a vitamin in 1940. Its status, however, is controversial. The body and intestinal bacteria can make inositol, but whether or not synthesis meets daily needs is unclear.

Inositol is found in the brain and nerve, muscle, skeletal, reproductive, and heart tissues. It is a component of cell membranes and functions in nerve transmission and the regulation of certain enzymes. It also might function in the manufacture, transportation, and function of fats.

Inositol deficiency in animals produces fat accumulation in the liver, nerve disorders similar to those observed in diabetics, and intestinal problems. Inositol might have a therapeutic function in the treatment of nerve disorders associated with diabetes. The metabolism of inositol is altered in chronic renal failure and multiple sclerosis, but increased dietary intake has not proven beneficial. Claims that inositol cures baldness were based on a few animal studies and have no relevance to hereditary hair loss in humans.

No deficiency or toxicity has been identified for inositol and this is unlikely as the substance is found in a variety of foods. Dietary intake averages approximately 1,000 mg a day. Inositol is added to infant non-cow's milk formulas as a preventive measure.

Lipoic Acid

Lipoic acid is a fat-soluble compound produced in the body and not considered a dietary essential for health. It is not a vitamin. Lipoic acid works with vitamin B_1, vitamin B_2, niacin, and pantothenic acid in the breakdown of carbohydrates, protein, and fats for energy. Dietary sources include liver and brewer's (nutritional) yeast.

Ubiquinone (Coenzyme Q)

Ubiquinone is named for its ubiquitous (widespread) distribution in plants and animals. It is a fat-soluble substance produced in the body and present in all cells, where it functions in the production of energy from carbohydrates. Ubiquinone is not a vitamin and no deficiencies or toxicities have been identified.

NON-VITAMINS

Laetrile

A biochemist named Ernst Krebs announced in 1952 he had developed a new drug that cured cancer. He called the drug laetrile and a few years later reclassified it as a vitamin (vitamin B_{17}). Krebs and his son produced and promoted the substance as a cancer preventative and cure, and claimed the Food and Drug Administration (FDA) and the medical association had joined efforts to keep the public away from this wonder drug.

Laetrile, or amygdalin, is obtained from apricot pits or almond kernels. Extensive testing of laetrile by the National Cancer Institute and other reputable organizations has found no benefits from its use in cancer prevention or treatment. In addition, laetrile does not meet the criteria to be called a vitamin as it has no known metabolic function and its removal from the diet does not produce deficiency symptoms. Laetrile contains 6% cyanide, is highly toxic, and potentially lethal. However, laetrile's greatest harm is that people with potentially curable cancer abandon conventional treatments and take laetrile until it is too late to benefit from effective therapy.

Pangamic Acid

Pangamic acid mistakenly has been called a vitamin (vitamin B_{15}). This substance is not essential to health, nor has a need, deficiency, or level of safe consumption been identified. Pangamic acid falsely has been credited with numerous functions including extension of cell life, stimulation of immune response, detoxification of pollutants, synthesis of proteins, protection of the liver, cure for fatigue, and regulation of hormones. Claims are unfounded that pangamic acid will cure fatigue, cancer, alcoholism, schizophrenia, heart disease, aging, senility, diabetes, hypertension, glaucoma, drug addiction, cirrhosis, hepatitis, jaundice, dermatitis, sciatica, brain dysfunction, autism, gangrene, sexual problems, or allergies.

Pangamic acid was originally obtained from apricot pits, but commercial products can contain anything. Analysis of pangamic acid samples reveals a variety of ingredients and no products sold commercially have been found by the Food and Drug Administration (FDA) to contain the substance alleged to be the original formula. The term vitamin B_{15} is meaningless and is used to describe anything the manufacturer wishes to include in the product.

CHAPTER 4

The Minerals

The human body reduced to its simplest form is a small pile of ashes. The carbon, hydrogen, oxygen, and nitrogen from protein-rich tissues and carbohydrate or fat stores have dissolved into the air or evaporated as water leaving only the minerals. These ashes, weighing approximately 5 pounds, might be small in size, but they play vital roles in all body tissues.

Minerals are involved in a variety of functions. They provide structure to bones and participate in muscle contraction, blood formation, building protein, energy production, and numerous other body processes. Some minerals, such as sodium, potassium, and calcium, have electrical "charges" that act something like a magnet to attach to other electrically charged substances and form complex molecules, conduct electrical impulses along nerves, or transport substances in and out of the cells. In the blood and other fluids, minerals regulate the pH balance of the body and the fluid pressure between cells and the blood. Minerals also bind to proteins and other organic substances and are found in red blood cells, all cell membranes, hormones, and enzymes—the catalysts of all bodily processes.

There are 22 minerals essential to human health and these nutrients are divided into two categories: major minerals and trace minerals. Major minerals are present in the body in amounts greater than a teaspoon, while a trace mineral totals less than a teaspoon. The terms "major" and "trace" do not reflect the importance of a mineral in maintaining optimal health, as a deficiency of either major or trace minerals produces equally harmful effects.

The major minerals include the following:

calcium	potassium
chloride	sodium
magnesium	sulfur
phosphorus	

The trace minerals include:

chromium	molybdenum
cobalt	nickel
copper	selenium
fluoride	silicon
iodine	tin
iron	vanadium
manganese	zinc

There are also trace amounts of arsenic, barium, bromine, cadmium, strontium, gold, silver, aluminum, bismuth, gallium, and other minerals in the body, but little is known about how, or if, these minerals affect health and maintenance of normal bodily processes.

In this chapter, the minerals are discussed individually, but should not be considered separate with respect to their absorption, function, or requirements. Minerals can work either together or against each other. Some minerals compete for absorption, so a large intake of one mineral can produce a deficiency of another. This is especially true of the trace minerals, such as iron, zinc, and copper. In other cases, some minerals can enhance the absorption of other minerals. For example, the proper proportion of magnesium, calcium, and phosphorus in the diet enhances the absorption and use of all three minerals. Absorption is also dependent on body needs; a person who is deficient in a mineral will absorb more of it than someone who is adequately nourished.

CALCIUM

Overview

Calcium is the most abundant mineral and the fifth most abundant substance in the body after carbon, hydrogen, oxygen, and nitrogen. The average healthy male body contains about 2½ to 3 pounds of calcium; the average healthy female body contains approximately 2 pounds. Of this calcium, 99% is located in the bones and teeth. The other 1% is in the blood and other body fluids and within all cells where it aids in the regulation of numerous body processes.

The mineral is absorbed in the small intestine with the help of vitamin D. Between 10% and 40% of dietary intake is absorbed, although women after menopause absorb as little as 7% of dietary intake. More calcium is absorbed when a person is deficient in the mineral; when intake is marginal; or when lactose (milk sugar) and adequate, but not excessive, amounts of protein, magnesium, phosphorus, and vitamin D are present. Calcium absorption is reduced with excessive intake of substances called *oxalates* and *phytates* that are found in foods such as spinach and unleavened whole wheat products; intake of alcohol, coffee, sugar, or drugs such as tetracycline, diuretics, and aluminum-containing antacids; or stress. People who exercise infrequently or who are bedridden absorb less and excrete more calcium and are more prone to bone disorders than are active people.

Functions

BONES AND TEETH. The primary function of calcium is in the development and maintenance of healthy bones and teeth. A constant supply of the mineral is required throughout life, especially during periods of growth, such as childhood, pregnancy, and lactation.

Calcium is found in two different forms in the bones. One form of calcium is bound tightly within the bone and is not easily removed. A second form of calcium can be easily removed from bone to aid in maintaining normal blood calcium levels. This exchangeable portion of calcium is a reserve that builds up when the diet is adequate in calcium. Calcium is removed from the less mobile portion of bone only when the calcium reserves are exhausted and dietary intake is poor. This can result in bone disorders, such as osteoporosis.

As with most tissues, bones are constantly being reformed. They are not static tissue. Throughout life, bones lose and gain calcium daily, which results in constant "remodeling" of bone tissue. In children, the gain in calcium outweighs the loss, and bone tissue increases in size and hardness. In later years or when dietary intake is poor, calcium loss might outweigh calcium gain and the bones become less dense and more susceptible to fracture. In the healthy adult who consumes an optimal diet, the process of bone maintenance is in balance with approximately equal amounts of calcium entering and leaving the bones each day. The "wives' tale" that a woman loses a tooth for each child is not true, as little calcium is lost from teeth even during times of calcium deprivation.

BLOOD CLOTTING. Calcium is necessary for the normal blood clotting mechanisms that begin the process of wound healing.

BLOOD PRESSURE. Adequate intake of calcium helps maintain normal blood pressure. In countries where the intake of calcium-rich dairy products is high, the incidence of hypertension is low. Calcium supplementation aids in the maintenance of normal blood pressure and increased calcium intake reduces blood pressure in some people with hypertension. (See pages 196–197 for more information on calcium and hypertension.)

CANCER. Calcium and vitamin D might offer some protection against cancer of the colon. People with colon cancer consume less calcium and vitamin D when compared to healthy people.

ENZYMES AND HORMONES. Calcium is essential for the production and activity of numerous enzymes and hormones that regulate digestion, energy and fat metabolism, and the production of saliva.

HEART DISEASE. Increased calcium intake, whether from supplements or from fermented dairy products such as yogurt, might lower blood cholesterol levels and reduce the risk for developing premature heart disease. The balance between calcium and magnesium is important in the prevention of heart disease. Heart disease rates increase when too much calcium is consumed in relation to magnesium.

MEMBRANES. Calcium aids in the transport of nutrients and other substances across cell membranes. The mineral also helps maintain all cell membranes and aids in the maintenance of connective tissue, the "glue" that holds body cells together.

MUSCLE CONTRACTION. Calcium and magnesium work together in the normal contraction of muscles, including the heartbeat. The normal balance between calcium, sodium, potassium, and magnesium maintains muscle tone.

NERVE TRANSMISSION. Calcium is essential for normal transmission of electrical impulses along nerves. The nerves become hypersensitive when blood calcium levels drop below normal and tetany (painful spasms of the muscles) can result. Calcium also aids in the release of neurotransmitters, the chemicals that transmit messages from one nerve cell to another.

PERIODONTAL DISEASE. Diseases of the gums are called periodontal diseases. Calcium supplementation or increased dietary intake of the mineral to 1,000 mg to 2,000 mg a day might reduce the incidence and progression of periodontal disorders. In contrast, a diet low in calcium might encourage the development of periodontal disease.

Deficiency

HYPERTENSION. Abnormally low levels of calcium inside and outside cells, reduced intake of calcium, and a low ratio of calcium to sodium are linked to increased risk for developing high blood pressure (hypertension). Increased intake of the mineral often alleviates or improves the condition.

OSTEOPOROSIS. Osteoporosis is the classic deficiency symptom of prolonged poor intake of calcium. Inadequate intake of calcium results in removal of calcium from the bone ("osteo" means bone, "porosis" means porous). The first bones to be affected are the backbone and jaw. (See pages 213–216 for more information on calcium and osteoporosis.)

TETANY. Very low levels of calcium in the blood can increase the sensitivity of the nerves and result in muscle spasms such as leg cramps, a condition called *tetany*. Pregnant women who consume little calcium or excess phosphorus are at greatest risk for developing tetany. Infants who are fed undiluted cow's milk also might develop tetany.

Daily Recommended Intake

Establishment of a Recommended Dietary Allowance is difficult as people can adapt to a wide range of calcium intakes. Some people in other parts of the world consume 200 mg of calcium daily and appear healthy. In the United States, osteoporosis is associated with calcium intake below 600 mg daily. The current adult RDA of 800 mg might not be adequate to prevent osteoporosis and evidence suggests that the daily intake should be increased to 1,000 mg to 1,200 mg for premenopausal women and 1,500 mg to 1,700 mg for postmenopausal women not taking estrogen. The daily need for calcium increases during pregnancy and lactation and during periods of rapid growth, such as childhood and adolescence.

The 1989 RDAs for calcium are:

	Calcium (mg)
INFANTS	
0–0.5 year	400
0.5–1 year	600
CHILDREN AND ADULTS	
1–10 years	800
11–24 years	1,200

	Calcium (mg)
25+ years	800
Pregnant	1,200
Lactating	1,200

Sources in the Diet

Dairy products, such as low-fat and non-fat milk, low-fat cheese, and low-fat yogurt are good dietary sources of calcium. They also contain lactose or milk sugar, which improves calcium absorption. Vitamin D-fortified milk is the only reliable dietary source of vitamin D, a nutrient essential for calcium absorption. Fatty selections within the dairy group, such as butter, sour cream, and cream cheese, are poor sources of calcium. Other good sources include dark green leafy vegetables, broccoli, canned fish with the bones, cottage cheese, cooked dried beans and peas, and hard tap water (Table 16).

Table 16.
THE CALCIUM CONTENT OF SELECTED FOODS

Food	*Amount*	*Calcium (mg)*
Yogurt, plain	1 cup	415
Sardines	3 ounces	372
Milk, non-fat	1 cup	302
Milk, non-fat, instant	1/3 cup	279
Cheese, cheddar	1 ounce	204
Salmon, canned, with bones	3 ounces	167
Tofu	1 cake	154
Cottage cheese, uncreamed	1 cup	146
Oysters	1/2 cup	113
Mustard greens, cooked	1/2 cup	97
Orange	1 medium	54
Broccoli, cooked	1/2 cup	50
Navy beans, cooked	1/2 cup	48
Apricots, dried	1/2 cup	44
Whole wheat bread	1 slice	24

Toxicity

Excessive intake of calcium, more than several grams each day, might raise blood levels of calcium above the normal range and increase the risk for calcium deposition into soft tissues, such as the kidneys or heart. Large intakes of calcium might reduce zinc and iron absorption, impair vitamin K metabolism, and encourage loss of calcium from bone.

Nutrient-Nutrient Interactions

- Calcium, magnesium, zinc, fluoride, and phosphorus work together in the formation and maintenance of bones and teeth.
- The ratio of calcium to phosphorus and calcium to magnesium is important in the absorption, use, and excretion of these minerals.
- Calcium requires vitamin D for absorption, consequently a vitamin D deficiency results in reduced calcium absorption.
- Calcium competes with zinc, manganese, magnesium, copper, and iron for absorption in the intestine, and a high intake of any one of these minerals could reduce the absorption of the others.
- Calcium might counteract the effects of sodium in the development of hypertension.
- Heart disease rates increase when too much calcium in relation to magnesium is consumed.
- Calcium absorption is reduced in the presence of excess dietary protein, fat, or phosphorus.

MAGNESIUM

Overview

More than half of the body's magnesium is in bone, one-fourth is in muscle, and the remainder is in body fluids and soft tissues, such as the heart and kidneys. The relatively large stores of magnesium in the bone provide a reservoir that can be used to guarantee an adequate blood supply of the mineral to the rest of the tissues when dietary intake is poor.

Functions

Magnesium is one of the most abundant minerals in soft tissues. It functions in the conversion of carbohydrates, protein, and fats to energy; the manufacture of proteins; the synthesis of the genetic material within each cell; and the removal of excess toxic substances, such as ammonia, from the body. Magnesium also functions in muscle relaxation and contraction, nerve transmission, the prevention of tooth decay, and the prevention of heart disease and arrhythmias (irregular heartbeat).

Magnesium and calcium have similar functions and can either encourage or antagonize each other. For example, excess intake of magnesium inhibits bone formation. The balance between these two minerals is reflected in their role in muscle contraction: calcium stimulates muscles and magnesium relaxes muscles. An excess intake of calcium produces symptoms that resemble magnesium deficiency.

HEART DISEASE. There is a high incidence of sudden death from heart attack in areas where people consume soft water; heart attack risk declines in hard water areas. The high concentration of magnesium in hard water might be responsible for these statistics as people dying from heart disease have unusually low levels of magnesium in their hearts.

An association exists in the balance between calcium and magnesium and the incidence of heart attack. Calcium and magnesium help regulate the constriction and relaxation of blood vessels. If too much calcium is present this balance might be affected, the arteries might constrict more than they relax and the blood and oxygen supply to the heart might be reduced. Prolonged constriction of the coronary arteries (arteries that supply the heart with blood and oxygen) could result in heart attack and hypertension.

Magnesium might reduce the pain and cramping of intermittent claudication, a condition caused by reduced blood flow to the legs. Magnesium levels are low in the muscles of patients with this disorder. Magnesium supplementation increases muscle concentrations of the mineral, reduces pain and cramping, and allows patients to walk without pain. (See pages 163 and 197 for more information on magnesium and heart disease.)

PREMENSTRUAL SYNDROME. Blood levels of magnesium are low in women with premenstrual syndrome. Some women who experience headache, dizziness, and craving for sweets sometimes respond to magnesium supplementation, whereas those with breast tenderness do not.

Deficiency

Poor magnesium intake affects all tissues, especially tissues of the heart, nerves, and kidneys. Heart failure caused by irregular heartbeat, which is a symptom of magnesium deficiency, is linked to insufficient intake of magnesium. Other symptoms of magnesium deficiency include loss of appetite, growth failure, muscle spasms, depression, hypertension, muscle weakness, convulsions, confusion, personality changes, nausea, lack of coordination, and gastrointestinal disorders. Loss of hair, swollen gums, and damage to the arteries resembling atherosclerosis are also symptoms of advanced magnesium deficiency. Deficiency symptoms can result from poor dietary intake, excessive vomiting or diarrhea, long-term use of diuretics, alcohol abuse, kidney disease, diabetes, or protein malnutrition.

Clinical deficiencies are rare, but marginal deficiencies might be more common. Many Americans do not consume the RDAs for magnesium and it is suspected that even the RDAs might not be optimal for many people. Lifestyle factors, such as physical or emotional stress, further increase the need for magnesium.

Daily Recommended Intake

Magnesium's complex interrelationship with other nutrients, such as calcium, protein, phosphorus, lactose, potassium, and calories, makes the establishment of RDAs difficult. A typical diet in the United States provides 120 mg of magnesium for every 1,000 calories and appears to prevent clinical deficiencies. This minimal amount will be inadequate to meet the increased demands of stress, disease, or poor absorption. The RDAs for children are only estimates based on the magnesium content of human milk and cow's milk. The 1989 RDAs reduced magnesium recommendations, despite evidence showing the importance of maintaining the calcium to magnesium ratio.

The 1989 RDAs compared to previous RDAs for magnesium:

Magnesium	Previous RDA	1989 RDA
INFANTS		
0–0.5 year	50	40
0.5–1 year	70	60
CHILDREN		
1–3 years	150	80
4–6 years	200	120
7–10 years	250	170
YOUNG ADULT MALES		
11–14 years	350	270
15–18 years	400	400
YOUNG ADULT FEMALES		
11–14 years	300	280
15–18 years	300	300
ADULTS		
Males 19+	350	350
Females 19+	300	280
Pregnant	450	320
Lactating	450	260–280

Sources in the Diet

The magnesium content of foods is variable. In general, good sources include nuts, cooked dried beans and peas, whole grain breads and cereals, soybeans, dark green leafy vegetables, and seafoods. Milk supplies about 22% of the magnesium in the American diet (Table 17).

Table 17.
THE MAGNESIUM CONTENT OF SELECTED FOODS

Food	Amount	Magnesium (mg)
Peanuts	¼ cup	63
Banana	1 medium	58
Beet greens	1 cup	58
Avocado	½	56
Peanut butter	2 Tbsp	56
Cashews	9 medium	52
Milk, low-fat	1 cup	40
Wheatgerm	2 Tbsp	40
Brewer's (nutritional) yeast	2 Tbsp	36
Collard greens	1 cup	31
Oysters	6 medium	27
Haddock, baked	3 ounces	20
Bread, whole wheat	1 slice	19
Bread, white	1 slice	5

Toxicity

The kidneys are efficient at excreting excess magnesium and it is unlikely that the mineral will accumulate to toxic levels. High levels of magnesium can develop in patients with kidney failure and in elderly people whose kidney functions are reduced. Symptoms of magnesium toxicity include weakness, lethargy, drowsiness, and difficulty breathing. High intake of magnesium might impair absorption and use of calcium.

Nutrient-Nutrient Interactions

- All chemical reactions that involve vitamin B_1 also require magnesium.
- Magnesium supplementation might prevent the deposition of oxalate stones in the kidneys during vitamin B_6 deficiency.
- Magnesium, calcium, and phosphorus function together in bone formation, muscle contraction, and nerve transmission.
- High intake of calcium might impair absorption of magnesium.

PHOSPHORUS

Overview

Phosphorus is second only to calcium as the most abundant mineral in the body; the average body contains approximately 1 to 1½ pounds. Phosphorus is essential to life but receives little attention as it is found in all foods of plant and animal origin, and a deficiency is rare to nonexistent in humans. More than 80% of the body's phosphorus is in bones and teeth. The other 20% is active in many metabolic processes and is found in every cell in the body.

Functions

A complete review of the roles of phosphorus in the body would require a list of all body processes. In addition to its contribution to the structure and function of bones and teeth, phosphorus also is a component of all soft tissues, including kidney, heart, brain, and muscles; is a substance fundamental to growth, maintenance, and repair of all body tissues; and is a part of the genetic code in all cells. Phosphorus is also necessary for the conversion of dietary carbohydrate, protein, and fat to energy and is a component of cell membranes. The mineral helps maintain the pH balance in the blood; is a component of many proteins, such as casein in milk; and helps activate the B vitamins. Phosphorus is also a component of the storage form of energy in the body and facilitates the absorption of nutrients such as glucose, which is the form of sugar found in the blood and used for energy in the body.

Deficiency

Excessive intake of phosphorus is much more common than a deficiency of the mineral. Long-term and excessive use of anticonvulsant medications or of antacids containing aluminum hydroxide reduces absorption of phosphorus and might result in deficiency symptoms. Patients placed on formula diets low in phosphorus are also at risk for developing phosphorus deficiency.

Daily Recommended Intake

The Recommended Dietary Allowances for phosphorus are arbitrary and are based on an estimate of the best ratio (1:1) for calcium and phosphorus. The average American diet contains 1,500 mg to 1,600 mg, or twice the adult RDA for phosphorus, and the ratio of calcium to phosphorus is often as low as 1:2.

The 1989 RDAs for phosphorus are:

	Phosphorus (mg)
INFANTS	
0–0.5 year	300
0.5–1 year	500
CHILDREN AND ADULTS	
1–10 years	800
11–24 years	1,200
25+ years	800
Pregnant	1,200
Lactating	1,200

Sources in the Diet

Protein-rich foods, such as meat, organ meats, fish, poultry, and eggs, are good sources of phosphorus. Milk is a good source of both calcium and phosphorus as it provides the two minerals in the best ratio. Fortified milk also contains vitamin D, which improves phosphorus and calcium absorption. Phosphorus is present as phytic acid in un-leavened whole grain breads and cereals, but it is unclear how well this form of phosphorus is absorbed. Food additives contribute as much as 30% of dietary phosphorus. Soft drinks contain as much as 500 mg of phosphoric acid per serving and can contribute to excessive phosphorus intake if consumed regularly (Table 18).

Table 18.
THE PHOSPHORUS CONTENT OF SELECTED FOODS

Food	Amount	Phosphorus (mg)
Liver	3 ounces	405
Yogurt, low-fat	1 cup	326
Chicken	3½ ounces	266
Milk, non-fat	1 cup	247
Haddock	3 ounces	210
Tuna, canned	3½ ounces	188
Soybeans, cooked	½ cup	166
Hamburger	3 ounces	159
Peanut butter	2 Tbsp	122
Egg	1 large	90
Bread, whole wheat	1 slice	57
Broccoli, cooked	½ cup	48
Orange	1 medium	33
Banana	1 medium	27
Carrots, cooked	½ cup	24

Toxicity

Overconsumption of phosphorus might occur in people who consume diets high in meat, convenience foods, and soft drinks and low in calcium-containing foods such as non-fat milk and dark green leafy vegetables. The effects of this imbalance in the ratio of calcium to phosphorus can contribute to faulty bone maintenance and osteoporosis.

Nutrient-Nutrient Interactions

- Phosphorus works with the B vitamins in energy metabolism.
- Vitamin D increases phosphorus absorption.
- The functions of calcium, magnesium, and phosphorus are closely related and disturbances in one mineral affect the other.

SULFUR

Overview

Sulfur is a component of all body tissues, especially those tissues that contain high amounts of protein such as hair, muscles, and skin. Insulin, the hormone that regulates blood sugar, also contains sulfur. Most of the sulfur in the body is bound to the sulfur-containing amino acids: methionine, cystine, and cysteine, which are building blocks of protein. Sulfur also is a component of vitamin B_1 and biotin.

Functions

Sulfur gives proteins their characteristic differences in shape, eg, it makes hair curly; is involved in the formation of bile acids important for fat digestion and absorption; is a constituent of bones and teeth; activates certain enzymes; and helps regulate blood clotting. Sulfur helps in the conversion of proteins, carbohydrates, and fats to energy because it is a component of vitamin B_1, biotin, and pantothenic acid; helps regulate blood sugar by being a constituent of the hormone insulin; and is a component of collagen, a protein in the connective tissue that holds cells together.

Deficiency

A deficiency of sulfur is unknown, although it is conceivable that a diet very low in protein would be inadequate in sulfur and could produce a deficiency. The protein deficiency, however, would be of greatest concern and the sulfur deficiency would be cured with increased protein intake.

Daily Recommended Intake

No Recommended Dietary Allowances or Safe and Adequate ranges have been established for sulfur. The American diet is high in protein and supplies adequate amounts of sulfur.

Sources in the Diet

Meat, organ meats, poultry, fish, eggs, cooked dried beans and peas, milk, and milk products are good sources of protein and sulfur.

Toxicity

No toxicity symptoms have been reported for sulfur. Excesses are excreted in the urine.

Nutrient-Nutrient Interactions

- The poisonous effects of arsenic are a result of its ability to bind to the sulfur portion of amino acids and inactivate them.
- Sulfur is a component of vitamin B_1, biotin, and the active form of pantothenic acid called *co-enzyme A*.

SODIUM, POTASSIUM, AND CHLORIDE

Overview

"You are the salt of the earth," "You are worth your weight in salt," and the word salary, which comes from the word salt (or sodium chloride), reflect the importance of these elements to mankind. Sodium, potassium, and chloride are so closely related in the body that they can be discussed together. These three elements are distributed throughout all body fluids, including the blood, lymph, the fluid between cells, and the fluid within each cell (intracellular fluid). Sodium and chloride are primarily found in fluids that surround cells and potassium is primarily found in fluids within cells.

The blood and other fluids require a narrow range of sodium concentration. When a person consumes a salty meal, the blood concentration of sodium increases, which stimulates thirst and more water is consumed to dilute the blood back to normal sodium levels. The extra water and sodium are then excreted by the kidneys. Water retention in many cases is a result of not drinking enough water to allow the kidneys to excrete excess fluid and sodium.

The blood becomes too diluted if blood levels of sodium drop and water is replaced without sodium, the lack of sodium outside the cells (extracellular) allows water to move from the blood into the cells. Symptoms of water intoxication develop, such as headache, muscular weakness, and poor memory.

IF SOME IS GOOD, IS MORE BETTER?

Many nutrients are found in the body within narrow ranges of concentration. Fluctuations from this normal range, either up or down, can result in disorders that can have a wide range of effects on body function. For example, vitamins A or D are essential nutrients, but if their concentrations in the body rise above or fall below acceptable limits deficiency or toxicity symptoms develop. For this reason, the oversimplified view that "if a little is good, more is better," or its opposite, "if high doses are bad, small doses also must be bad" can be dangerous.

Consider the reasoning behind the following beliefs:

- Some fiber is good for you, so you should eat as much fiber as possible.
- Too much sugar is bad for you, so you should not eat any sugar.
- Chlorine is a poison so we should not consume any salt because it contains the related compound chloride.
- High doses of fluoride can cause mottling of teeth, so we should not drink fluoridated water.
- Protein is an essential nutrient, so we should supplement the diet with protein powders.

The simple black and white nature of these statements makes them easy to believe; however, the reasoning implied in these beliefs leads people to the wrong conclusions. Moderate intake of fiber is wise to prevent heart disease, hypertension, and cancer, but excessive intake of fiber can result in mineral deficiencies and gastrointestinal upsets. It is true that a diet high in sugar is linked to malnutrition or obesity, but moderate intake of sugar in conjunction with a nutritious diet of whole grain breads, fresh fruits and vegetables, lean meats or dried beans, and non-fat dairy foods is harmless.

Functions

Sodium, potassium, and chloride function to maintain the normal balance and distribution of fluids throughout the body. They also function in the maintenance of normal pH balance, the maintenance of normal muscle contraction and relaxation, and the maintenance of normal nerve transmission and function.

Potassium is important in the regulation of the heartbeat. The reduction in blood levels of potassium and abnormal blood sugar levels characteristic of people on very-low-calorie diets might be alleviated with potassium supplements.

Potassium also might help regulate normal blood pressure and prevent hypertension. Populations with high potassium intake have a low incidence of hypertension, and when potassium-containing foods are added to the diets of hypertensives, their blood pressures drop. The ratio of potassium to sodium also might be important in the development of hypertension. An increase in potassium and a decrease in sodium in the American diet might provide the proper ratio between these two elements that would prevent hypertension.

Chloride is a component of hydrochloric acid or stomach acid and so aids in the digestion of foods. Excessive vomiting causes loss of chloride from the stomach, which upsets the pH balance of the body, causing a range of disorders from dehydration to coma.

A chlorine compound is used to kill harmful bacteria in public water supplies that would otherwise spread disease. The addition of chlorine to water is an important public health measure and has eliminated numerous waterborne diseases such as typhoid fever. The related compound, chloride, in the diet is harmless.

Deficiency

SODIUM. A deficiency of sodium is uncommon and is usually a result of starvation or severe fasting, vomiting, perspiration, or diarrhea. In the rare occurrence of sodium deficiency, fluids move from the blood into the cells, which results in muscle weakness and twitching, poor concentration and memory loss, dehydration, and loss of appetite. A liter of perspiration contains only 1 gram of sodium. Therefore, it is much more important to replace fluids than to take sodium tablets when dehydrated, as more water than sodium is lost in perspiration.

POTASSIUM. Potassium deficiency can occur with chronic diarrhea, vomiting, diabetic acidosis, kidney disease, or prolonged use of laxatives or diuretics. Symptoms of a potassium deficiency include slowed growth, bone fragility, paralysis, sterility, muscle weakness, mental apathy and confusion, kidney damage, and damage to the heart. Sudden death that can occur during fasting, anorexia nervosa, or starvation is often a result of heart failure caused by potassium deficiency. Dehydration is dangerous because the potassium deficiency that occurs numbs the person's desire for water. Excessive use of laxatives and diuretics, vomiting and diarrhea, or chronic low intake of water combined with profuse perspiration can lead to dehydration and potassium deficiency.

CHLORIDE. A deficiency of chloride would result in an upset in the body's pH balance, called *alkalosis*. This imbalance between acid and alkaline produces vomiting, sweating, and diarrhea. Other symptoms of chloride deficiency include muscle weakness, loss of appetite, lethargy, and, in infants, failure to thrive. Deficiency is uncommon as the element is consumed in salt (sodium chloride).

Daily Recommended Intake

SODIUM. Sodium intake reflects habit, taste, and custom, not need. A daily intake of between 200 mg and 500 mg maintains fluid balance in the body; however, intakes vary between 2,300 mg and 20,000 mg of sodium daily. No RDA has been established for sodium. The Senate Select Committee on Nutrition and Human Needs and the US Dietary Goals recommend a reduction in sodium intake to no more than 2,000 mg a day, the equivalent of 1 teaspoon of salt.

The 1989 Estimated Minimum Requirements of Healthy People for sodium are:

Sodium (mg)	
INFANTS	
0.0–0.5 year	120
0.5–1 year	200
CHILDREN	
1 year	225
2–5 years	300
6–9 years	400
10+ years	500

POTASSIUM. The typical adult intake of potassium is between 800 mg and 1,500 mg.

The 1989 Estimated Minimum Requirements of Healthy People for potassium are:

Potassium (mg)	
INFANTS	
0.0–0.5 year	500
0.5–1 year	700
CHILDREN	
1 year	1,000
2–5 years	1,400
6–9 years	1,600
10+ years	2,000

CHLORIDE. Interest in the nutritional requirements of chloride have been minimal because the element is so easily obtained from the diet.

The 1989 Estimated Minimum Requirements of Healthy People for chloride are:

Chloride (mg)	
INFANTS	
0.0–0.5 year	180
0.5–1 year	300
CHILDREN	
1 year	350
2–5 years	500
6–9 years	600
10+ years	750

Sources in the Diet

SODIUM AND CHLORIDE. Sodium and chloride are in most foods, but by far the largest amounts are in table salt. A pinch of salt contains 267 mg of sodium; a teaspoon of salt sprinkled on a meal provides over 2,000 mg of sodium. Processed and convenience foods, olives, pickles, sauerkraut, catsup, sandwich meats, beef broth, soy sauce, baking powder, monosodium glutamate (MSG), and numerous food additives contain large amounts of sodium. Meat, chicken, fish, grains, vegetables, fruits, nuts, milk and milk products, and seeds contain moderate amounts of sodium and chloride. A diet of unprocessed, natural foods with no added salt would provide more than the daily recommendation for sodium and chloride.

POTASSIUM. Potassium is found in a variety of foods including fruits, vegetables, meat, milk, and grains. Lean meats contain 300 mg to 500 mg of potassium per serving. Potatoes, avocados, bananas, apricots, orange juice, and other dried or fresh fruits or cooked dried beans and peas are excellent sources of potassium (Table 19).

Table 19.
THE SODIUM AND POTASSIUM CONTENTS OF SELECTED FOODS

Food	Amount	Sodium (mg)	Potassium (mg)
Asparagus	5 spears	2	278
Avocado	½ medium	4	604
Bacon	2 slices	440	90
Banana	1 medium	2	550
Beans, red cooked	⅔ cup	3	340
Beef broth	1 serving	784	107
Big Mac	1	963	387
Bouillon	1 cube	960	0
Bread, whole wheat	1 slice	121	63
Cantaloupe	¼ melon	12	251
Carrots, raw	1 large	47	341
Cheeseburger	1	823	303
Crackers, saltines	2	66	7
Egg	1 medium	59	62
Fish, no added salt	3 ounces	70	380
French Fries, no added salt	Small order	170	361
Ham, cured	3 ounces	860	332
Lettuce, romaine	3½ ounces	9	264
Meat, poultry	3 ounces	100	221
Milk, non-fat	1 cup	128	408
Olives	2 large	150	5
Orange	1 medium	2	300
Peanuts, roasted	2½ ounces	2	740
Peanuts, salted	2½ ounces	460	700
Peas, fresh	½ cup	9	380
Peas, frozen	½ cup	100	160
Peas, canned	½ cup	230	180
Pickles	1 large	1,428	200
Pie, apple	1 piece	482	128
Potato, baked	1 medium	6	755
butter	2 tsp	81	2
salt	1 tsp	2,000	0
Pudding, chocolate	½ cup	161	168
Salad dressing	1 Tbsp	120	5
Soup, freeze-dried	1 pkg	1,350	131
Soup, creamed, canned	1 cup	996	166
Soup, chicken low-sodium	1 cup	48	149
Soup, chicken	1 cup	754	40

Toxicity

SODIUM. Diets in the United States contain excessive amounts of sodium, as much as 15 times the recommended daily intake. A diet high in sodium is linked to hypertension and restriction of sodium lowers blood pressure in many people with hypertension. There are no known benefits to excessive sodium intake and consumption of a low-sodium diet throughout life is not only harmless, but might prevent the development of hypertension.

POTASSIUM. Dietary intake of potassium in excess of 18,000 mg can cause high concentrations of the element in the blood, disturbances in heart and kidney function, and alterations in fluid balance. Blood levels of potassium can escalate as a result of excessive intake of salt substitutes that contain potassium, kidney failure, acidosis, major infections, hemorrhages in the gastrointestinal tract, and severe breakdown of muscle.

Nutrient-Nutrient Interactions

• Potassium supplementation in patients with hypertension might increase magnesium requirements.

CHROMIUM

Overview

The average body contains about 600 mcg of chromium with the highest concentration occurring during infancy.

Functions

The main function of chromium is as a component of glucose tolerance factor (GTF), a substance that works with insulin to facilitate the uptake of blood sugar (glucose) into the cells and regulate blood sugar levels. GTF contains niacin; the amino acids glycine, glutamic acid, and cysteine; and chromium. The chromium-insulin combination also stimulates the synthesis of protein.

Deficiency

DIABETES. Poor dietary intake of chromium results in limited availability of GTF and impaired insulin activity. The blood sugar remains elevated, the person exhibits glucose intolerance, and a diabetes-like condition similar to that seen in adult-onset diabetics develops.

Other symptoms of chromium deficiency also resemble diabetes. In both conditions, the person experiences numbness and tingling in the toes and fingers, an increase in blood sugar, nerve disorders in the arms and legs, glucose intolerance, and reduced muscle coordination. In many people, these symptoms disappear when chromium intake is increased. (See pages 173–174 for more information on chromium and diabetes.)

HYPOGLYCEMIA. Hypoglycemia is the opposite of diabetes. Instead of the elevated blood sugar (hyperglycemia) characteristic of diabetes, hypoglycemics experience low blood sugar. Hypoglycemia is not a disease, but a symptom of an abnormality in the body's use of sugar and is found in diabetes as well as other conditions. Reactive hypoglycemia occurs after consumption of a meal high in carbohydrates when blood sugar drops below normal levels as a result of insulin. Supplementation with 200 mcg of chromium improves the symptoms of hypoglycemia in some individuals and chromium might be effective in the management of this disorder.

CARDIOVASCULAR DISEASE. Poor dietary intake of chromium might be associated with elevated blood cholesterol levels and increased risk for developing cardiovascular disease (CVD). (See page 162 for more information on chromium and heart disease.)

In the United States, blood and tissue levels of chromium decrease as a person ages; at the same time, the risk for developing diabetes and cardiovascular disease increases. In contrast, people in primitive cultures have chromium levels two to three times higher than most Americans, their chromium status does not decline with age, and these degenerative disease are infrequent to nonexistent.

As many as 90% of all American diets are low in chromium. Even well-designed diets contain only 25 mcg/1,000 calories. At this level of intake, it would take 8,000 calories each day to obtain the upper dietary limit considered safe and adequate. A person who consumes 2,000 calories or less, or who consumes a diet high in refined white breads and rice and processed or convenience foods, and low in whole grain breads and cereals and other nutrient-dense foods would not meet even the lower level of intake for chromium. In addition, a diet that contains high amounts of sugar or strenuous exercises increases urinary loss of chromium and might contribute to a chromium deficiency.

Daily Recommended Intake

There is limited information on chromium requirements for humans. The 1989 Safe and Adequate Ranges for chromium are:

	Chromium (mcg)
INFANTS	
0–0.5 year	10–40
0.5–1 year	20–60
CHILDREN	
1–3 years	20–80
4–6 years	30–120
CHILDREN AND ADULTS	
7+ years	50–200

Sources in the Diet

The best dietary source of chromium is brewer's (nutritional) yeast grown on a chromium-rich medium. Other good sources include whole grain breads and cereals, pork kidney, molasses, lean meats, and cheeses. Little information exists on the chromium content of vegetables. Refined and processed foods are low in the mineral. Hard tap water can supply between 1% and 70% of the daily intake. Inorganic chromium, such as chromic chloride, is not as well absorbed as the form of chromium found in foods, nutritional yeast, and chromium picolinate (Table 20).

Table 20.
THE CHROMIUM CONTENT OF SELECTED FOODS

Food	Amount	Chromium (mcg)
Grains and Cereals		
Buckwheat, raw	½ cup	38
Whole wheat cereal, raw	1 cup	3
All bran	1 cup	14
Puffed rice	1 cup	10
Wheatgerm	2 Tbsp	1.4
Orange juice	²/₅ cup	13
Molasses	2 Tbsp	4.4
Sugar	2 Tbsp	0
Cheese	1 ounce	4.4

Toxicity

Excess intake or tissue accumulation of chromium can inhibit, rather than enhance, the effectiveness of insulin.

Nutrient–Nutrient Interactions

- Chromium combines with the B vitamin niacin to form glucose tolerance factor (GTF).

COBALT

Functions

The only known function of cobalt is as a constituent of vitamin B_{12}. In this capacity, cobalt aids in the formation of normal red blood cells, maintenance of nerve tissue, and normal formation of cells.

Deficiency

A deficiency of cobalt is equivalent to a deficiency of vitamin B_{12} and can cause anemia, nerve disorders, and abnormalities in cell formation. Strict vegetarians who do not consume foods of animal origin can develop vitamin B_{12} and cobalt deficiencies over 3 to 6 years of poor dietary intake.

Daily Recommended Intake

The dietary intake of cobalt is based on the body's need for vitamin B_{12}, or 2 mcg of vitamin B_{12} each day. There is no known need for cobalt alone. There are no RDAs or Estimated Safe and Adequate ranges for cobalt.

Sources in the Diet

Information is limited on the dietary sources of cobalt as consumption of the mineral alone is thought to be of little importance. Organ meats, such as liver and kidneys, oysters, and clams are excellent sources of cobalt and muscle meats are good dietary sources because these foods supply the mineral as part of vitamin B_{12}. Vegetables, fruits, and other foods of plant origin contain cobalt, but as these sources do not provide the mineral as part of vitamin B_{12} it is of little use.

Toxicity

Toxicity is rare; however, large doses of inorganic cobalt (cobalt not combined with vitamin B_{12}) might stimulate thyroid and bone marrow function, resulting in excess production of red blood cells (polycythemia). Cobalt is used as an anti-foaming agent in the processing of some beer. Consumption of large amounts of this beer could cause polycythemia and heart disorders.

Nutrient-Nutrient Interactions

• See the section on vitamin B_{12}, page 57.

COPPER

Overview

This essential trace mineral is found in all tissues, but is most concentrated in the brain, heart, kidney, and liver. The copper concentration in bones and muscles is moderate to low, but because these tissues comprise a large portion of the body, one-half of the total copper content of the body is found here. Only about 30% of dietary intake is absorbed.

Functions

Copper facilitates the activity of several enzymes and in this capacity is involved in the development and maintenance of the cardiovascular system, including the heart, arteries, and other blood vessels; the skeletal system; and the structure and function of the nervous system, including the brain. Copper is also important in the development and maintenance of red blood cells (and their protein hemoglobin) and normal hair and skin color.

Copper is a component of the antioxidant enzyme superoxide dismutase and might protect cell membranes from potential damage by highly reactive oxygen fragments. In this antioxidant role, copper might function to prevent the development of cancer. (See pages 126–128 for more information on antioxidants.)

Copper releases iron from storage and increases the intestinal absorption of iron, aids in the formation of connective tissue, breaks down fats in fat tissue, and is necessary for the normal functioning of insulin. Copper also aids in the conversion of dietary protein, carbohydrate, and fat to energy; and contributes to the synthesis of hormone-like compounds called *prostaglandins* that regulate a variety of body functions including heartbeat, blood pressure, and wound healing.

Deficiency

A clinical deficiency of copper is rare, but has been observed in children with severe protein malnutrition, chronic diarrhea or other malabsorption problems, or iron-deficiency anemia. Marginal copper deficiencies might be more common and are found in patients consuming hospital diets. Copper is stored in the liver, so a deficiency develops slowly even in the presence of a low-copper diet. Because copper is necessary for the normal development and maintenance of blood, bone, nerves, connective tissue, and other tissues, a deficiency of this essential trace mineral can cause a variety of disorders.

ANEMIA. As blood levels of copper drop, iron is poorly absorbed, red blood cells are not produced, and anemia develops. Supplementation with both iron and copper is required in the treatment of this form of anemia.

HAIR AND SKIN. A copper deficiency causes loss of color from the skin and hair. This results from poor formation of melanin, the copper-dependent pigment that gives color to hair and contributes to a suntan.

HEART DISEASE. Copper deficiency causes extensive damage to the heart and arteries, abnormal electrocardiograms, and heart attacks, and is associated with high blood pressure. (See page 163 for more information on copper and heart disease.)

MENKES' SYNDROME. Menkes' syndrome is a genetic defect in copper absorption. Infants show stunted growth, defective skin pigmentation, kinky or steely hair, abnormal development of the arteries and bones, and progressive mental deterioration. Premature death is typical.

NERVOUS SYSTEM. Impaired energy production and reduced enzyme activity that results from a copper deficiency interferes with the proper functioning of the central nervous system. This impairment causes poor concentration, poor coordination, numbness and tingling, and a variety of nervous system disorders.

RESISTANCE TO INFECTION. A low copper intake can result in a reduction in white blood cells and increased susceptibility to colds, infections, and disease. The ratio of zinc intake to copper intake also influences the immune system and resistance to infection; a person is more susceptible to disease when copper intake is high and zinc intake is low.

SCOLIOSIS. Scoliosis is a condition that can strike young people, especially girls, and women and results in defects in muscular growth, connective tissue formation, and skeletal development. The cause of scoliosis has not been determined. Studies on skeletal defects in animals show a relationship between the severity of spinal abnormalities and the degree of dietary copper restriction; an increased intake of copper reduces the risk for developing scoliosis. Copper might aid in the treatment of scoliosis by its role in the development of connective tissue that provides the framework for normal bone development. This preliminary information does not prove that copper deficiency causes scoliosis, but does suggest that diet plays a role in the development of the disorder.

TISSUE FORMATION. A copper deficiency results in poor formation of collagen, the protein component of connective tissue. Connective tissue provides the framework for numerous other tissues and faulty formation results in bone deformities, damaged blood vessels, reduced resiliency of skin and other internal and external linings of the body, and heart failure.

Daily Recommended Intake

Typical diets in the United States provide between 0.8 mg and 3.0 mg of copper daily.

The 1989 Safe and Adequate Ranges for copper are:

		Copper (mg)
INFANTS		
	0–0.5 year	0.4–0.6
	0.5–1 year	0.6–0.7
CHILDREN		
	1–3 years	0.7–1.0
	4–6 years	1.0–1.5
	7–10 years	1.0–2.0
	11+ years	1.5–2.5
ADULTS		1.5–3.0

Sources in the Diet

Copper is found in a wide variety of unprocessed foods including whole grain breads and cereals, shellfish, nuts, organ meats, poultry, cooked dried beans and peas, and dark green leafy vegetables. Milk and milk products are poor sources of the mineral. Drinking water that runs through copper pipes can contribute substantial amounts of the mineral to the diet (Table 21).

Table 21.
THE COPPER CONTENT OF SELECTED FOODS

Food	Amount	Copper (mg)
Oysters	6 medium	14.2
Lobster	1 cup	2.45
Liver, cooked	3 ounces	2.4
Avocado	1 half	0.5
Potato, baked	1 medium	0.36
Soybeans, cooked	½ cup	0.3
Banana	1 medium	0.26
Fish, cooked	3 ounces	0.16
Chicken, meat only	3½ ounces	0.14
Spinach, cooked	½ cup	0.13
Peas, green, cooked	½ cup	0.12
Bread, whole wheat	1 slice	0.06
Carrots, cooked	½ cup	0.06
Cheddar cheese	1 ounce	0.03
Cottage cheese	½ cup	0.01

Toxicity

Copper toxicity is rare. Patients with ulcerative colitis might accumulate copper in the tissues. This excess of copper might aggravate the symptoms of the intestinal disorder, including impaired healing and reduced resistance to infection. Daily intakes of more than 20 mg can cause nausea and vomiting.

Wilson's disease is an inherited disorder characterized by excessive accumulation of copper in the tissues, liver disease, mental retardation, tremor, and loss of coordination. Copper deposits in the cornea of the eye produce an apparently harmless ring configuration. Treatment of Wilson's disease includes a low-copper diet and the medication penicillamine that binds to copper and increases its excretion.

Nutrient-Nutrient Interactions

- The balance between iron, zinc, and copper is important in the absorption and use of both minerals. Excessive intake of one mineral might result in a secondary deficiency of the other nutrient, or increased risk for developing heart disease, high blood pressure, increased susceptibility to infection, or a variety of disorders.
- Cadmium, molybdenum, and sulfate alter copper absorption.
- Copper facilitates the absorption and use of iron.
- Excessive calcium intake inhibits the absorption of copper.
- Blood levels of copper are elevated when there is a niacin deficiency, although the significance of this association is unknown.

FLUORIDE

Overview

The average body contains approximately 2.6 grams of fluoride, and the largest accumulation is in the bones and teeth.

Functions

DENTAL. The main function of fluoride is to protect developing and mature teeth from decay. One milligram of fluoride for every liter of water (1 part fluoride for every million parts water or 1 ppm) reduces dental cavities by 70%. Fluoride's effects are especially pronounced if fluoride ingestion is started during the early years when teeth are still forming.

BONE. Bones are more stable and resistant to degeneration and osteoporosis when the diet is adequate in fluoride. Some elderly patients show a reduction in urinary excretion of calcium, improved bone strength, and a reduction in the symptoms of osteoporosis when their intake of fluoride is adequate. However, fluoride supplementation might increase the number of hairline fractures in bone, and the use of this mineral in the treatment of osteoporosis is controversial.

Fluoride also might aid in wound healing and enhance iron absorption.

Deficiency

DENTAL. The incidence of dental caries is high in areas of the United States where the water is not fluoridated and fluoride intake is low.

Daily Recommended Intake

No RDAs have been established for fluoride. However, it is recommended that water supplies be fortified with the mineral to a level of 1 ppm to provide an adult with 1.5 mg to 4.0 mg daily.

The average daily intake of fluoride is between 0.2 mg and 4.4 mg.

The 1989 Estimated Safe and Adequate Ranges for fluoride are:

	Fluoride (mg)
INFANTS	
0–0.5 year	0.1–0.5
0.5–1 year	0.2–1.0

	Fluoride (mg)
CHILDREN AND ADOLESCENTS	
1–3 years	0.5–1.5
4–6 years	1.0–2.5
7+ years	1.5–2.5
ADULTS	1.5–4.0

Sources in the Diet

The best dietary source of fluoride is fluoridated water. The fluoride content of food depends on the fluoride content of the soil in which the food is grown. Other sources of fluoride include unintentional ingestion of fluoridated toothpaste or use of fluoridated water in food processing. A cup of tea provides 0.3 mg of fluoride. Bottled fluoridated water or fluoride tablets can be used by people who live in areas where the water is not fluoridated. Topical application of fluoride to the teeth is not as effective in preventing cavities as is ingested fluoride.

Toxicity

Mottling, pitting, and dulling of the teeth has been observed in areas where fluoride is a natural ingredient in the water at levels of 2 ppm to 6 ppm. Intakes greater than 8 ppm can cause fluorosis of the bones that produces arthritis-like symptoms. Fatal poisoning can occur if fluoride is ingested in amounts greater than 2,500 times the recommended intake. Chronic ingestion of 50 mg/day can occur with some forms of air or environmental pollution and results in bone and tooth deformities. The levels used in the fluoridation of water pose no harmful effects to health and greatly reduce the incidence of tooth decay and possibly periodontal disease. (See Box on page 88.)

Nutrient-Nutrient Interactions

- Fluoride works with calcium, phosphorus, magnesium, and vitamin D in the formation and maintenance of healthy bones and teeth.

IODINE

Overview

More than 60% of the approximately 20 mg to 30 mg of iodine in the body is found in the thyroid gland. The remaining 40% is distributed throughout the body, especially in the ovaries, muscles, and blood. Besides dietary intake, iodine also can be absorbed through the skin.

Functions

The only known function of iodine is as a component of the thyroid hormones. These hormones regulate the rate of metabolism, growth, reproduction, nerve and muscle function, the synthesis of proteins, the growth of skin and hair, and the use of oxygen by cells. One of these hormones, thyroxin, regulates the rate at which the body uses energy from food and thus is an important regulator of body weight.

Deficiency

Poor iodine intake is associated with the development of endemic or simple goiter, a condition called *hypothyroidism*. During an iodine deficiency, the activity of the thyroid hormones remains normal until the body stores of the mineral are exhausted. A center in the brain called the *pituitary gland* recognizes the lack of iodine and diminished thyroid gland function and signals to the thyroid gland to increase its activity. The thyroid gland enlarges or swells as a result of this increased activity and the swelling that occurs at the front of the neck is called a goiter. Young women between the ages of 12 and 18 years old and boys between the ages of 9 and 13 years old living in areas where the iodine content of the soil is poor are the most prone for developing goiter. Iodine deficiency during pregnancy causes cretinism, extreme and irreversible mental and physical retardation.

Substances in foods called *goitrogens* also can cause goiter. Goitrogens are natural inhibitors of the thyroid gland and are found in raw cabbage, turnips, peanuts, cauliflower, rutabagas, mustard seeds, soybeans, and cassava. Prolonged consumption of large amounts of these raw foods when the diet is low in iodine could produce goiter; cooking deactivates these compounds. Some drugs act as goitrogens, such as thiourea, thiouracil, sulfonamide, and disulfiram.

Goiter can be prevented and treated with the inclusion of adequate amounts of iodine in the diet. A person who consumes a low-iodine diet and who lives in an area of the country where the soil is low in this mineral should consume iodized salt. A person who must severely restrict the intake of salt should consider iodine supplements, unless fresh saltwater fish is included frequently in the weekly diet.

Daily Recommended Intake

The 1989 RDAs for iodine are:

	Iodine (mcg)
INFANTS	
0–0.5 year	40
0.5–1 year	50
CHILDREN	
1–3 years	70
4–6 years	90
7–10 years	120
ADOLESCENTS AND ADULTS	
11+ years	150
Pregnant	175
Lactating	200

Sources in the Diet

Fresh saltwater shellfish and seafood, iodized salt, and foods grown on iodine-rich soil are good sources of the mineral. The iodine content of milk depends on the iodine in the cows' diets. A teaspoon of iodized salt contains 420 mcg of iodine. Half of the salt sold in the United States is iodized. Many of the "natural" brands of sea salt do not contain iodine. Some bakeries use iodine as a dough stabilizer and a slice of this bread contains as much as 150 mcg of iodine. Milk processed in equipment cleaned with related compounds called *iodates* also contributes to the daily intake. Iodine comes in a variety of forms and its presence in foods is difficult to measure.

Toxicity

Doses greater than 25 times the recommended daily intake can produce "iodide goiter," a hyperactive, enlarged goiter, which is similar to the effect noted in an iodine deficiency. It does not appear that intakes of iodine below 25 times the RDA is a public health concern at this time.

Hyperthyroidism or Graves' disease is an overactive thyroid. Hyperthyroidism is not a result of overconsumption of iodine, but rather develops as a result of disruption in the regulatory mechanisms that control thyroid hormone function. The person is anxious, nervous, loses weight, has an increased metabolic rate, cannot tolerate heat, and the eyeballs protrude.

Nutrient-Nutrient Interactions

There is no evidence at this time that iodine interacts with other nutrients.

IRON

Overview

The adult body contains between ¹/₂ to 1 teaspoon of iron, with more than 65% of that iron used in hemoglobin, enzymes, and other functions. The remaining 35% is stored for future use.

Functions

OXYGEN TRANSPORTATION. Iron is the oxygen-carrying component of the blood. Four particles (atoms) of iron are bound to each protein molecule, called *hemoglobin*, in each red blood cell. When the blood passes through blood vessels in the lungs, oxygen binds to iron and is carried to all the tissues of the body. After releasing oxygen to the tissues, iron binds to the cellular waste product carbon dioxide and carries it to the lungs for exhalation.

An iron-containing molecule within each cell, called *myoglobin*, has a similar function to hemoglobin. Myoglobin transports the newly-arrived oxygen within the cell to be used to convert substances to energy and for all normal cell activities. Iron is therefore the main determinant of how much oxygen reaches and is used by all body tissues, including the brain, muscles, heart, and liver.

RESISTANCE TO INFECTION. Iron strengthens the immune system and increases resistance to colds, infections, and disease.

Deficiency

ANEMIA. Iron deficiency anemia is the classic symptom of poor iron intake. It is the most common form of anemia, and might be the most prevalent nutrient deficiency in the United States. Anemia is the final stage of iron deficiency. Prior to a reduction in red blood cells, the tissue stores have been depleted, mental capacity has diminished, and other symptoms of marginal iron deficiency have developed. (See pages 140–143 for more information on anemia.)

HEART DISEASE. Iron deficiency has an adverse effect on the heart. An electrocardiogram (EKG), a measurement of heart function, shows irregularities in heartbeat and function in people who are iron-deficient. These abnormalities disappear when the person is supplemented with iron.

MENTAL SKILLS. An iron deficiency might affect the ability to comprehend or understand new information. Children who are iron-deficient do not perform as well in school or on intelligence tests than do children who consume adequate amounts of iron. The iron-deficient children also show impairment in attention span, learning and memory, and hand-eye coordination and might be hyperactive. These symptoms appear prior to signs of iron deficiency anemia and can be treated with iron supplements. Iron deficiency might also affect job performance, mood, and memory, and increased intake of iron might improve an iron-deficient adult's ability to work effectively and efficiently. Cravings for nonfood items, such as ice, clay, or starch, is common in iron deficiency. This symptom is called *pica*, and iron supplementation cures these cravings in some cases.

People at risk for developing iron deficiency anemia include infants, children less than 2 years old, teenage girls, pregnant women, premenopausal women, the elderly, and possibly female endurance athletes; pregnant teenagers are at very high risk. It is estimated that between 10% and 50% of people in these categories are iron deficient. However, everyone is a possible candidate for deficiency.

Poor dietary intake of iron is a primary cause of the deficiency. For example, menstruating females compared to men require almost twice the iron to replace monthly losses. In addition, females frequently follow weight-loss diets and often consume less food and less iron than do males. The average well-balanced diet in the United States supplies 6 mg of iron/1,000 calories. It would take 2,500 calories to meet the RDA for women, but the average intake is 1,600 calories or less.

Daily Recommended Intake

The RDAs take into account that only about 10% of dietary intake is absorbed. It is impossible for a woman during pregnancy and lactation to consume enough food to meet her iron requirement and a supplement that contains 30 mg or more of elemental iron is usually recommended.

The 1989 RDAs for iron are:

	Iron (mg)
INFANTS	
0–0.5 year	6
0.5–1 year	10
CHILDREN	
1–10 years	10
YOUNG ADULTS AND ADULTS	
Males 11–18 years	12
Males 19+ years	10
Females 11–50 years	15
Females 51+ years	10
Pregnant	30
Lactating	15

Sources in the Diet

Excellent sources of iron include organ meats, lean red meats, dried fruits, cooked dried beans and peas, dark green leafy vegetables, fish, poultry, prune juice, and oysters. Good sources include whole grain breads and cereals, green peas, strawberries, tomato juice, brussels sprouts, winter squash, blackberries, nuts, and broccoli. The iron in supplements and fortified foods is poorly absorbed, but does contribute to daily needs (Table 22).

Table 22.
THE IRON CONTENT OF SELECTED FOODS

Food	Amount	Iron (mg)
Liver, cooked	3 ounces	7.5
Oysters, raw	½ cup	6.6
Heart, beef, cooked	3 ounces	5.0
Dried apricots	½ cup	3.6
Molasses, blackstrap	1 Tbsp	3.2
Beef, ground, cooked	3 ounces	3.0
Raisins	½ cup	2.6
Navy beans, cooked	½ cup	2.6
Spinach, cooked	½ cup	2.4
Lima beans, cooked	½ cup	2.4
Split peas, cooked	½ cup	2.1
Chicken, meat only	3½ ounces	1.4

Table 22. (*continued*)
THE IRON CONTENT OF SELECTED FOODS

Food	Amount	Iron (mg)
Potato, baked	1 medium	1.1
Whole wheat bread	1 slice	0.8
Banana	1 medium	0.8
Avocado	½ medium	0.7
Broccoli, cooked	½ cup	0.7
Orange	1 medium	0.6
Apple	1 medium	0.4
Milk	1 cup	0.1
Cheese	1 ounce	0.05

The way in which a food is prepared will affect its iron content. Acidic foods, such as spaghetti sauce and tomato-based soups, cooked in cast iron cookware can increase the iron content of the meal 300-fold. Foods should be cooked for a short amount of time in a minimum amount of water to maximize iron intake. Iron leaches from food during prolonged cooking and is lost if the cooking water is discarded.

The iron in meats is called *heme iron* and it is better absorbed than the nonheme iron in vegetables, fruits, beans, and whole grain items. The iron in foods of plant origin is better absorbed if it is eaten at the same meal with a small amount of meat (heme iron) or vitamin C-rich foods. For example, only about 2% of the iron in nuts is absorbed if they are eaten alone. When nuts are consumed in a meal with chicken, which contains heme iron, and a salad that contains vitamin C, as much as 7% to 10% of the iron in nuts is absorbed. For infants, breastmilk is a better source of absorbable iron than is cow's milk.

Toxicity

Under normal circumstances, iron intake is regulated by need and dietary excesses are not absorbed. Accumulation of iron is possible, however, as the body cannot excrete excesses once they are absorbed. Hemosiderosis results from ingestion and absorption of excess iron. Iron is deposited in tissues, but at a level that is not harmful. Hemochromatosis is a more severe form of iron toxicity, where large amounts of iron are deposited in the liver, spleen, and other tissues, causing pronounced impairment in function and tissue damage. These conditions are rare and are usually associated with a genetic disorder that results in abnormal absorption of the mineral.

Nutrient-Nutrient Interactions

- Vitamin C increases the absorption of iron.
- Vitamin B$_6$ is necessary for the formation of the iron-containing protein in red blood cells called hemoglobin.
- Excess consumption of calcium, copper, or magnesium carbonate could reduce the absorption of iron.
- Iron competes with calcium, manganese, and zinc for absorption in the intestine and excess intake of one of these minerals could produce a deficiency of the others.

MANGANESE

Overview

Information on manganese is limited, since the first report of a manganese deficiency occurred as recently as 1972.

Functions

The known functions of manganese are not specific and other minerals, such as magnesium, apparently can function in its place. Manganese participates in the formation of connective tissues, fats and cholesterol, bones, blood clotting factors, and proteins. It also is important in the digestion of proteins. Manganese might function as an antioxidant in some body process.

Deficiency

Inadequate intake of manganese is associated with impaired fertility, growth retardation, birth defects, bone malformations, seizures, and general weakness.

Daily Recommended Intake

Average intake of manganese ranges from 2 mg to 9 mg/day. This intake prevents known clinical deficiency symptoms, but it is unknown whether it also prevents a marginal deficiency.

The 1989 Estimated Safe and Adequate Ranges for manganese are:

	Manganese (mg)
INFANTS	
0–0.5 year	0.3–0.6
0.5–1 year	0.6–1.0
CHILDREN	
1–3 years	1.0–1.5
4–6 years	1.5–2.0
7–10 years	2.0–3.0
ADOLESCENTS AND ADULTS	
11+ years	2.5–5.0

Sources in the Diet

Excellent sources of manganese include spinach, tea, whole grain breads and cereals, raisins, blueberries, wheat bran, pineapple, cooked dried beans and peas, and nuts. Moderate amounts are obtained from dark green leafy vegetables and dried fruits (Table 23).

Table 23.
THE MANGANESE CONTENT OF SELECTED FOODS

Food	Amount	Manganese (mg)
Tea	1 cup	0.4–2.7
Raisins	1 small box	0.201
Spinach, cooked	½ cup	0.128
Carrots, cooked	½ cup	0.120
Broccoli, cooked	½ cup	0.119
Orange	1 medium	0.052
Green peas	½ cup	0.051
Wheat bran	1 cup	0.048
Apple	1 medium	0.046
Milk	1 cup	0.046
Chicken, meat only	3½ ounces	0.021

Toxicity

Excessive dietary intake of manganese could interfere with iron absorption and result in iron-deficiency anemia.

Nutrient-Nutrient Interactions

- Calcium, iron, copper, manganese, and zinc compete for absorption in the small intestine and high intake of one of these minerals reduces the absorption of the other two.

• Manganese functions with vitamin K in the formation of blood clotting factors.

MOLYBDENUM

Overview

All tissues contain small amounts of molybdenum, with the largest amounts found in the liver, kidney, bone, and skin. These concentrations are sensitive to dietary intake and increase or decrease by raising or lowering the amount consumed in the diet.

Functions

Molybdenum is a component of the enzyme xanthine oxidase that aids in the formation of uric acid (a normal breakdown product of metabolism), is important in the mobilization of iron from storage, and is necessary for normal growth and development.

Deficiency

A deficiency of molybdenum causes stunted growth, anemia, loss of appetite, weight loss, and shortened life span in animals. Deficiency symptoms have not been reported in humans.

Daily Recommended Intake

The estimated average daily intake in the United States is between 45 mcg and 500 mcg.

The 1989 Estimated Safe and Adequate ranges for molybdenum are:

	Molybdenum (mcg)
INFANTS	
0–0.5 year	15–30
0.5–1 year	20–40
CHILDREN	
1–3 years	25–50
4–6 years	30–75
7–10 years	50–150
ADOLESCENTS AND ADULTS	
11+ years	75–250

Sources in the Diet

The molybdenum content of vegetables, fruits, and grains depends on the content of the soil in which they are grown. Plants grown on molybdenum-rich soil can contain as much as 500 times the molybdenum as plants grown on depleted soil. Hard tap water is a good source of the mineral. Lean meat, whole grain breads and cereals, cooked dried beans and peas, dark green leafy vegetables, and organ meats are good dietary sources.

Toxicity

Toxicity symptoms vary between species and age groups and depend on the form of molybdenum consumed. Prolonged intake of more than 10 mg is associated with goutlike symptoms, such as pain and swelling of the joints in humans.

Nutrient-Nutrient Interactions

- Excessive intake of copper might interfere with the absorption of molybdenum.
- Molybdenum works with vitamin B_2 in the conversion of food to energy.
- Molybdenum is important in iron metabolism.

SELENIUM

Overview

In the 1960s, selenium was identified as an essential mineral. The highest concentrations of selenium are found in the liver, kidney, heart, and spleen.

Functions

The most important known function of selenium is as a component of the antioxidant enzyme glutathione peroxidase. This selenium-dependent enzyme protects red blood cells and cell membranes from damage by highly reactive oxygen fragments. Selenium also works closely with, and in some cases can replace, the antioxidant vitamin E.

CANCER. Leukemia and cancers of the colon, rectum, breast, ovaries, and lung are less likely to develop in people who consume a selenium-rich diet. The anti-cancer effects of selenium are enhanced in the presence of vitamin E and a deficiency of the vitamin might reduce the effectiveness of selenium. Some evidence also shows that selenium might enhance the effectiveness of the immune system and the body's natural defense system that combats the development of cancer. (See pages 154–155 for more information on selenium and cancer.)

RHEUMATOID ARTHRITIS. Selenium as a component of the antioxidant enzyme glutathione peroxidase reduces the quantity of damaging compounds, such as hydrogen peroxide, that initiate or promote in-flammation associated with rheumatoid arthritis. Selenium also is involved in the production of hormone-like substances called pros-taglandins that regulate the inflammation process. It has not been proven, however, whether selenium supplementation is a consistent and effective treatment for rheumatoid arthritis.

Deficiency

BIRTH DEFECTS. Animal studies show that a selenium deficiency dur-ing pregnancy could have irreversible effects on the baby's develop-ment and growth, and have detrimental effects on the formation of the immune system.

CANCER. People with low blood levels of selenium are at increased risk for developing cancer. Healthy people have the highest selenium concentrations in their blood and people with cancer, such as cancers of the breast, ovaries, pancreas, cervix, and uterus, have the lowest concentrations. These blood levels reflect dietary intake; as selenium intake drops, the risk for developing cancer increases.

DOWN'S SYNDROME. Patients with Down's syndrome have low blood levels of selenium, which might contribute to the free radical damage to nerves characteristic of this condition. (See pages 126–128 for more information on free radicals and antioxidant nutrients.)

FIBROCYSTIC BREAST DISEASE (FBD). FBD is a condition characterized by painful breast lumps. Women with low blood levels of selenium have a higher risk for developing FBD than do healthy women.

HEART DISEASE. People at risk for heart disease who have low levels of selenium in their blood might benefit from selenium supplementa-tion. People who consume selenium-poor diets have weakened and damaged hearts, a condition called *cardiomyopathy*, which may be the reason for their increased risk of premature heart attacks. A form of heart disease, called *Keshan's disease* that affects primarily children is effectively treated with selenium supplementation. (See page 163 for more information on selenium and heart disease.)

Other symptoms of selenium deficiency include muscle weakness and tenderness, anemia, and damage to the pancreas.

Daily Recommended Intake

The 1989 RDAs for selenium are:

	Selenium (mcg)
INFANTS	
0–0.5 year	10
0.5–1 year	15
CHILDREN	
1–6 years	20
7–10 years	30
ADOLESCENTS AND ADULTS	
Males 11–14 years	40
Males 15–18 years	50
Males 19+ years	70
Females 11–14 years	45
Females 15–18 years	50
Females 19+ years	55
Pregnant	65
Lactating	75

Sources in the Diet

The selenium content of food is dependent on the selenium content of the soil in which the food is grown and can vary 200-fold. Grains, such as whole wheat, brown rice, and oatmeal are excellent sources if the grain was grown on selenium-rich soil. Poultry, low-fat dairy products, lean meat, organ meats, and fish are also good sources. Some of the selenium content is lost when foods are washed, cooked, stored improperly, or processed or refined (Table 24).

Table 24.
THE AVERAGE SELENIUM CONTENT OF FOOD CATEGORIES

Food Category	Amount	Selenium (mcg)
Organ meats	4 ounces	149.6
Seafood	4 ounces	37.9
Lean meat and chicken	4 ounces	22.7
Whole grain cereals and bread	1 serving	12.3
Low-fat dairy products	1 serving	3.6
Vegetables	1 serving	1.6
Fruit	1 serving	0.5
Sugar	1 tsp	0.2

Toxicity

Selenium can be very toxic. Children raised in selenium-rich areas of the country have a higher incidence of tooth decay and tooth loss. Large doses of either the inorganic forms of selenium or nutritional yeast fortified with inorganic selenium might cause cancer. Other symptoms of selenium toxicity include hair loss, white streaking of the fingernails, tenderness and swelling of the fingers, fatigue, nausea, and vomiting. These toxicity symptoms appear in individuals whose daily intakes are greater than 750 mcg.

Doses two to three times the RDA appear to be harmless. The organic forms of selenium, such as selenomethionine and selenocysteine, are better absorbed and less likely to cause toxic symptoms than the inorganic forms of the mineral, such as sodium selenite and selenate. The organic forms of selenium are available in selenium-rich nutritional yeast, whole grain products, and some supplements.

Nutrient-Nutrient Interactions

- Selenium and vitamin E work closely as antioxidants in preventing damage to cell membranes and possibly in the prevention of cancer.
- Large doses of vitamin C interfere with the absorption and use of inorganic selenium, such as sodium selenite.

ZINC

Functions

Zinc is a component of numerous enzymes in the body and functions in the detoxification of alcohol in the liver, the mineralization of bone, the digestion of protein, and the conversion of calorie-containing nutrients to energy. It also functions in the production of proteins, the proper functioning of insulin in the regulation of blood sugar, the maintenance of the genetic code, normal taste, wound healing, and the maintenance of normal blood levels of vitamin A and use of the vitamin by the tissues. Zinc is also important in the maintenance of the immune system and normal blood cholesterol levels, normal growth and development, the production of hormone-like substances called prostaglandins that regulate numerous body processes including blood pressure and heart rate, and the normal functioning of the oil glands of the skin.

ANOREXIA NERVOSA. Although the onset of the disorder might be related to social pressures, the progression of anorexia might be partially attributed to altered taste perception and metabolic upsets. Zinc improves taste perception and improves weight gain in patients with anorexia.

CANCER. Zinc might aid in the prevention and treatment of cancer. The effect of zinc on the immune system strengthens the body's defense against abnormal cell growth associated with cancer development. This essential trace mineral is also important in normal cell growth and development, which would aid in the prevention of any disease associated with abnormal cell growth. Zinc improves taste perception in cancer patients undergoing radiation therapy and aids in the maintenance of normal weight and nutrient intake during treatment.

RESISTANCE TO INFECTION. Zinc has a beneficial effect on the immune system and the body's natural defense against colds, infection, and disease. Zinc also inhibits the growth of disease-causing bacteria and in moderate doses might reduce tooth decay caused by bacteria in the mouth. Zinc also might reduce some of the symptoms of the common cold.

Deficiency

Symptoms of a zinc deficiency include anemia, slowed growth, reduced taste perception, birth defects, poor healing of wounds, sterility, poor alcohol tolerance, spontaneous abortion, delayed sexual maturation, glucose intolerance, mental disorders, dermatitis, and hair loss. Even mild deficiencies of zinc result in slowed growth, poor wound healing, delayed maturation, and inflammatory bowel disorders.

Children who consume a diet low in zinc are shorter and exhibit mental impairment as compared to children who consume a zinc-rich diet. Vegetarians also have low levels of zinc in the blood and vegetarian children tend to be short for their age.

Several dietary factors affect zinc absorption and can contribute to a zinc deficiency. A high fiber diet that contains excessive amounts of phytates in unleavened whole grain products contributes to a zinc deficiency, especially when the diet is low in zinc. Phytates bind to zinc and reduce absorption of the mineral. Leavening agents, such as baker's yeast, deactivate phytates. Overconsumption of foods or supplements fortified with iron or copper, but not zinc, can produce a secondary deficiency of the latter.

Zinc deficiency is not uncommon, especially in preschool children, hospital patients, low-income families, and elderly populations. Athletes and vegetarians also might be at risk for marginal zinc intake.

Lean meat is the best dietary source of zinc and anyone who consumes limited amounts of meat while consuming adequate to large amounts of refined grains, dairy products, and convenience foods, could be at risk for zinc deficiency.

Daily Recommended Intake

Healthy adult men require about 12.5 mg of zinc daily and it is assumed women require somewhat less because of their lower body weights. A well-balanced diet contains between 10 mg and 15 mg of zinc per day.

The 1989 RDAs for zinc are:

	Zinc (mg)
INFANTS	
0–1 year	5
CHILDREN	
1–10 years	10
ADOLESCENTS AND ADULTS	
Males 11+ years	15
Females 11+ years	12
Pregnant	15
Lactating, 1st 6 mo	19
Lactating, 2nd 6 mo	16

Sources in the Diet

Oysters, lean meat, poultry, fish, and organ meats are the best dietary sources of zinc. Whole grain breads and cereals are good sources of zinc. The zinc in breastmilk is better absorbed than the zinc in infant formula or cow's milk (Table 25).

Table 25.
THE ZINC CONTENT OF SELECTED FOODS

Food	Amount	Zinc (mg)
Oysters	6 medium	124.9
Turkey, dark meat only	3 ounces	3.7
Liver, cooked	3 ounces	3.3
Lima beans, cooked	½ cup	2.7
Pork, lean, cooked	3 ounces	2.6
Wheatgerm	2 Tbsp	1.8
Turkey, light meat only	3 ounces	1.8

Table 25. (*continued*)
THE ZINC CONTENT OF SELECTED FOODS

Food	Amount	Zinc (mg)
Yogurt, plain	1 cup	1.3
Almonds	¼ cup	1.2
Milk, nonfat	1 cup	0.9
Potato, baked	1 medium	0.4
Lentils, cooked	½ cup	0.18
Spinach, cooked	½ cup	0.17
Orange juice	6 ounces	0.13

Toxicity

Even moderate intakes of zinc, eg 25 mg/day, can impair copper absorption. Zinc in doses greater than 150 mg might interfere with the normal functioning of the immune system and reduce the body's defense against disease. Long-term ingestion of 80 mg to 150 mg of zinc lowers HDL-cholesterol and thus might increase risk for heart disease. Zinc in quantities 10 to 30 times the RDA for several months can cause low blood levels of copper and low levels of white blood cells. Doses of zinc sulfate that exceed 2 grams a day can cause nausea, stomach upset, and vomiting.

Nutrient-Nutrient Interactions

- High intakes of zinc can inhibit copper absorption and result in copper deficiency.
- High dietary intake of zinc might reduce iron absorption and encourage iron depletion from body storage.
- Adequate zinc intake might aid in vitamin D and calcium metabolism and reduce bone loss associated with marginal calcium intake.
- Zinc assists in the transportation of vitamin A in the blood.
- Zinc deficiency increases the amount of dietary vitamin E necessary to maintain normal blood and tissue levels of this fat-soluble vitamin.

ADDITIONAL TRACE MINERALS

Aluminum, arsenic, boron, cadmium, lead, mercury, nickel, silicon, tin, and vanadium are trace minerals found in the tissues of humans.

The biological usefulness of these minerals is poorly understood and some of these minerals are toxic.

ALUMINUM

Aluminum, once thought to be a harmless mineral, might be related to serious bone and brain disorders. A high intake of aluminum affects the absorption and use of calcium, phosphorus, magnesium, selenium, and fluoride and might be implicated in the development of bone deterioration. Muscle weakness and aching also is related to aluminum intake.

Abnormal levels of aluminum in the body are associated with nerve damage and brain disorders, such as Alzheimer's disease. Alzheimer's disease affects people in their middle to later years and is characterized by progressive and irreversible loss of memory and body function. Rats injected with aluminum learn at a slower rate and deposit aluminum in their brains in a pattern that resembles Alzheimer's patients. Whether the accumulation of aluminum is the cause or a result of Alzheimer's disease is unclear.

Sources of aluminum include food additives (such as sodium aluminum phosphate used as an emulsifier in processed cheese, cake mixes, frozen doughs, pancake mixes, and self-rising flours), table salt (contains sodium silicon aluminate or aluminum calcium silicate to retard clumping), and white flour (contains potassium alum to whiten the flour). Acidic foods, such as spaghetti sauce, cooked in aluminum pans dissolve the mineral into the food and increase the aluminum content of the diet. The mineral leaches from aluminum coffee pots into the coffee; the newer the pot or the longer the brewing time, the higher the aluminum content of the beverage. Aluminum-containing antacids, antiperspirants, and other products add to the daily intake of aluminum. Antacids average 35 mg to 208 mg of aluminum per dose; heavy users of antacids can ingest up to 5,000 mg. Hemorrhoidal preparations, vaginal douches, and lipstick also contain aluminum.

ARSENIC

The role of arsenic in the body is unknown, although this mineral is found throughout the body and is essential for the growth and development of other animals. Estimated daily intake of arsenic is 0.4 mg to 0.9 mg, an amount far below levels known to be toxic.

BORON

Boron is found in numerous tissues in the body. This trace element may play a role in bone health. No deficiency symptoms have been identified for this mineral.

CADMIUM

Cadmium is not excreted from the body and can accumulate over time to toxic levels. The estimated daily intake is 13 mcg to 24 mcg, of which very little is absorbed. Excessive intake occurs when soft water leaches cadmium from pipes. Cigarette smoke, air pollution, and the air near zinc refineries also provide a source of cadmium. Symptoms of cadmium toxicity include anemia, muscle wastage, hypertension, and liver and kidney damage.

LEAD

Lead is a toxic mineral that produces nerve damage, anemia, muscle wastage, lethargy, and mental impairment. Lead is ingested from a variety of sources including fresh and canned food, water, lead-based paint, plants grown in soil contaminated with lead, lead-glazed pottery, and air pollution.

MERCURY

Mercury salts are used in medicine, agriculture, and industry, and accumulation of toxic levels is possible. Mercury alters the shape and function of proteins, such as hormones, antibodies, hemoglobin in red blood cells, and all enzymes. The consequences of mercury toxicity are widespread. Ingestion of a toxic dose of mercury causes immediate gastrointestinal disturbances including a metallic taste in the mouth, thirst, nausea, vomiting, pain in the abdomen, and bloody diarrhea. A common first aid for mercury poisoning is to drink a protein-rich beverage such as milk. The mercury acts on the protein in the milk rather than the proteins that line the mouth, throat, stomach, and intestine. Vomiting is induced to remove the mercury and milk.

The body accumulates mercury in the kidneys, nerves, blood, liver, bone marrow, spleen, brain, heart, skin, and muscles. The developing infant is very susceptible to mercury toxicity during pregnancy. Some fish, such as tuna, are high in mercury and should be consumed in moderation, especially during pregnancy and breastfeeding.

Most people in the United States have dental fillings that contain mercury amalgams and the stability of this mercury has been questioned. Some evidence shows that mercury in the mouth might dissolve and over time migrate into the blood. This source of mercury might suppress the immune system and the body's natural defense against infection and disease.

NICKEL

No established role for nickel has been identified, although the mineral is found in association with the genetic code within each cell and might help activate certain enzymes. Nickel is probably involved in the activity of hormones, cell membranes, and enzymes. Low blood levels of nickel are observed in people with vitamin B_6 deficiency, cirrhosis of the liver, and kidney failure. The significance of these low blood levels is not known. In contrast, elevated blood levels of nickel are associated with the development of cancer, heart attack, thyroid disorders, psoriasis, and eczema.

The average daily intake of nickel is between 0.17 mg and 0.70 mg and the best dietary sources include whole grain breads and cereals and vegetables. A diet high in meat and other foods of animal origin and fat might be low in nickel.

SILICON

Silicon's primary function is in the development and maintenance of bone, and a silicon deficiency causes weak and malformed bones of the arms, legs, and head. Silicon is also important in the formation of connective tissue, the protein webwork in bone in which calcium is embedded. Silicon levels are high in people with atherosclerosis, but it is not known whether or not the mineral is related to the development or progression of cardiovascular disease. The daily diet contains ample amounts of silicon and the mineral is well absorbed. Dietary sources include whole grain breads and cereals, vegetables, and cooked dried beans and peas.

TIN

Tin is essential for some species and functions in normal growth and development, but no essential role has been identified in humans. High intakes of tin might destroy red blood cells. Elevated tissue and blood levels of tin can be a result of leakage of the metal into canned foods. Tin absorption is poor and it is not clear how much of the daily intake of 1.5 mg to 3.5 mg actually crosses the intestinal lining and enters the blood.

VANADIUM

Vanadium is essential for some animals and a deficiency can cause growth retardation, bone deformities, and infertility. However, no role for vanadium has been identified in humans. The average human body contains 20 mg of vanadium, which probably is involved in cholesterol metabolism and hormone production. Preliminary reports show that vanadium might protect against the development of breast cancer and might slow the growth of tumors.

Daily intake of vanadium is estimated at 2 mg to 4 mg for a well-balanced diet. Good dietary sources of vanadium include whole grain breads and cereals, nuts, root vegetables, liver, fish, and vegetable oils.

SECTION 2

VITAMINS AND MINERALS IN THE PREVENTION AND TREATMENT OF DISEASE

CHAPTER 5

Vitamins, Minerals, and Disease

INTRODUCTION

Modern history of nutrition begins with disease. The novelty and excitement of nutrition started at the turn of the century with the discovery of the first vitamin and its cure of a deficiency disease. In these early stages of research, vitamins and minerals were only investigated for their roles in curing specific diseases. The attempts were successful and common diseases that crippled, blinded, or killed, such as scurvy and pellagra, were miraculously erased. Clinical vitamin and mineral deficiency diseases were discovered and a "well-balanced" diet was believed to be one that prevented the onset of overt disease. Today, clinical nutrient deficiency diseases are uncommon in the United States and when they do occur they are usually a result of long-term medication use or another disease that limits food intake or nutrient use.

As the science of nutrition continues to develop and more sophisticated techniques for assessing nutritional status are discovered, the association between vitamins and minerals and disease expands beyond the realm of overt clinical deficiencies. Many conditions once thought to be the natural consequence of aging are now considered the result of lifelong poor eating habits. For example, a strong relationship exists between marginal dietary intake of vitamins and minerals and the development, progress, and cure of chronic disorders such as infectious diseases, disorders of the stomach and intestine, bone diseases, heart and blood vessel diseases, diseases of the liver, and cancer. Marginal vitamin and mineral intake is also related to wound healing, stress, the healing of burns, the strength of the immune system, and the aging process. (See pages 13–16 for more information on marginal nutrient deficiencies.) In addition, overconsumption of foods high in fat or sugar results in obesity and disorders related to obesity.

The science of nutrition expanded beyond just the prevention of disease with the discovery of a relationship between the intake of specific nutrients and behavior, intelligence, and mental health. For example, women were told for years that the changes in their emotions and bodies experienced the week before menstruation were "all in their heads." Marginal nutrient deficiencies have since been associated with these symptoms and increased intake of certain vitamins and minerals, such as vitamin B_6 and magnesium, might lessen the severity and frequency of premenstrual symptoms in some women. It appears that the "balanced diet" once thought to be a solution to clinical nutrient deficiency diseases is actually one that meets the unique nutrient needs of each individual for optimal health of both body and mind.

In less than a century, the study of vitamins and minerals has grown from a small arena of clinical nutrient deficiencies to include the role of nutrients in the prevention and treatment of chronic disease, the dietary and pharmacological role of vitamins and minerals in behavior and intelligence, and the function of nutrients in fundamental metabolic systems, such as the antioxidant and immune systems that affect the very basis of life and health.

THE ANTIOXIDANTS

The story of antioxidants begins with free radicals. Free radicals are highly reactive compounds formed by radiation; found in air pollution, ozone, and cigarette smoke; consumed in rancid fats; and produced during the normal breakdown of proteins in the body. Fragments of oxygen, such as peroxides and superoxides, are the most commonly identified free radicals.

Free radicals have an "extra" electrical charge that causes them to seek out other substances in the body in order to neutralize themselves. This initial reaction neutralizes the free radical, but in the process another one is formed. A chain reaction begins and thousands of free radical reactions can occur within seconds of the first reaction unless the extra free radical is deactivated.

The fatty membranes that surround cells are the prime targets for free radical attack. The shape and function of the fats in membranes are changed when a free radical attacks them. The damaged membrane is no longer able to transport nutrients, oxygen, and water into the cell or regulate the removal of waste products. Extensive free radical damage can cause the membrane to rupture and release its cellular components. These cellular components can further damage the surrounding tissues. Free radicals also attack nucleic acids that comprise the genetic code within each cell. Nucleic acids regulate normal cell formation and the growth and repair of damaged or aging tissues. The damage caused by free radicals has been linked to premature aging. Although why a body ages is only partially understood, all theories agree that at some point the body's cells become unable to replenish their components and as one cell dies, other cells dependent on the dying cell also are lost. The accumulation of cellular debris within a cell also is associated with aging. Finally, the cells' inability to correctly replenish necessary proteins because of damage to the genetic code is common in aging. Free radicals contribute to all of these processes.

Free radical damage also is associated with age-related diseases. Free radical damage to nucleic acids might initiate growth of abnormal cells, which is the first step in the development of cancer. The initial stages of atherosclerosis and heart disease, where the lining of the arteries are damaged and cholesterol begins to accumulate in the damaged area, are thought to be caused by free radical attack to the cell membranes of the tissues that line the blood vessels. Free radicals also are associated with inflammation, drug-induced damage to organs, suppression of immunity and increased susceptibility to infection and disease, and increasing the symptoms of other disorders, such as muscular dystrophy, arthritis, and Parkinson's disease. In addition, diseased tissues are more susceptible to free radical damage, so damage escalates during illness.

Oxygen might have its harmful side but it is still the most important "nutrient" for life; a person can survive for only a few moments without it. The body has developed a complex antioxidant system to defend itself from oxygen fragments and other free radicals. An antioxidant is any compound that fights against (anti) the destructive effects of free-radical oxidants. This antioxidant system is comprised of enzymes, vitamins, and minerals. Antioxidants act as scavengers and prevent the formation of free radicals or bind to and neutralize these reactive substances before they damage tissues.

Many nutrients, such as selenium, copper, manganese, and zinc are considered antioxidants because they work in conjunction with an antioxidant enzyme and are necessary for the enzyme to function properly. The antioxidant enzyme is not produced or is ineffective when the diet does not supply adequate amounts of the related vitamin or mineral. Other nutrients, such as vitamin C, vitamin E, and beta carotene apparently function as antioxidants independent of an enzyme.

More information is needed on how free radicals affect tissues and the functions of antioxidants in inhibiting free radical activity. The evidence shows, however, that a diet low in fat and high in the antioxidant nutrients might aid in the prevention of some diseases and premature aging. During conditions that expose the body to high amounts of free radicals, such as exposure to air pollution, radiation, and herbicides, poor diet, cigarette smoking, high dietary intake of vegetable oils, and the inflammatory diseases, the need for antioxidant nutrients is even more critical.

VITAMINS, MINERALS, AND THE IMMUNE SYSTEM

The body is under constant attack. Air, food, water, other people, and all aspects of the environment expose a person to bacteria, viruses, and other microscopic organisms. Some of these microorganisms are useful to the body and help maintain health. For example, a bacteria called *Lactobacillus acidophilus* found in some yogurts can live in the small intestine and reduces the risk for developing gastrointestinal disorders or possibly high blood cholesterol levels. Other microorganisms, however, promote infection and disease.

One of three things can happen when a microorganism, such as a bacteria, invades the body: 1) the bacteria can die; 2) the bacteria can cause the body's defense system, called the immune response, to activate even though there are no obvious signs of disease or infection; or 3) the microorganism can survive, multiply, and produce observable signs of infection or disease that even can result in death to the infected person. Swelling, inflammation, and increased body temperature are symptoms of infection. Diseases related to invasion of the body by microorganisms include infections associated with acquired immune deficiency disease (AIDS), herpes simplex, and possibly cancer.

The immune system is the body's defense against invasion by foreign substances, such as microorganisms. It is a complex network of specialized tissues, organs, cells, and chemicals whose primary purpose is to recognize and destroy a foreign invader. The lymph nodes and vessels, spleen, bone marrow, thymus gland, and tonsils are examples of organs and tissues that participate in the immune system. The cells and secretions of the immune system include specialized white blood cells called T and B lymphocytes, a chemical called interferon produced by T lymphocytes, chemicals called antibodies produced by B lymphocytes, and scavenger cells (monocytes and macrophages) that engulf and destroy microorganisms and other foreign substances. In addition, the skin and mucous membranes that line all internal and external surfaces of the body form a natural barrier against invasion by unwanted substances.

A well-functioning immune system recognizes unwanted microorganisms, abnormal and potentially cancerous cells, or any foreign substance in the body and destroys them, thus preventing the development of infection and disease. In contrast, the body's defenses are weak and a variety of disorders are possible when the immune system is not functioning at its best.

Poor nutrition is one of the most frequent reasons that the immune system malfunctions. All immune system processes are affected during malnutrition: the size, structure, and composition of the immune system organs are altered, the white blood cells are reduced in number and strength, and the chemicals produced by these cells are altered. Low intake of one or more vitamins and minerals with or without generalized malnutrition reduces ability to fight off infection and increases risk for developing immune-related diseases. In contrast, adequate intake of several vitamins and minerals and consumption of a low-fat diet enhances the immune system and reduces risk for developing diseases or infections.

The trace minerals and vitamins associated with the immune response include copper, iron, selenium, zinc, vitamin A and beta carotene, vitamin E, vitamin C, and the B vitamins, especially folic acid, vitamin B_6, and pantothenic acid. Limited evidence shows that intake of magnesium, nickel, and tin might also affect the strength of the immune system.

The immune system can be strengthened or stimulated to an optimal level, beyond which further attempts to activate this system apparently have an adverse effect. While moderate doses of some nutrients stimulate the body's defense system, larger doses impair the immune response. For example, some evidence shows that vitamin C in doses greater than several grams a day and zinc in doses greater than 150 mg/day might interfere with the immune response and place a person at increased risk for developing disease or infection.

IN CONCLUSION

Nutrition, the study of nourishment, is the "new kid on the block" in the scientific community. The word "vitamin" was first used in 1911 and essential minerals were still being discovered in the 1970s, whereas other sciences such as medicine, physics, and astronomy have been active for centuries. The expanding role of vitamins and minerals in the prevention and treatment of disease has created more questions than answers, and this limited supply of accurate information, coupled with the enthusiasm and interest in nutrition, leaves gaps that are often filled with inaccurate information and confusion. This chapter attempts to clarify many of the confusing issues related to vitamins, minerals, and disease by presenting the most reliable information based on current research.

ACNE

Overview

Acne is an inflammatory disease of the oil-producing (sebaceous) glands of the skin. There are many types of acne, but acne vulgaris is the most common; it usually begins during puberty and rarely lasts beyond the 25th year.

Nutrition and Acne

Certain foods have been blamed as the cause of acne and it has been suggested that chocolate, soft drinks, sugar, greasy foods, nuts, milk, salt, or iodine should be eliminated from the diets of children with acne. None of these foods, however, have been shown to increase the symptoms of acne. Poor nutrition will affect the body's immune system and increase the likelihood of the child developing a number of disorders or infections, but the addition of a small amount of chocolate to an otherwise healthy diet will not cause acne. A child might show allergic-like symptoms to certain foods that cause skin disruptions. Elimination of the food from the diet will not produce immediate relief from symptoms and it can take up to 2 months before results are seen.

Stress, and its associated increase in certain hormones, is related to the development and severity of acne. Relaxation, in the form of vacations or recreation, usually relieves some or all of the symptoms of acne. Sunshine and swimming are also relaxing and the sun inhibits bacterial growth, while the water cleanses the skin.

VITAMIN A. The synthetic form of vitamin A called retinoic acid (Retin-A) has been confused with the vitamin for the treatment of acne. There is no evidence that vitamin A (retinol or beta carotene) is an effective treatment for acne and consumption of large doses of this fat-soluble vitamin can cause toxic symptoms, such as joint pain, nausea, itching, cracking and drying of the lips and skin, hair loss, and cracks at the corners of the mouth. An individual should not self-medicate with retinoic acid without the advice and supervision of a pharmacist or physician.

ZINC. Zinc supplementation might be effective in the treatment of acne. Zinc maintains normal blood levels of vitamin A and aids in the normal functioning of the oil-producing glands of the skin. These functions combined with the typical adolescent diet low in zinc could explain why zinc is sometimes effective in the treatment of this disorder. Some people show fewer skin blemishes and their skins are less oily when zinc supplements are added to their diets.

Dietary Recommendations

A low-fat, high-fiber, nutrient-dense diet adequate in all vitamins and minerals and low in sugars and refined and convenience foods should be consumed. The diet should contain a variety of fruits, vegetables, whole grain breads and cereals, cooked dried beans and peas, low-fat or non-fat dairy products, and lean meats, chicken, and fish and should contain ample amounts of zinc-rich foods. (See pages 117–118 for dietary sources of zinc.)

The most important prevention and treatment for acne is thorough daily cleansing of the skin to keep it free from dirt and oil. Antibiotics, such as tetracycline, reduce the numbers of bacteria that break down the plugged oils and these medications are effective in the treatment of acne for some people. Retinoic acid is available by prescription and might help prevent the formation of or release the plug of oils or reduce the formation of excess oils in acne. Benzoyl peroxide is also used in the treatment of this skin disorder. The blemishes should never be squeezed or poked, as this will cause more scarring than the acne. Regular exercise, effective stress management, avoidance of alcohol and tobacco, and moderate exposure to sunshine are also important for health and the prevention and treatment of acne.

ACRODERMATITIS ENTEROPATHICA

Overview

Acrodermatitis enteropathica is an inherited zinc-deficiency disorder in infants characterized by loss of hair, dermatitis, diarrhea, psychological disturbances, and chronic illness called "failure to thrive." The parents and family members of the infant have low blood levels of zinc. The cause of acrodermatitis enteropathica is unknown; however, a defect in the body's ability to absorb zinc has been suggested.

Nutrition and Acrodermatitis Enteropathica

Acrodermatitis enteropathica was first noted in infants fed cow's milk. All symptoms of the disorder disappeared when the infants were placed on breastmilk. The zinc in cow's milk is poorly absorbed, whereas the zinc in breastmilk is easily digested and absorbed by the infant's developing gastrointestinal tract.

ZINC. Small daily supplements of zinc usually reverse all symptoms of this disorder and return the infant to health.

ACQUIRED IMMUNODEFICIENCY SYNDROME (AIDS)

Overview

Acquired immunodeficiency syndrome (AIDS) is a devastating, progressive disease characterized by suppression of the immune response, the body's natural defense system against disease and infection, and a high incidence of a type of cancer called *Kaposi's sarcoma*. The person does not die from AIDS, but from secondary infections, such as pneumonia or cancer. (See pages 128–129 for more information on the immune system.)

Nutrition and AIDS

Many patients with AIDS show muscle and tissue wastage and the increased incidence of infections and tumors that often follows weight loss. Poor nutrition, which negatively affects the body's ability to defend itself against infection and disease and which results in weight loss and damage to tissues, could predispose a person to infection that causes or increases the symptoms of AIDS. Long-term low intake of certain vitamins and minerals might suppress the immune system. People with a suppressed immune system who are exposed to the AIDS virus might not be able to fight the infection. Poor nutrition plays an additional role in the progress of the disease and risk of infection after the person has developed AIDS.

Malnutrition is common in AIDS patients. Signs of malnutrition are observed in patients in both the early and advanced stages of the disease and poor dietary intake probably interferes with treatment or encourages the progression of the disease.

Information is limited on specific nutrients and their association or impact on the prevention and treatment of AIDS. Zinc and selenium levels are low in the blood of AIDS patients and these deficiencies might contribute to a poorly functioning immune system and increased susceptibility to disease. Deficiencies of fatty acids, such as eicosapentaenoic acid (EPA) and gamma linolenic acid (GLA) might contribute to the development of AIDS and Kaposi's sarcoma; however, this is purely speculative at this time.

Dietary Recommendations

Until further information is available on dietary requirements for the prevention and treatment of AIDS, a low-fat, high-fiber, nutrient-dense diet should be consumed, adequate in all vitamins and minerals and low in sugars and refined and convenience foods. The diet should contain a variety of fruits, vegetables, whole grain breads and cereals, cooked dried beans and peas, low-fat or non-fat dairy products, and lean meats, chicken, and fish. Calorie intake should be adequate to maintain normal body weight. A multiple vitamin-mineral supplement that supplies at least 100% of the USRDA for all vitamins and minerals including magnesium, selenium, and zinc, as well as regular exercise, effective stress management, avoidance of alcohol and tobacco are important considerations in the treatment of AIDS.

ALLERGIES

Overview

Food allergy is an adverse reaction to a food that results in the activation of the immune system. For an adverse reaction to be labeled a food allergy, it must be proven that the person reacts to a specific food, the symptoms must recur two or more times when the food is consumed (preferably without the patient knowing he or she is ingesting the suspected food), and changes in the immune system must be observed.

More commonly, people misdiagnose food intolerances as food allergies. People can have a "simple" intolerance to a food that results from a genetic defect in an enzyme or other metabolic peculiarities not related to the allergic response. An example is lactose intolerance, where a person is missing a digestive enzyme (lactase) that aids in the breakdown and absorption of lactose or milk sugar. The bloating, flatulence, diarrhea, and discomfort that results from drinking milk is not an allergic response, but is a result of the accumulation of gas and fluids from the presence of undigested sugar in the intestine.

Pseudo-intolerances to food also are mistaken for food allergies. Personal preferences against or avoidance of a food or foods results in the person avoiding the food because it "does not agree with him or her." Dislike for a food is not a food allergy and avoidance of an entire food group can result in vitamin and mineral deficiencies.

One-third of the adults in the United States avoid a food because of a related adverse reaction, such as headaches, nausea, vomiting, skin irritations, or indigestion. Although these might be allergic symptoms, more than likely they are signs of food intolerance, pseudo-intolerance, or other psychological associations with food.

The development of food allergies depends on individual variation in heredity, intestinal absorption of nutrients, immune response, and exposure to foods. Food allergies are most common in premature infants and in children during the first few years of life when the immature digestive tract allows semi-digested food particles to pass into the blood stream. Breastfeeding for the first 6 to 12 months of a child's life reduces the incidence of food allergies in the newborn. Food allergies are more likely to develop in children of allergic parents than in children with no family history of food allergies. Infants and children with food allergies often outgrow the allergies. This is especially true for allergies to milk and eggs and is less true for allergies to peanuts and fish. New allergies can develop at any age; however, the incidence of food allergies decreases with age and although approximately 20% of people experience food allergies at some point in their lives, only about 1% to 5% of allergies persist into adulthood.

There are two types of food allergies: the immediate or obvious type and the delayed type. Only 5% of diagnosed food allergies are the immediate type where a person experiences an allergic reaction within minutes of eating a food. For example, the individual allergic to shrimp will develop allergic symptoms, such as hives, asthma, or a migraine headache, within approximately 30 minutes of eating the shellfish.

The delayed type of food allergy is more common, less obvious, more chronic, and very difficult to detect and correct. Adverse reactions to a food might take up to 5 days to appear and can occur in unrelated tissues such as the respiratory tract in the form of bronchitis, asthma, or inflammation of the sinuses (sinusitis).

Symptoms blamed on food allergy are extensive and diverse, although actual documented symptoms of food allergies are restricted to the respiratory tract, the digestive tract, and the skin. Any gastrointestinal disorder can result from an allergic reaction to a food, including faulty absorption of food, diarrhea, vomiting, swelling and tenderness of the mouth and throat, or rectal bleeding. Classic skin complaints include burning and itching of the skin, rash, hives, or small bruises (hemorrhages) below the skin. Some forms of dermatitis also are attributed to food allergies. Headaches, blood in the urine, inflammation and reddening of the whites of the eye (conjunctivitis), and joint pain also can occur as a result of food allergy. In all of the above allergic reactions, symptoms can be mild to severe; the most severe symptoms are anaphylactic reactions, which can cause severe itching and hives, perspiration, constriction of the throat, breathing difficulties, lowered blood pressure, shock, and in rare cases respiratory failure and death. The frequency and severity of other disorders, such as rheumatoid arthritis, bed-wetting, and migraine headaches, have been associated with food allergies; however, evidence supporting these claims are not conclusive.

The diagnosis of food allergies is complicated and the result of a single test does not determine a conclusive diagnosis of the condition. Diagnosis is based on the accumulation of evidence based on a thorough history of the individual's symptoms, foods thought to aggravate, previous medical and emotional history, and a medical exam to identify any possible underlying disorders that might explain or contribute to the allergic-like symptoms.

Several popular tests for food allergies have been developed, but their accuracy and usefulness are questionable. Cytotoxic testing takes a suspected food component, mixes it with a sample of the person's blood, and records changes in the white blood cells (immune response). Sublingual testing takes a drop of the suspected food component, places it under the individual's tongue, and records signs of an allergic reaction. In the provocative and neutralization testing, extracts of the suspected food are injected under the skin and allergic symptoms are recorded. None of these tests produce reliable results. The radioallergosorbent extract test (RAST) and the skin test are the most reliable diagnostic tests for food allergy and are performed by a physician or physician's assistant.

Nutrition and Allergies

FOODS. The most common causes of food allergies are eggs, milk, and wheat. It is a specific protein in wheat—called gluten—that triggers the allergic response. Although corn is low in gluten, some people also are sensitive to corn. Other common foods include nuts, citrus fruits, fish, shellfish, chocolate, and tomato-based products. Some fiber or laxative preparations, especially those that contain psyllium, might cause an allergic reaction in some individuals (Table 26).

Table 26.
FOOD INTOLERANCES AND THEIR SYMPTOMS

Food Or Food Ingredient	Symptoms
Chocolate, aged cheese, red wine, brewer's (nutritional yeast, canned fish	Migraine headaches
Fermented cheese, fermented foods (sauerkraut), pork sausage, canned tuna, sardines	Migraine headaches, skin rash or itching
Shellfish, strawberries, tomatoes, peanuts, alcohol, pineapple	Itching, eczema
Milk	Bloating, flatulence, diarrhea, abdominal pain
Coffee, tea, cola	Nerve disorders or high blood pressure
Legumes, berries, apples	Diarrhea, abdominal pain, flatulence
Monosodium glutamate (MSG)	Asthma, dizziness, headaches
Metabisulfites	Asthma, itching, fluid retention, congestion of the nose
Food additives and colorings	Asthma, itching, headaches, gastrointestinal disorders, hyperactivity, behavioral problems

ADDITIVES. No evidence exists that food additives are responsible for widespread food allergies, but a few additives, such as sulfiting agents, monosodium glutamate (MSG), the preservatives called benzoates, and yellow azo food dyes do produce symptoms in some people.

Sulfiting agents, including sodium or potassium metabisulfite, sulfur dioxide, and sodium or potassium bisulfite, have been used for years to keep fruits and vegetables looking fresh, especially in restaurants. They have become a greater concern with the increased popularity of salad bars and the higher exposure to sulfiting agents used to maintain a bright appearance to the fresh vegetables. Some people develop an allergic-type reaction to sulfiting agents and experience a wide range of symptoms from nausea and diarrhea to asthma, anaphylactic shock, unconsciousness, and even death. The Food and Drug Administration (FDA) banned the use of sulfiting agents on fruits and vegetables intended for raw use and foods and beverages must be labeled when sulfites are included in "detectable amounts" (10 ppm or more). All wine and some beers contain sulfites. Other foods that typically contain these preservatives include frozen and dried potatoes, vinegar and cider, maraschino cherries, lemon and grape juices, dried fruits and vegetables, some canned seafood soups, baking mixes, seafood (especially shrimp), fruit drinks, and colas. Sulfiting agents are sometimes listed on the label as "vegetable freshener," "potato whitening agent," "whiteners," or "whitening agents."

Tartrazine, or FD&C yellow dye #5, causes allergic reactions in some people. It is difficult to avoid this coloring as it is found in a variety of processed foods, such as orange drinks, cake mixes, cheese curl snacks, macaroni and cheese dinners, gelatin, instant pudding, and lemon candies. Reported allergic symptoms to this additive include asthma, burning and itching of the skin, fluid retention, and nasal congestion.

The most effective treatment for most food allergies is to avoid the offending food. Alternative foods, such as soy-based formulas instead of cow's milk for infants, can be found in some cases. Simple foods used in uncomplicated recipes are easy to avoid, but foods that are common ingredients in a variety of items are more difficult to identify and substitute or avoid. For example, wheat flour is found in a variety of processed foods and recipes, including cakes, bread, pies, gravies, soups, and salad dressings. A person must learn to read food labels and become familiar with the normal composition of standard foods such as mayonnaise, catsup, and peanut butter. The degree of strictness in avoiding a food will depend on individual sensitivity to the food; some individuals with food allergies suffer extreme allergic reactions to trace amounts of the offending food, while others can consume average amounts if the food is eaten with other foods. Often the offending food can be reintroduced 6 months to several years after removal from the diet with no allergic symptoms. In other cases, the way in which a food is prepared can alter the reaction. For example, the person might tolerate the food cooked, but cannot eat it raw.

Cross-reactions are possible with foods from the same grouping; if a person is allergic to peanuts, it is possible that other legumes also will be poorly tolerated. Other related foods that might produce cross-reactions include shrimp and crab or cow's milk and goat's milk.

The elimination-challenge test is useful when food allergies are suspected, but the offending foods have not been identified. The person is placed on a restricted, simple diet that excludes all foods suspected to cause allergies. After several days, one food at a time is introduced back into the diet and signs of allergy are recorded. The final diet is based on all foods that do not produce allergic symptoms. The elimination-challenge test can take several weeks to complete and should be conducted with the supervision of a registered dietitian (R.D.) or physician (M.D.). Reintroduction of a food can cause immediate or delayed allergic reactions that should be monitored closely by a skilled professional. Self-diagnoses are often wrong and can result in unnecessary avoidance of nutritious foods.

Limited evidence is available for the use of vitamins, minerals, or other nutrients in the treatment of allergies. Vitamin C might reduce some of the nasal congestion associated with the allergic reaction. Fish oils reduce the symptoms of inflammatory disease, but it is unclear whether they are effective in the treatment of allergies.

ALZHEIMER'S DISEASE

Overview

Alzheimer's disease is characterized by a slow, progressive, irreversible loss of memory. Basic body functions, such as the ability to eat and bladder control, are lost as the disease progresses. Alzheimer's disease usually affects older people, but cases also are reported in young and middle-aged people. It is the cause of dementia and slow death in thousands of Americans each year.

Nutrition and Alzheimer's Disease

Poor nutrition is related to Alzheimer's disease, but it is unclear whether it is a cause or an effect. Early damage to brain cells located in the region of appetite control might explain changes in food intake. A poor diet and vitamin-mineral intake might predispose an individual to Alzheimer's. It is certain that once the disease has reached advanced stages the patient loses interest in or the ability to choose or consume nutritious foods and the resultant malnutrition can increase the symptoms or speed the progression of the disease. Long-term rejection of food, either by pushing food out of the mouth by tongue movements, rejecting foods, or loss of memory of how to eat results in protein-calorie malnutrition and wasting of the body and nervous system. Long-term use of many medications further depletes the body of vitamins and minerals. (See Chapter 6.)

ALUMINUM. Dietary intake and abnormal accumulation of aluminum in the brain are associated with a variety of brain and nervous system disorders. In addition, aluminum tends to deposit in the brain cells most affected by Alzheimer's disease. This association does not prove that aluminum causes Alzheimer's; however, there is a strong relationship between the toxic mineral and this degenerative brain disease. The intake of aluminum has increased since the development of aluminum cookware, utensils, and foil. The mineral dissolves from aluminum pots into the food or beverage. For example, coffee brewed in aluminum pots contains more aluminum than does coffee brewed in glass pots; the longer the brewing time or the newer the pot, the greater the amount of aluminum in the beverage. Other sources of aluminum are medications and sundries, such as aluminum-containing antacids and antiperspirant deodorants. If aluminum intake is a contributor to Alzheimer's disease, prevention would include avoidance of all aluminum-containing substances and the treatment would include medications that bind to the mineral, reduce its absorption, and increase its excretion.

CHOLINE. Choline and its dietary source lecithin have shown varying effectiveness in the treatment of memory loss and Alzheimer's disease. The attempts to use this vitamin B-like substance are based on the observation that a particular neurotransmitter called *acetylcholine*, which contains choline and is responsible for the transfer of messages related to memory, is not produced in sufficient amounts in the brains of patients with Alzheimer's disease. Symptoms, such as slowed speech, shaking, and palsy-like movements, appear when acetylcholine production in the brain is inadequate. Supplementation with choline or purified soya lecithin (containing 90% phosphatidylcholine) sometimes has improved brain function in patients with memory loss. In other cases, however, increased intake of choline or lecithin raises blood levels of choline, but has no affect on acetylcholine levels or brain function. If choline or lecithin are effective in the treatment of memory loss, they are probably useful only in the beginning or mild stages and are then only useful in prolonging the onset of more advanced stages of the disease.

VITAMIN B_{12}. It is estimated that over 70% of older persons who are deficient in vitamin B_{12} also have Alzheimer's disease. Blood levels of the vitamin are significantly lower in Alzheimer patients than in patients suffering from other brain or memory disorders. It is not known whether the vitamin deficiency causes or results from deterioration of brain tissue. One of the functions of vitamin B_{12} is to maintain healthy nerve tissue, and this might be how a deficiency of the vitamin contributes to the progression of Alzheimer's disease.

Other vitamins and minerals are likely to be low in the diets of patients with age-related memory loss. Patients with dementia compared to patients the same age but without memory loss consume less vitamin C, vitamin E, and niacin and have lower levels of folic acid in their blood. The relationship between these nutrients and the initiation or progression of Alzheimer's disease is unknown.

Dietary Recommendations

Limited information is available on dietary recommendations for the prevention or treatment of Alzheimer's disease. Until more is known, a low-fat, high-fiber, nutrient-dense diet should be consumed, adequate in all vitamins and minerals and low in sugars and refined and convenience foods. The diet should contain a variety of fruits, vegetables, whole grain breads and cereals, cooked dried beans and peas, low-fat or non-fat dairy products, and lean meats, chicken, and fish. A multiple vitamin-mineral supplement that contains at least 100% of the USRDA for vitamin B_{12}; a calcium supplement; regular exercise; effective stress management; and avoidance of aluminum cookware, aluminum-containing medications and sundries, alcohol, and tobacco might be important for the prevention and treatment of Alzheimer's disease.

ANEMIA

Overview

Anemia is a reduction in the number or size of red blood cells or in the amount of hemoglobin within the cells. Red blood cells carry oxygen from the lungs to the tissues and transport carbon dioxide from the tissues back to the lungs to be exhaled. Any condition that reduces the oxygen-carrying capacity of the red blood cells reduces the oxygen supply to the tissues, including the internal organs, the muscles, and the brain.

Symptoms of anemia include lethargy, weakness, poor concentration, or being out of breath after minor physical effort. A pale complexion is sometimes observed in the anemic person. Increased susceptibility to colds and infection might be an early warning of anemia. A desire to eat non-food items such as chalk, ice, or dirt (a condition called pica) also might indicate anemia. In the later stages of anemia, the fingernails become thin and flat, the tongue becomes smooth and waxy, and stomach disorders are possible.

Anemia can result from severe blood loss from excessive bleeding or chronic low-grade blood loss from a bleeding ulcer or repeated blood donations. Anemia also can be nutritional in origin and can result from a dietary deficiency of iron, vitamin B_{12}, folic acid, vitamin B_6, vitamin C, vitamin E, or copper. The deficiency can result from poor dietary intake, impaired absorption, or faulty use of the nutrient within the body.

Nutrition and Anemia

IRON. Iron gives red blood cells their capacity to carry oxygen. Iron is attached to the protein hemoglobin in red blood cells. It is the iron that binds to oxygen in the lungs and releases oxygen to the tissues. The manufacture of red blood cells decreases when the body does not have an adequate amount of iron. The few red blood cells that are formed are small and pale in color.

Iron deficiency is the most prevalent nutritional deficiency in the United States and occurs most frequently in infants, young children, teenagers, women of childbearing age, pregnant and lactating women, and the elderly. Adult males are at low risk for iron deficiency because their daily needs are low and their food intake is high. If iron deficiency is diagnosed in this population it is often an indication of internal bleeding from another condition, such as stomach ulcers or cancer.

Anemia is the later stage of iron deficiency. The iron in muscles and other body stores has been depleted for months before the red blood cells are affected. Prior to a reduction in red blood cells, moderate to severe iron deficiency in children and adults can result in irritability, headaches, loss of appetite, clumsiness, lethargy, poor school performance, and hyperactivity. Teenagers show poor attention span and reduced perception that interferes with learning abilities. (See pages 105–108 for more information on iron and anemia.)

SELENIUM. Selenium deficiency might result in or aggravate the symptoms of anemia. Blood selenium levels are low in anemic animals and selenium supplements correct the anemia. Selenium's role as a component of the antioxidant enzyme glutathione peroxidase, which protects red blood cell membranes from free radical damage, might be an explanation for the mineral's association with anemia.

VITAMIN B_2. Increased intake of vitamin B_2 combined with iron supplements is more effective in the treatment of anemia than is iron alone.

VITAMIN B_{12} AND FOLIC ACID. Poor dietary intake of either vitamin B_{12} or folic acid results in a form of anemia called *macrocytic* or *megaloblastic* anemia. In contrast to the pale, small red blood cells common to iron deficiency anemia, the red blood cells are large, fragile, and limited in numbers. The results are the same; however, in both forms of anemia the oxygen-carrying capacity of the blood is reduced and lethargy, poor concentration, and other symptoms of anemia develop. (See pages 53–60 for more information on folic acid, vitamin B_{12}, and anemia.)

VITAMIN E. Vitamin E might be beneficial in the prevention and treatment of certain forms of anemia. Patients with kidney disease who are on dialysis often suffer from anemia. The cause of this anemia is unknown; however, the type of anemia resembles the "hemolytic" or fragile-cell anemia characteristic of a vitamin E deficiency. Supplementation with vitamin E increases the number of red blood cells and reduces the rate of red blood cell destruction in some patients.

OTHER VITAMINS AND MINERALS. Copper, vitamin C, and vitamin B_6 are related to the formation of hemoglobin and red blood cells, and a deficiency of any one of these nutrients results in anemia.

Copper is required in such minute amounts that normal dietary intake usually provides an ample supply of the mineral; however, long-term, inadequate intake of copper will result in abnormal use of iron and anemia. Copper-deficiency anemia is most common in infants fed cow's milk or copper-deficient infant formula rather than breastmilk.

Vitamin C is necessary for optimal absorption and use of iron. One of the symptoms of vitamin C deficiency is anemia related to the vitamin's role in iron metabolism.

Vitamin B_6 deficiency results in an anemia that resembles iron-deficiency anemia. The blood levels of iron are adequate but hemoglobin and red blood cells are not formed in the absence of vitamin B_6. Treatment consists of a therapeutic trial dose of 50 mg to 200 mg of vitamin B_6 each day; the anemia should respond within a few weeks if vitamin B_6 is the cause. This treatment should be followed only with the supervision of a physician.

Dietary Recommendations

Iron deficiency and iron deficiency anemia can be prevented and successfully treated with an increase in dietary iron, supplemental iron, or both. Attention span, school and work performance, and susceptibility to infection improve when the iron content of the diet is increased. Anemia might take longer to treat.

Infants and young children might develop iron deficiency anemia after weaning as a result of a prolonged milk-based diet and by overconsumption of foods low in iron. Poor food choices combined with the normal decline in appetite after the first year of life can result in chronic low iron intake.

Excess consumption of iron in supplement form has its drawbacks. Large doses of iron can cause stomach upsets and constipation. Doses of 3 to 10 grams of iron can be fatal in children. Iron also competes with other trace minerals, such as zinc and copper, for absorption from the intestine and increased intake of one can cause secondary deficiencies of the other minerals. For example, iron-fortified formulas might produce low blood levels of zinc in infants. This nutrient-nutrient interaction adds support to the argument that the "one nutrient-one disorder" approach to vitamin-mineral fortification or supplementation might be an oversimplification of a much more complex and integrated process of nutrient status. An iron supplement for anemia might be an incomplete therapy that causes secondary deficiencies of other nutrients.

A low-fat, high-fiber, nutrient-dense diet should be consumed, adequate in all vitamins and minerals and low in sugars and refined and convenience foods. The diet should contain a variety of iron-rich fruits, vegetables, whole grain breads and cereals, cooked dried beans and peas, and lean meats, chicken, and fish. Although red wine contains four to five times as much iron as white wine, the iron is poorly absorbed. A multiple vitamin-mineral supplement that contains at least 100% of the USRDA for all vitamins and minerals, including copper, iron, selenium, vitamin B_2, vitamin B_6, vitamin B_{12}, folic acid, vitamin C, and vitamin E; as well as regular exercise, effective stress management, moderate use of alcohol, and avoidance of tobacco are important for the prevention and treatment of anemia.

ARTHRITIS

Overview

Arthritis is inflammation of the joints, which can be long-term (chronic) or short-term (acute). Rheumatoid arthritis and osteoarthritis are the most common forms of arthritis, and the symptoms of rheumatoid arthritis are the most severe.

Rheumatoid arthritis is a chronic, disabling, and crippling disease characterized by inflammation of the lining of the joints. The small joints of the hands and feet are the most common sites for rheumatoid arthritis, but any joint can be affected. The causes of rheumatoid arthritis are unclear and are possibly a combination of a disturbance in the body's immune response, infection, heredity, or an as yet unidentified factor.

Osteoarthritis differs from rheumatoid arthritis in that it is a degeneration of the cartilage rather than inflammation of the lining of a joint. The joints most likely to be affected by this degenerative diseases are the joints of the feet and toes, the thumb joint, and the joints of the weight-bearing bones, such as the knees, hips, ankles, and backbone. Osteoarthritis is the most common form of arthritis and is found in most people in their later years. There is no single cause of osteoarthritis and this joint disorder is probably a result of physical stresses experienced throughout life, especially injuries or other diseases of the joints and obesity.

Nutrition and Arthritis

It is common for people with rheumatoid arthritis to be poorly nourished. The inflammatory process of arthritis changes the lining of the intestine and reduces the absorption of some nutrients, while increasing the daily nutrient requirements. Nutritional status is further depleted if the person is on long-term medication therapy that increases nutrient needs or causes peptic ulcers and gastritis, which reduces the desire to eat. Finally, the crippling and pain of rheumatoid arthritis can interfere with the purchase, preparation, and consumption of food.

Poor dietary intake of certain vitamins and minerals as well as weight loss and muscle wastage are associated with rheumatoid arthritis, although it is unclear whether poor nutrition is a cause or a result of the disease. Joint pain and stiffness increase when the patient is malnourished and deficiencies of folic acid, vitamin C, vitamin D, vitamin B_6, vitamin B_{12}, iron, magnesium, and zinc are found in patients with rheumatoid arthritis. In addition, children with arthritis have abnormal blood levels of certain trace minerals, including iron, zinc, and copper. Enriched and fortified foods, convenience and snack foods, and other foods common in the diets of children are not typically good sources of zinc, copper, and other trace minerals and the poor dietary intake might contribute to the development or severity of rheumatoid arthritis. Low blood levels of copper are probably a result of the disease, however, rather than a cause.

In adults, blood levels are low and symptoms improve with the increased dietary intake of calcium, selenium, zinc, and vitamin E. The antioxidant nutrients, such as selenium and vitamin E, might be effective because of their ability to stop free radical damage to joint linings which in turn causes the accumulation of fluids, swelling, and associated pain. The addition of several antioxidant nutrients to the diets of patients with rheumatoid arthritis might be beneficial in the prevention and treatment of this disease. Now, however, medications are the most effective treatment for rheumatoid arthritis, and no dietary therapy is widely accepted.

FISH OILS. Eicosapentaenoic acid (EPA), the fatty acid found in fish oils, might be useful in the treatment of rheumatoid arthritis. People with arthritis who take EPA supplements report improvements in morning stiffness. Evidence linking fish oils to improvements in rheumatoid arthritis is limited and no dietary recommendations can be made at this time.

FOOD INTOLERANCE. Food intolerances have been blamed for some cases of rheumatoid arthritis. Improvements in pain, number of painful joints, duration of morning stiffness, and grip strength are experienced when foods likely to be poorly tolerated, such as wheat cereals or milk, are eliminated from the diet. These improvements in symptoms are maintained as long as the patient follows the restricted diet and symptoms return when a patient returns to previous eating habits.

Dietary Recommendations

Rheumatoid arthritis is linked to poor nutritional status and good nutrition counteracts the adverse effects of medication therapy. For example, supplementation with calcium and vitamin D can help prevent the bone loss associated with the use of steroids prescribed in the treatment of rheumatoid arthritis. Increased intake of vitamin C can offset the adverse effects of aspirin on the absorption of vitamin C.

Weight loss and maintenance of ideal body weight is recommended for patients with either rheumatoid arthritis or osteoarthritis. Symptoms of osteoarthritis often subside with a return to a healthy weight.

Until more is known about diet and rheumatoid arthritis, a low-fat, high-fiber, nutrient-dense diet, adequate in all vitamins and minerals and low in sugars, refined and convenience foods is a healthy and safe preventive measure. The diet should contain a variety of fruits, vegetables, whole grain breads and cereals, cooked dried beans and peas, low-fat or non-fat dairy products, and lean meats, chicken, and fish. A multiple vitamin-mineral supplement that contains no more than 100% of the USRDA for the trace minerals as well as regular exercise, effective stress management, and avoidance of alcohol and tobacco are important for the prevention and treatment of arthritis. In addition, the patient with either rheumatoid arthritis or osteoarthritis should lie down at least once during the day to rest the joints and remove the weight from them. Massage and heat also can reduce pain.

Although adequate intake of vitamins and minerals is essential to the health of the person with arthritis, overconsumption of nutrients might be harmful. Large amounts of iron might increase the symptoms of arthritis. Large doses of vitamin D cause calcium to be deposited in tissues, such as the kidney and heart. The damage caused by calcification of soft tissue is irreversible.

ASTHMA

Overview

The causes of asthma are not clear. The disorder might be inherited as several members within a family usually suffer from asthma. In some cases, asthma is a result of food allergies. Psychological and emotional influences also contribute to the asthma attacks.

Nutrition and Asthma

VITAMIN B_6. Increased intake of vitamin B_6 might reduce the symptoms of asthma. Some people who consume 100 mg of vitamin B_6 daily report a reduction in occurrence, severity, and duration of asthmatic attacks. Asthma patients have lower blood levels of vitamin B_6 than do healthy adults and although supplementation might not raise these levels, it does appear to improve symptoms. Supplementation with large doses of vitamins or minerals should be supervised by a physician.

VITAMIN C. Blood levels of vitamin C decrease temporarily during an asthmatic attack, while blood levels of the stress hormone cortisone increase. It is not known whether an increased dietary intake of vitamin C might aid in the prevention of the asthmatic attack.

SELENIUM. Blood levels of selenium are low in patients with asthma and these low levels might worsen the inflammation associated with the disorder.

VEGETARIAN DIET. A strict vegetarian or vegan diet (avoidance of all foods of animal origin) might aid in the treatment of asthma. Improvements in the frequency and severity of asthmatic attacks are reported by people placed on a strict vegetarian diet. In addition, medications usually prescribed for asthma, such as cortisone, are dropped 50% to 90% and some people are able to discontinue medication on the vegetarian diet.

Dietary Recommendations

Some food allergies produce asthma-like symptoms. (See pages 133–138 for more information on food allergies.) For example, some people are sensitive to the flavor enhancer monosodium glutamate (MSG), the coloring agent FD&C yellow dye #5, salicylates, or the meta-bisulfites preservatives and develop asthma-like symptoms whenever these food additives are consumed. The asthma symptoms develop within minutes to hours after the food is ingested, so it is possible to identify the offending food and eliminate it from the diet. Specific dietary recommendations for asthma are not available (Table 27).

Table 27.
SALICYLATES IN FOODS

Food Groups	Contain Salicylates
Beverage	Tea, root beer, birch beer
Meat	Corned beef, meat processed with vinegar
Milk	None
Vegetable	Cucumbers, green peppers, tomatoes, potatoes
Fruit	Apples, apple cider, apricots, blackberries, boysenberries, cherries, currants, dewberries, gooseberries, huckleberries, maraschino cherries, grapes, melons, nectarines, peaches, raisins, raspberries, prunes, plums
Cereals and Breads	None
Fat	Salad dressing, mayonnaise, avocado, olives

A low-fat, high-fiber, nutrient-dense diet adequate in all vitamins and minerals and low in sugars and refined convenience foods, and any food suspected to cause allergic reactions is a healthy and safe protective measure. The healthful diet should contain a variety of fruits, vegetables, whole grain breads and cereals, and cooked dried beans and peas, low-fat or non-fat dairy products, and lean meats, chicken, and fish should be consumed in moderation. A strict vege-tarian diet also can be designed to meet all vitamin and mineral needs. Regular exercise, effective stress management, and avoidance of alcohol and tobacco are important in the prevention and treatment of asthma.

BRUISING

Overview
A bruise is a surface injury to the skin where the small blood vessels that reside below and within the skin are broken. Bruises that develop without an injury can be a sign of numerous disorders, including

leukemia, low blood levels of platelets (cell fragments responsible for blood clotting), or nutrient deficiencies.

Nutrition and Bruising

Nutrients necessary for the normal healing of bruises and wounds include protein, vitamin A, vitamin B_{12} and other B vitamins, vitamin C, vitamin E, folic acid, calcium, and copper. In addition, chronic use of alcohol or some medications depletes the body of these nutrients and impairs the healing of wounds and bruises. A physician should be consulted if the diet is adequate in nutrients and the bruising persists.

VITAMIN C. The classic symptom of scurvy, the vitamin C deficiency disease, is tiny hemorrhages below the skin called *petechial hemorrhages*. Vitamin C is necessary for the formation of collagen, the protein portion of connective tissue. This tissue holds the body's cells together, while improper formation causes other tissues to fall apart. Consequently, a vitamin C deficiency causes the blood vessels to become fragile and blood leaks into the surrounding tissues, causing small bruises.

Dietary Recommendations

A low-fat, high-fiber, nutrient-dense diet should be consumed, adequate in all vitamins and minerals and low in sugars and refined and convenience foods. The diet should contain a variety of fruits, vegetables, whole grain breads and cereals, cooked dried beans and peas, low-fat or non-fat dairy products, and lean meats, chicken, and fish. Regular exercise, effective stress management, and moderate consumption of alcohol, and avoidance of tobacco are important in the prevention and treatment of bruises.

BURNS

Overview

A widespread burn is one of the most severe injuries to the body. Repair of damaged tissues and changes in the nervous system and hormone regulation associated with burns can double normal energy (calorie) requirements. Excessive loss of protein, water-soluble vitamins, and minerals caused by the injured tissue increases the daily need for these nutrients. Simultaneous infection further increases protein and nutrient needs. In addition, burn patients often lose their appetites and the maintenance of good nutritional status is challenging.

Nutrition and Burns

The dietary management of patients with severe burns should be supervised by a dietitian and a physician. It will include the replacement of fluids and electrolytes (eg, sodium, chloride, potassium, and other nutrients) and adequate intake of calories and nutrients based on ideal body weight, percentage of body burned, and a nutritional assessment. The daily need for all vitamins and minerals also increases during the healing process.

CALCIUM. Blood levels of calcium are low in patients with burns that cover more than 30% of their bodies. Loss of calcium is exaggerated when the patient is unable to move or exercise. Calcium supplementation and early initiation of exercise might be necessary to prevent bone loss.

ZINC. Low blood levels of zinc are seen in patients with severe burns. Zinc supplementation is recommended to treat post-burn loss of appetite and impaired wound healing.

Dietary Recommendations

Nutritional support for the patient with severe burns will include increased intake of protein, calories, vitamins, minerals, fluids, and electrolytes. Frequent feedings, use of supplementary feedings in the form of tube feedings or intravenous solutions, and sterile serving containers also might be recommended.

Nutrition for the treatment of minor burns does not vary from dietary recommendations for the healthy adult. A low-fat, high-fiber, nutrient-dense diet should be consumed, adequate in all vitamins and minerals and low in sugars and refined and convenience foods. The diet should contain a variety of fruits, vegetables, whole grain breads and cereals, cooked dried beans and peas, low-fat or non-fat dairy products, and lean meats, chicken, and fish. Regular exercise, effective stress management, and avoidance of alcohol and tobacco are important for the healing of burns.

CANCER

Overview

Cancer is a group of diseases characterized by the uncontrolled growth and spread of abnormal cells. The abnormal cells trespass into surrounding tissues, interfere with the tissues' ability to function, and eventually damage or destroy the healthy cells. Cancer cells also can break loose, travel through the blood and lymph, lodge in tissues in other parts of the body, and develop into new cancers. This ability to form secondary cancers is called *metastasis* (Table 28).

Table 28.
THE 7 WARNING SIGNS OF CANCER

1. C hange in bowel or bladder habits
2. A sore that does not heal
3. U nusual bleeding or discharge
4. T hickening or lump in breast or elsewhere
5. I ndigestion or difficulty in swallowing
6. O bvious change in wart or mole
7. N agging cough or hoarseness

Cancer develops in two stages: an initiation stage where the normal, healthy cell or its genetic code is altered and a promotion stage where the abnormal cell is encouraged to multiply. Both stages are necessary for cancer to develop. The initiation stage happens quickly and frequently and is caused by a substance called a *mutagen* or a *carcinogen*. The promotion stage, where a substance called a *promoter* is in contact with the abnormal cell, is more lengthy, allowing the slow growth of cancer to go undetected for up to 30 years. Cancer will not develop unless the cell exposed to a mutagen or carcinogen is subsequently in contact with something that will promote its growth. In addition, the strength of the immune system might have an important role in the prevention or development of cancer (Figure 2).

Nutrition and Cancer

Nutritional excesses and deficiencies are associated with the development of cancer. It is estimated that as much as 70% of all cancers are diet-related, which makes diet second only to tobacco as the most influential factor in the development of cancer.

Many substances in food act as mutagens or promoters. For example, the food additives called nitrites, found in processed meats such

Figure 2

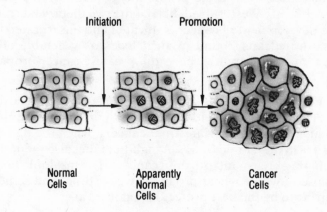

Initiation   Promotion

Normal
Cells

Apparently
Normal
Cells

Cancer
Cells

The two stages of cancer growth are initiation and promotion.

as bacon and bologna, are converted in the body to nitrosamines, which are potent carcinogens. Alcohol does not initiate cancer, but it promotes the growth of a pre-existing abnormal cell. Other dietary mutagens include aflatoxin (a mold that forms on peanuts), heavy metals such as lead, polychlorinated biphenyl (PCB), and pesticides such as malathione and DDT. Examples of suspected dietary promoters are saccharin, excess dietary fat, and excessive use of coffee or caffeine.

On the other hand, the diet also contains many substances that prevent the development or progression of cancer. A diet low in fat and alcohol, and high in fiber, vitamin A or beta carotene, vitamin C, vitamin E, selenium, and several other nutrients and substances found in food inhibits the initiation and promotion of several types of cancer.

BODY WEIGHT. People who maintain a healthy or ideal body weight, as compared to people who are 20% or more above their ideal body weight, live longer and are at a lower risk for developing cancers, especially cancers of the prostate, uterus, gallbladder, kidney, cervix, stomach, colon, and breast.

DIETARY FAT. No other dietary change has as profound an effect on lowering the risk for developing cancer than does reducing dietary fat intake. Numerous studies show that a typical American diet that provides more than 30% to 35% of its calories from fat is strongly linked to and perhaps is a cause of cancer of the breast, ovaries, uterus, colon, and prostate. The risk for developing these cancers is low in countries where people consume a low-fat diet. However, their risk for cancer increases when these people move to the United States and consume the fatty Westernized diet. Of the two dietary fats associated with the development of cancer (saturated and unsaturated fats), the polyunsaturated fats, found in such foods as vegetable oils, salad dressings, and mayonnaise, have the greatest cancer-promoting effects.

FIBER. A low-fat, high-fiber diet is a person's best safeguard against cancer. People have an 8-fold increase in the risk for certain forms of cancer, such as colon and intestinal cancers, when the diet is low in fiber, as it is in the United States. A high-fiber diet also reduces the risk for developing breast and prostate cancers. The insoluble fibers, such as cellulose in whole wheat products, wheat bran, and some vegetables, appear to be the best protectors against cancer.

VITAMIN A AND BETA CAROTENE. A diet high in vitamin A or the building block for vitamin A, called *beta carotene*, found in fruits and vegetables protects a person against cancer, especially cancers of the mouth, larynx, esophagus (throat), breast, cervix, bladder, and lungs. In contrast, a person who consumes a diet low in vitamin A or beta carotene is at increased risk for developing cancer.

Vitamin A and beta carotene apparently protect against cancer by their inhibition of both the initiation and promotion stages. Beta carotene also might aid in the prevention of cancer by:

1. inhibiting the growth of abnormal cells
2. strengthening the immune response so cancer cells are less likely to grow
3. fortifying cell membranes so they are less vulnerable to attack or damage, and
4. altering cell production so abnormal cells are less likely to develop.

Vitamin A also aids in the prevention of tissue damage caused by radiation.

The most common cancers in the United States are cancers of epithelial tissue, the tissue that lines the inside and outside of the body. Skin, mucous membranes, and the tissues that line the lungs, mouth, throat, stomach, colon, prostate, cervix, and uterus are examples of epithelial tissues. One of the main functions of vitamin A is to aid in the development and maintenance of these tissues. A deficiency of vitamin A produces changes in these tissues that resemble the initial changes in cancer. Tissues low in vitamin A are more prone to

develop cancer than are tissues with a high concentration of the vitamin.

Beta carotene is more effective than vitamin A in preventing lung
cancer. Lung cancer rates are lower in cigarette smokers who also
consume a diet high in fruits and vegetables than in smokers who
avoid these foods. The risk for lung cancer rises when the intake of
beta carotene is low. Both vitamin A and beta carotene help prevent
the precancerous changes in the mouth observed in people who chew
tobacco. Daily requirements for beta carotene might increase with
excessive exposure to sunshine.

People with precancerous conditions also might benefit from adequate vitamin A intake. Benign breast disease is characterized by pain
and breast lumps and is associated with a 2-fold increase in risk for
developing breast cancer. Symptoms of breast pain and lumps are
reduced in some individuals when the vitamin A content of the diet is
increased. There is no evidence, however, that the vitamin or beta
carotene will cure the disorder.

Vitamin A or beta carotene also might assist in the treatment of
cancer. Vitamin A-rich foods or vitamin A supplements, when taken in
conjunction with chemotherapy or radiation therapy, might improve
the cancer patient's outcome for recovery and reduce damage to
healthy tissue caused by chemotherapy or radiation. A combination of
vitamin A and the amino acid arginine might slow the growth of
tumors and improve the survival time of the cancer patient.

FOLIC ACID. Folic acid's main function in the maintenance of the
genetic code of cells and the regulation of normal cell division and
growth might explain this B vitamin's link to a reduced risk for developing cancer. A microscopic view of cells shows a folic acid deficiency
produces changes in the cell's structure that resemble the beginning
of cancer. Preliminary evidence shows folic acid prevents the conversion of a normal cell to a precancerous cell and might convert damaged cells back to normal ones.

VITAMIN B$_6$. Vitamin B$_6$ might have a secondary effect on the prevention of cancer by strengthening the immune system and aiding the
body in its efforts to resist cancer. Limited evidence also shows this B
vitamin might protect against the initiation of cancer.

VITAMIN C. The risk for developing cancer of the stomach, throat, and
possibly bladder is reduced when the diet is high in vitamin C-rich
foods, while these cancers are more prevalent in people who consume
little vitamin C. Nitrosamines are potent cancer-causing substances
found in cigarette smoke and formed in the stomach from food additives called nitrites. Vitamin C neutralizes these carcinogens and

protects the tissues that are in contact with them, such as the stomach, the colon, and the bladder.

Vitamin C might have other anti-cancer actions. The vitamin might strengthen the cells' resistance to invasion by abnormal growth, enhance the immune response, or protect cell membranes from free radical damage that could result in cancer. (See pages 126–128 for information on free radicals.)

VITAMIN D. Vitamin D might prevent or slow the growth of certain forms of cancer, such as cancers of the breast or colon and non-Hodgkin's lymphoma. The likelihood of developing colon cancer is higher in areas where people have limited exposure to sunlight (the necessary factor for the production of vitamin D in the skin) than in areas where the sun shines frequently. In addition, people who consume a diet low in vitamin D are at higher risk for developing colon cancer than are people who consume ample amounts of the vitamin.

VITAMIN E. A diet high in vitamin E is linked to a reduced risk for developing cancers, whereas low blood levels of vitamin E increase the risk for developing cancer. In addition, tumor formation, growth, and numbers decrease and animals live longer when given vitamin E supplements. Women with low levels of vitamin E in their blood have a 5-fold increase in risk for breast cancer when compared to women with normal to high blood levels of vitamin E. Risk for breast cancer is reduced when vitamin E is added to the diet. People with lung cancer also show depleted vitamin E stores in their tissues when compared to tissues of healthy people.

Vitamin E works with other antioxidants, such as selenium, to prevent free radical damage to cell membranes or the cell's genetic code that could otherwise lead to abnormal cell growth or function. The antioxidant properties of vitamin E might explain the vitamin's ability to reduce the incidence of cancers of the stomach, bowel, and bladder. A deficiency of the vitamin allows increased tissue damage by nitrites, while adequate intake of the vitamin reduces the formation of nitrosamines from dietary nitrites. (See pages 126–128 for information on antioxidants.)

Another proposed way that vitamin E might protect against cancer is the vitamin's ability to protect the body's genetic code. Cancer often begins as an alteration in the genetic code that regulates the shape, function, and characteristics of each cell. Vitamin E might protect the genetic code from alterations that initiate the growth of abnormal cells. In addition, abnormal cells might be converted back to normal cells when a person consumes adequate amounts of vitamin E.

The multifaceted nature of cancer combined with the different forms of vitamin E make the link elusive. Some studies find no association while others show a preventive effect from vitamin E supplementation that depends on the form of vitamin E or intake of other nutrients such as selenium. Vitamin E succinate might be the most potent form of the vitamin.

VITAMIN K. In laboratory studies, tumor cell growth is curtailed when vitamin K is present. The cancers responsive to vitamin K therapy included breast, ovary, colon, stomach, bladder, liver, and kidney cancers.

IRON. A diet low in iron might increase a person's risk for developing cancer. This trace mineral probably exerts its effect by strengthening the immune system. However, excessive iron intake also is linked to an increased risk for developing cancer.

SELENIUM. Increased intake of selenium might reduce the risk for developing cancer. People who live in areas of the country where the selenium content of the soil is high have a low incidence of cancer, especially cancers of the digestive tract, lungs, breast, and lymph system. The incidence of cancer is lower in countries where the people consume a selenium-rich diet than in countries where the selenium content of the diet is poor. Blood levels of selenium are low in cancer patients with Hodgkin's disease, leukemia, and cancers of the breast, lymph system, stomach and intestine, colon, bladder, and genital tract. People with low blood levels of the mineral have a 2-fold greater risk of developing cancer than do people with adequate blood selenium levels.

Selenium might protect an individual from developing cancer by its antioxidant capabilities, its effect on the immune system, or its ability to neutralize the toxic effects of certain metals. Selenium works with vitamin E in the protection of cell membranes and the cell's genetic code from free radical damage that could lead to abnormal cell shape, function, or growth. Selenium also might strengthen the immune response and improve a person's defense against abnormal cell growth. Finally, selenium helps detoxify cadmium and mercury, two minerals that cause cancer.

The form of selenium might be important in the prevention or treatment of cancer. The organic form of the mineral called *selenomethionine* or *selenocysteine* is apparently more potent and less toxic than the inorganic forms, such as sodium selenite.

VANADIUM. The trace mineral vanadium might aid in the prevention of cancer. Limited evidence shows supplementation with vanadium in animals limits the initiation of tumors and reduces the number of tumors that form.

ZINC. Zinc is related to the prevention of cancer because of its contribution to the formation and regulation of the cells' genetic code, the maintenance of a strong immune system, and the healing of damaged tissues. Patients with cancer have low blood levels of zinc and the progression of the disease is accelerated when zinc levels are low. Zinc supplements also might improve appetite in cancer patients.

CALCIUM. Calcium's protective effect against cancer is limited to the large intestine. The mineral's close dietary association with vitamin D makes it difficult to isolate either nutrient as the one that affects cancer rates. However, it appears calcium binds to cancer-promoting fats in the intestine and reduces their ability to initiate the cancer process.

OTHER DIETARY FACTORS. The frequent inclusion of cruciferous vegetables (vegetables in the cabbage family, such as broccoli, Brussels sprouts, kohlrabi, cauliflower, and cabbage) might reduce a person's risk for developing cancer, especially cancers of the stomach, colon, and respiratory tract. The protective effect is caused by substances called *indoles* in the vegetables. These vegetables have added benefits as they also provide ample amounts of vitamin A, folic acid, vitamin C, and fiber.

A diet that supplies most of its protein from vegetable sources rather than meats or dairy products might reduce the risk for developing cancer, such as prostate, pancreatic, and lymph cancers. Vegetarians are less likely than meat-eaters to develop cancer. People who consume a large part of their food intake as meat, cheese, eggs, and milk have a 4-fold increased risk for developing prostate cancer as people who consume primarily vegetable protein from cooked dried beans and peas, whole grain breads and cereals, and tofu.

The omega 3 fatty acids, such as gamma linolenic acid (GLA) found in Evening Primrose Oil and eicosapentaenoic acid (EPA) found in fish oil might aid in the prevention of cancer and might suppress the growth of tumors.

A high intake of sugar and alcohol is associated with an increased risk for some types of cancer, especially cancers of the intestinal tract. These effects are accented when combined with a high-fat, low-fiber diet. Artificial sweeteners, especially saccharin and cyclamates, also are linked to the development of cancer.

Old or damaged peanuts and peanut butter contain a naturally-occurring contaminant called *aflatoxin* that is one of the most potent cancer-causing substances known to occur in the food supply. The amount of aflatoxin allowed in commercial peanuts is limited by the Food and Drug Administration (FDA) to no more than 20 ppb (parts per billion).

Limited evidence shows that some commonly eaten foods might contain cancer-causing substances if eaten in excessively large amounts. For example, commercial mushrooms might contain cancer-causing substances. When these substances are isolated from the mushrooms and are fed in large amounts to laboratory animals some cause atherosclerosis and heart disease while others cause cancer. Chili, a main ingredient in Indian curry, might be a mutagen capable of converting a normal, healthy cell into an abnormal, potentially cancerous one. Chili is suspected as a contributor to the development and promotion of oral and throat cancer in India. Other naturally-occurring cancer-causing substances include safrole in oil of sassafras and black pepper; psoralen in celery, parsley, figs, and parsnips; catechol in coffee; gossypol in cottonseed oil; and certain alkaloids in herbs, herbal teas, and honey. However, the amount of these carcinogens in the normal diet is minute and consumption of a wide variety of foods will reduce their impact as well as increase dietary intake of other food substances that protect the body against cancer.

More than 3,000 additives are intentionally added to foods; another 12,000 chemicals migrate unintentionally into the food supply. Intentional additives provide color, texture, taste, consistency, or retard spoilage in processed foods. Unintentional additives, such as vinyl chloride, slip into foods during harvesting, processing, packaging, or storage. Some of these additives might encourage the growth of cancer. For example, butylated hydroxytoluene, better known as BHT, is a preservative used to prolong shelf life that also might promote the formation of tumors. The FDA attempts to regulate the amount of hazardous substances in food and has established guidelines for the ingredients that can be added to foods. Any additive suspected to cause cancer must be removed from the food supply; however, only a portion of the substances added to foods have been adequately tested for their ability to cause cancer.

The method used to cook foods might increase the risk for developing cancer. Frying, barbecuing, or broiling fatty meats and fish at high temperatures can convert the fats and proteins into cancer-causing substances. Benzo[a]pyrenes are formed from fats when meats are cooked over a grill. The amount formed will depend on the temperature of the cooking and the length of time the meat is exposed to the flame. The risk for cancer is reduced when perforated foil is placed over the grill to interfere with the fats contacting the flame or the food is cooked for a short amount of time with no charring of the meat.

Smoked foods, such as ham, sausage, fish, or oysters absorb tar during processing. This tar, like the tar in cigarette smoke, contains several cancer-causing substances that could be harmful to health if consumed in large amounts. Commercially available liquid smoke is less hazardous.

Dietary Recommendations

The anti-cancer diet primarily consists of whole grain breads and cereals, fresh fruits and vegetables, cooked dried beans and peas, and small amounts of non-fat or low-fat dairy products, chicken, and fish. Foods are steamed, baked, poached, stewed, or lightly broiled, and fat is limited by avoiding gravies, sauces, creams, and other fats. At least two servings of dark green or orange vegetables should be included in the daily diet to obtain adequate amounts of beta carotene and folic acid. One or more servings of citrus fruits will provide vitamin C. Frequent inclusion of vegetables from the cabbage family also is recommended. Adequate daily intake of fiber can be obtained from 6 servings of whole grain breads and cereals, 4 servings of fresh fruit and vegetables, and 1 serving of cooked dried beans and peas.

Calorie intake should be adequate to maintain ideal body weight. Salt-cured, smoked, and nitrite-containing foods should be avoided or consumed in limited amounts. Contaminated, moldy, or spoiled foods should be avoided, in particular old peanuts that might harbor aflatoxin. A multiple vitamin-mineral preparation that contains all the vitamins and minerals, especially vitamin A, vitamin C, folic acid, vitamin E, selenium (as selenomethionine), and zinc, at a level 100% to 300% of the USRDA will supplement the anti-cancer diet. Large doses of vitamins or minerals are discouraged as preliminary evidence suggests that certain nutrients, such as vitamin C, iron, and zinc, consumed in large amounts might promote the development of cancer by inhibiting the immune response and increasing the body's susceptibility to infection and disease (Table 29).

Table 29.
DIETARY GUIDELINES FOR THE PREVENTION OF CANCER*

1. Avoid obesity.
2. Cut down on total fat intake.
3. Eat more high-fiber foods, such as whole grain cereals, fruits, and vegetables.
4. Include foods rich in vitamins A and C in your daily diet.
5. Include cruciferous vegetables in your diet.
6. Eat moderately of salt-cured, smoked, and nitrite-cured foods.
7. Keep alcohol consumption moderate, if you do drink.

*Established by the American Cancer Society, Inc, 90 Park Avenue, New York, NY 10016.

Regular exercise; effective management of stress; avoidance of all tobacco (cigarettes, pipes, cigars, and chewing tobacco); avoidance of second-hand tobacco smoke; moderate consumption of alcohol; and avoidance of radiation, air and water pollution, and carcinogens at home or on the job are important factors in an anti-cancer lifestyle.

Although the diet and environment contain cancer-causing substances, they also contain cancer-preventing factors. It is impossible to avoid all cancer-causing substances, but it is possible to reduce the body's exposure to them and to increase factors that will aid in the prevention of cancer initiation and promotion.

CARDIOVASCULAR DISEASE (CVD)

Overview

Cardiovascular disease is a general term for any disease of the heart (cardio) and blood vessels (vascular). Diseases in this category include:

Atherosclerosis. Fat-clogged arteries.

Coronary artery disease. Atherosclerosis of the arteries that supply blood, oxygen, and nutrients to the heart.

Heart attack or myocardial infarction. Damage to the heart caused by reduced or blocked blood supply.

Stroke. Damage to brain tissue that results from reduced or blocked blood supply.

Hypertension. High blood pressure.

Congestive heart failure. Poor blood circulation and pooling of blood and fluid in the ankles and feet caused by a weakened heart.

Despite the association between CVD and advancing age, the occurrence of heart disease in the United States is not a natural consequence of aging. Atherosclerosis and other forms of CVD are rare to nonexistent in some countries, even in the elderly. The incidence of CVD increases, however, when these people migrate to the United States and assume the Westernized diet high in fat, salt, sugar, and cholesterol and low in fiber. In many cases, the suffering and death from CVD could be avoided if a person made a few changes in diet, exercise, and other lifestyle habits. The sooner these changes are made, the better; however, it is never too late to begin.

Atherosclerosis is the underlying cause of most heart disease.

Several factors are related to the initiation and progression of the atherosclerotic process. These include:

- Elevated blood cholesterol
- Elevated low density lipoprotein-cholesterol (LDL-cholesterol), one of the carriers of cholesterol in the blood
- Reduced high density lipoprotein-cholesterol (HDL-cholesterol), another of the carriers of cholesterol in the blood
- Cigarette smoking
- Hypertension
- A sedentary lifestyle
- Obesity
- Excessive and prolonged stress
- A family history of CVD
- Male gender after 35 years old or female gender after menopause.

The most important indicator of cardiovascular disease is blood cholesterol levels. The risk for developing atherosclerosis increases with increasing levels of blood cholesterol and anything that lowers blood fat levels lowers the risk for developing CVD. The average blood cholesterol level for adults in the United States is approximately 240 mg% and Americans have a 50–50 chance of developing heart disease. The heart disease risk is much lower or nonexistent in countries where the average blood cholesterol level is 150 mg%.

LIPOPROTEINS. How cholesterol is packaged in the blood has an important effect on the risk for developing CVD. Fat-soluble cholesterol cannot float freely in the watery medium of the blood and must be packaged in carriers called lipoproteins. Lipoproteins are ideal for transporting fats because they have a water-soluble exterior that dissolves easily in the blood and a fat-soluble interior that can hold cholesterol and other fats. Different lipoproteins transport fats to different places within the body and some are associated with an increased risk for developing CVD, while others lower a person's risk.

A person's risk for developing CVD is high when a large portion of cholesterol and triglycerides are packaged in low-density or very low density lipoproteins (LDL-cholesterol and VLDL-cholesterol). A person's risk for developing CVD is low when a large portion of cholesterol is packaged in high density lipoproteins (HDL-cholesterol). A blood cholesterol below 200 mg%, a ratio of total cholesterol to HDL-cholesterol that is 3.5:1 or lower, and an LDL-cholesterol level below 130 mg% are indicators that a person's risk for CVD is low; blood cholesterol above 200 mg%, LDL-cholesterol above 130 mg%, or a ratio above 4.5:1 indicates a high risk for developing CVD. Recently, a new lipoprotein, called Lipoprotein (a) or Lp (a) also has been implicated in CVD risk.

Nutrition and Cardiovascular Disease

The incidence of cardiovascular disease has escalated in the United States population as the consumption of fat, cholesterol, salt, and sugar have increased and the intake of fresh fruits and vegetables and whole grain breads and cereals have decreased.

FATS AND CHOLESTEROL. The increased dietary intake of cholesterol, from such foods as meat, dairy products, fats, and eggs, raises blood cholesterol levels; in general, the more fat and cholesterol in the diet, the higher the blood cholesterol levels and the greater the risk for developing CVD. The saturated fats found primarily in beef, pork, and other red meats; fatty dairy products; hydrogenated vegetables, such as shortening and margarine; coconut and palm oils used in snack foods; and eggs, and dietary cholesterol found only in foods of animal origin are the greatest contributors to the development of atherosclerosis and CVD. Unsaturated fats found in olive oil and avocados and polyunsaturated fats found in vegetable oils and salad dressings do not increase blood cholesterol levels and probably do not increase a person's risk for developing CVD.

Special fats called omega 3 fatty acids or eicosapentaenoic acid (EPA) and docosahexaenoic acid (DHA) found in fish oils reduce blood cholesterol and LDL-cholesterol, raise HDL-cholesterol, interfere with the abnormal clumping of blood cell fragments associated with CVD, and reduce a person's risk for developing atherosclerosis.

FIBER. Some forms of fiber, such as pectin in fruits and the fibers in alfalfa, cooked dried beans, oat bran, and guar gum reduce blood cholesterol and LDL-cholesterol. Other fibers, such as wheat bran, have little or no effect on blood cholesterol levels.

VITAMIN D. Large doses of vitamin D are linked to increased risk for developing premature atherosclerosis and heart disease.

VITAMIN E. The evidence linking the antioxidant vitamin E with CVD is not conclusive. Vitamin E might aid in the prevention of heart disease by interfering with the abnormal clumping of blood cell fragments called platelets associated with the development of atherosclerosis. Vitamin E sometimes is effective in reducing the symptoms of intermittent claudication, the pain and tension in the legs that results from poor blood flow in patients with heart disease. Vitamin E also might protect blood vessel walls and lipoproteins from free radical damage that would initiate the development of atherosclerosis and heart disease.

VITAMIN B$_1$. Abnormal heart function and enlargement of the heart result from severe vitamin B$_1$ deficiency; however, no other evidence exists linking this vitamin to heart disease.

NIACIN. Large daily doses of niacin might decrease blood cholesterol and LDL-cholesterol levels, increase HDL-cholesterol levels, and reduce the risk for developing CVD. Cholesterol-lowering medications are more effective when combined with niacin.

VITAMIN B$_6$. Low levels of vitamin B$_6$ are found in patients who are recovering from a heart attack, but it is unclear whether the low levels are a cause or a result of the disease. Inadequate intake of vitamin B$_6$ might encourage the formation of atherosclerosis and increase the risk for developing CVD.

FOLIC ACID. Folic acid might reduce the production of some substances that encourage the formation of atherosclerosis. However, information is limited on the effects of folic acid on the prevention or treatment of heart disease.

BIOTIN AND PANTOTHENIC ACID. Blood cholesterol levels increase and cardiovascular problems develop when the body is deficient in either biotin or pantothenic acid. However, deficiencies of these B vitamins are rare to nonexistent in the United States population.

VITAMIN C. Cholesterol production in the liver and conversion of cholesterol to bile acids for excretion require vitamin C. Supplementation with vitamin C might lower blood cholesterol and LDL-cholesterol and increase HDL-cholesterol and might remove cholesterol from deposits in artery walls. This latter function, however, is controversial and more information is required before recommendations can be made for vitamin C in the prevention or treatment of CVD.

CALCIUM. Adequate intake of calcium from dietary sources or from supplements might aid in lowering blood cholesterol levels and reduce a person's risk for developing CVD. The risk for heart disease might increase, however, when large amounts of calcium are consumed in the presence of a magnesium deficiency.

CHROMIUM. Consumption of a diet low in chromium is associated with elevated blood cholesterol and increased risk of developing cardiovascular disease. Patients with advanced heart disease have low levels of chromium in their tissues and reduced levels of chromium in the blood might be a good indicator of advancing heart disease. In contrast, blood cholesterol levels drop, HDL-cholesterol levels rise, and risk for developing CVD decreases when chromium is added to the diet.

COPPER. Copper is important in the development and maintenance of healthy arteries and other blood vessels. A deficiency of this trace mineral produces the same type of damage to the blood vessels and heart as does a heart attack. One study showed that dietary intake resembling the copper intake in the American diet produced copper depletion in the heart tissue and heart disease. Low blood levels of copper are associated with high blood cholesterol levels and increased risk for developing CVD. The ratio of zinc to copper also might be important in the regulation of blood cholesterol.

IRON. Iron deficiency is related to irregular heart beat and abnormal heart function, which disappear when the diet is supplemented with iron.

MAGNESIUM. Magnesium relaxes blood vessel walls and the heart muscle, while a deficiency results in irregular heart beat, blood vessel wall spasms, high blood pressure, as well as damage and decay of the heart. A magnesium deficiency increases the risk for atherosclerosis, angina or chest pain associated with heart attack, and irregular heart beat called cardiac arrhythmias. Blood levels of magnesium are low in heart attack patients and these low levels are reported prior to, during, and following a heart attack. Supplementing the patient with magnesium returns the heart beat to normal and reduces the chances of experiencing a heart attack. In addition, the doses of antiarrhythmic medications given to patients suffering from a heart attack can be reduced with magnesium is given. Magnesium also might reduce the pain and cramping of intermittent claudication that is related to reduced blood flow in heart disease.

SELENIUM. The risk for heart disease, atherosclerosis, and death from heart disease increases when blood levels of selenium are low. People who consume diets low in selenium develop heart damage called cardiomyopathy, which might explain the increased risk for heart attack observed in these people. One study found a 6- to 7-fold increased incidence of premature heart attacks in patients with low blood levels of selenium. Selenium also might protect against free radical damage to blood vessel walls that initiates the development of atherosclerosis and heart disease.

ZINC. Zinc supplementation might reduce the risk for developing heart disease by changing lipoprotein concentrations, ie, decreasing LDL-cholesterol and increasing HDL-cholesterol. However, large doses of zinc, exceeding 50 mg a day, lowers the HDL-cholesterol level and thus increases the risk for developing heart disease.

Dietary Recommendations

Dietary guidelines established by the American Heart Association, the National Cholesterol Education Committee, and the U.S. Senate Select Committee in their report "The U.S. Dietary Goals" for the prevention of cardiovascular disease include maintaining ideal body weight, reducing fat intake to 30% of total calories or less, reducing cholesterol intake to 300 mg/day or less, increasing fiber and complex carbohydrates, and reducing intake of salt and sugar.

In practical terms, these guidelines mean that Americans should increase their consumption of whole grain breads and cereals, cooked dried beans and peas, and fresh fruits and vegetables. These foods contain little or no fat, cholesterol, salt, or sugar; are limited in calories; and contain ample amounts of fiber. In addition, evidence shows that a vegetarian diet might lower a person's risk for heart disease.

Americans should reduce their consumption of refined and processed sugars and foods high in sugar, such as processed snack foods, desserts, ice cream, soda pop, and fruit canned in heavy syrup. Diets high in sugar contribute to either obesity or malnutrition and might increase a person's risk for developing CVD.

Additionally, individuals should reduce their consumption of foods high in fats, such as fatty cuts of beef, pork, sausage and luncheon meats, dairy products, butter, margarine, oils, salad dressing, mayonnaise, pie crusts, gravies, sauces, and foods cooked in fats and oils. Lean meat intake should be limited to no more than 6 ounces a day. Meat consumption is linked to an increased risk for developing cardiovascular disease, despite its fat content. Even if the cut is lean it still contains similar amounts of cholesterol to that found in fatty cuts.

Low-fat and non-fat dairy products should be chosen. The only exception to this guideline is whole milk for infants and children less than 2 years old. Consumption of foods high in cholesterol, such as egg yolks, organ meats, fatty or lean beef and pork, should be reduced. Consumption of salt and salted foods, such as processed or convenience foods, snack foods, fast foods, canned soups, or soy sauce, and alcohol also should be reduced.

The low-fat, low-cholesterol, low-sugar, low-salt, high-fiber diet will aid in the maintenance of ideal body weight and is similar to the diet recommended for the prevention of cancer, hypertension, diabetes, and many other degenerative disorders. In addition, frequent inclusion of fish, such as salmon and herring, might further protect the heart against disease. A multiple vitamin-mineral supplement that contains vitamin E, vitamin C, the B vitamins, chromium, copper, iron, magnesium, selenium, zinc, and other nutrients; regular aerobic exercise; avoidance of tobacco; moderate intake of alcohol;

effective coping with stress; and prevention of diabetes and hypertension will help in the prevention and treatment of heart and blood vessel diseases.

CARPAL TUNNEL SYNDROME (CTS)

Overview

Carpal tunnel syndrome is a disorder of the hands and wrists. The area (tunnel) that encloses the bones of the wrist (carpus) becomes inflamed and constricts the nerves that are embedded within the area. Carpal tunnel syndrome often occurs in people who have repetitive motion jobs, such as computer operators and assembly line workers.

Nutrition and Carpal Tunnel Syndrome

A vitamin B_6 deficiency might encourage the development or increase the symptoms of CTS. Patients with CTS are more likely than healthy people to have vitamin B_6 deficiencies and often the symptoms of CTS are relieved by vitamin B_6 supplementation. In many cases, patients no longer require surgery when vitamin B_6 is added to the diet.

Vitamin B_6 is important in the development and maintenance of healthy nerve tissue and a deficiency can result in inflammation of the nerve tissue similar to that observed in CTS, which might partially explain the vitamin's effectiveness in CTS. People with CTS might either consume inadequate amounts of vitamin B_6 or have unusually high requirements for the vitamin.

Dietary Recommendations

Dietary recommendations for the prevention or treatment of carpal tunnel syndrome are limited. Consuming a diet low in fat, high in fiber, vitamins, and minerals and low in sugars, refined and convenience foods, and fast foods is wise. The diet should contain a variety of fruits, vegetables, whole grain breads and cereals, cooked dried beans and peas, low-fat or non-fat dairy products, and lean meats, chicken, and fish. A multiple vitamin- mineral supplement that contains vitamin B_6 as well as regular exercise, effective stress management, avoidance of alcohol and tobacco, and moderate exposure to sunshine are important for optimal health and might be useful in the prevention and treatment of CTS. Vitamin B_6 intake should not exceed 100 mg a day as large doses of this nutrient can be toxic.

THE COMMON COLD

Overview

The common cold is the most widespread infectious disease. It is caused by a virus that is easily spread from one person to another and is resistant to the body's natural defense system.

Nutrition and the Common Cold

All nutrients related to the strengthening of the immune system are important in the prevention of the common cold or any other infection. (See page 128 for more information on nutrition and the immune system.) In particular, vitamin C and zinc might aid in the prevention and treatment of the common cold.

VITAMIN C. Some studies show that vitamin C does not reduce the frequency or duration, but might reduce the severity of a cold. Other studies show that vitamin C is effective in preventing the common cold or shortening its duration, but has no effect on the severity of symptoms. In many cases, people report fewer colds when they take either a vitamin C tablet or a placebo they think is vitamin C.

There might be some truth to the vitamin C-common cold connection despite the contradictory evidence. Adequate vitamin C intake might stimulate the immune system in older adults or other people with poorly functioning immune systems. The vitamin strengthens the immune system by increasing the production or activity of white blood cells, which are responsible for destroying foreign invaders such as viruses and bacteria. There is a reduction in white blood cell formation and impaired wound healing when vitamin C is deficient in the diet, and the body's resistance to infection and disease improves when vitamin C intake is increased. Vitamin C appears to be more effective for women than men in reducing the symptoms of the common cold.

ZINC. Zinc might alter the duration of the common cold by inhibiting the growth of bacteria and by stimulating the immune system. People who consume diets low in zinc are more susceptible than well-nourished people to infection and show signs of immune system impairment. The addition of zinc to the diet increases the amount and activity of white blood cells. People diagnosed with poorly functioning immune systems have low levels of zinc in their blood; when they increase their intake of zinc their immune system is strengthened and they are more resistant to infection. This evidence shows that reduced amounts of zinc in the blood might contribute to a malfunctioning immune system.

Zinc also has a direct effect on slowing the growth of microorganisms, such as the viruses responsible for the common cold. Certain viruses do not survive in an environment rich in zinc. This effect is the basis for zinc lozenges as a common anticold treatment. The use of zinc lozenges was promoted after one study showed that people with cold symptoms who were treated with zinc gluconate lozenges experienced a reduction in symptoms, such as sore throat and fever, as compared to people who were not treated with the lozenges. The results of this one study have not been supported by further research.

Zinc is an excellent example of how the "some is good, more is better" myth is incorrect. Although adequate intake of zinc appears to stimulate the immune system and protect the body against colds and infections, excess intake of zinc can suppress the immune system and possibly increase a person's risk for infection. In addition, zinc intake in excess of 150 mg to 200 mg in the presence of low to moderate copper intake can reduce the absorption and use of copper and contribute to a secondary copper deficiency.

Dietary Recommendations

A low-fat, high-fiber, nutrient-dense diet should be consumed, adequate in all vitamins and minerals and low in sugars and refined and convenience foods. The diet should contain a variety of fruits, vegetables, whole grain breads and cereals, cooked dried beans and peas, low-fat or non-fat dairy products, and lean meats, chicken, and fish. A multiple vitamin-mineral supplement and a vitamin C supplement as well as regular exercise, effective stress management, avoidance of alcohol and tobacco, and outdoor activity are important for optimal health and the prevention of the common cold.

In addition, several glasses of fluids, such as fruit juice, water, herb teas, or bottled mineral water, several servings of fresh fruits and vegetables, moderate exercise such as a 15 minute walk, and extra sleep and relaxation each day are important for the treatment of and speedy recovery from the common cold.

CYSTIC FIBROSIS

Overview

Cystic fibrosis is the most common genetic disease that causes death in the United States and is the most common cause of lung disease in children. The primary symptoms of cystic fibrosis are chronic lung disease, abnormal functioning of the pancreas that results in poor digestion of food and gastrointestinal discomfort, and very high concentrations of salt in the sweat. The pancreas produces many important enzymes necessary for normal digestion and absorption of foods. In cystic fibrosis, the pancreas does not function properly and these digestion enzymes are in short supply or lacking. People with mild forms of cystic fibrosis might not experience this poor absorption and subsequent malnutrition. The pancreas also produces the hormone insulin that regulates blood sugar, and it is common for people with cystic fibrosis to have high blood sugar levels and the symptoms of diabetes.

Nutrition and Cystic Fibrosis

The maintenance of optimal nutritional status is very important for people with cystic fibrosis. Adequate intake of all vitamins, minerals, protein, calories, and fiber improves height and weight, allows the formation of normal fat deposits that protect internal organs from damage, and encourages the normal development of puberty and growth. Optimal nutrition also improves the resistance to lung infections common in this disease. It is very important that the planning and monitoring of a nutritious diet for the person with cystic fibrosis be supervised by a physician and dietitian (Table 30).

Table 30.
GENERAL DIETARY GUIDELINES FOR THE CYSTIC FIBROSIS PATIENT

Nutrient	Dietary Guidelines
Calories	Adequate intake of calories to maintain ideal body weight and promote growth.
Protein	Two to four times the RDA for age; 12% to 15% of total calorie intake.
Carbohydrate	Most easily digested of three calorie-containing nutrients (protein, fat, and carbohydrate).
Fat	Fat often poorly absorbed. Intake varies according to tolerance.
Fat-soluble vitamins	Two to three times the RDA for age. Provided in water-soluble form.
Water-soluble vitamins	Intake equal to the RDA. Antibiotic therapy requires increased intake of vitamin B_2 (riboflavin).
Minerals	Intake equal to the RDA.
Pancreatic enzymes	Given at meals. Dosage and timing considered to prevent diarrhea and avoid constipation.

People with cystic fibrosis either have a good appetite, absorb and use nutrients well, and show normal growth and development; have a good appetite, do not absorb or use nutrients well, and show signs of malnutrition and stunted growth; or have a poor appetite, eat poorly, and do not gain weight or develop normally.

PROTEIN, CARBOHYDRATE, AND FAT. Patients with cystic fibrosis might not digest protein well and artificial diets or modified protein diets are often used. Most carbohydrates, such as breads, cereals, noodles, and rice, are well tolerated, but milk sugar (lactose) might need to be eliminated from the diet. Fat is poorly absorbed in cystic fibrosis patients with abnormal pancreatic function. Much of the dietary fat is excreted, resulting in diarrhea. A low-fat diet, or the use of special fats that do not require the presence of enzymes for digestion and absorption can be used. Essential fatty acids, such as linoleic acid, are likely to be deficient as a result of poor dietary intake or absorption.

VITAMINS AND MINERALS. The lack of fat-digesting enzymes increases the likelihood that the fat-soluble vitamins will not be absorbed and blood levels of vitamins A, D, E, and K are often low in the blood and tissues of people with cystic fibrosis. Deficiencies of the fat-soluble vitamins are found even when people receive supplements. It is possible that some of the manifestations of cystic fibrosis are a result of vitamin A deficiency. Not only vitamin A, but its protein carrier in the blood and zinc, necessary in the transportation of vitamin A, are low in the body.

Limited information is available on the water-soluble vitamins and cystic fibrosis. Vitamin B_{12} deficiency has been identified in patients, as has a vitamin B_2 deficiency.

Information on mineral status in cystic fibrosis also is limited. Blood levels of copper are elevated in advanced stages of the disease and some evidence exists that blood levels of zinc and iron are low. Some people with cystic fibrosis have low blood levels of selenium and vitamin E that implies a link between the body's antioxidant system and the development or progression of the disease. Children with cystic fibrosis show improved growth and reduced numbers of lung infections when the diet is adequately supplemented with vitamins, minerals, and other nutrients.

Dietary Recommendations

Every nutrient is a concern for patients with cystic fibrosis, but the degree of dietary control will vary with each person. Calories might have to be increased to 50% to 100% more than the normal requirement for age, and protein intake may need to be doubled. Fat intake should be low (30% of calories) or divided in small doses throughout the day; administration of pancreatic enzymes with meals is usually necessary. New foods should be introduced into the diet one at a time to assess the person's tolerance.

The low intake or poor absorption of food justifies a multiple vitamin-mineral that supplies all the vitamins and minerals in amounts equal to or slightly greater than 100% of the USRDA. A supplement that supplies vitamins A, D, E, and K in a water-soluble form is usually recommended. Vitamin B_{12} and vitamin B_2 might be required in amounts exceeding the normal requirements.

DERMATITIS

Overview

Dermatitis is a general term for inflammation of the skin. Usually dermatitis results from chafing of the skin, allergies, long-term medications, or nervous irritability. Symptoms of dermatitis include rash, itching, burning, dryness, blemishes, or other skin disorders, and treatment or cure will depend on the cause of the skin irritation.

Nutrition and Dermatitis

Poor dietary habits combined with deficiencies of several vitamins are related to skin disorders and dermatitis. The skin is a primary site for nutrient deficiency symptoms as skin cells are produced, die, and are replaced by new cells every few days. The short lifespan of skin cells allows deficiencies of nutrients to develop quickly.

VITAMIN A. Changes in skin texture result from vitamin A deficiency. The skin becomes bumpy, scaly, and rough resembling "goose flesh" or "alligator skin." The skin on the forearms and thighs is the first to be affected, but in advanced stages the entire body is involved.

VITAMIN B_2. A deficiency of vitamin B_2 results in soreness and burning of the mouth and lips and dermatitis characterized by simultaneous dryness and greasy scales.

NIACIN. Early symptoms of niacin deficiency include skin eruptions and dermatitis. The dermatitis of pellagra is a scaly, dark pigmentation that develops on areas of the skin exposed to sunlight, heat, or mild irritation.

VITAMIN B_6. Dermatitis is one symptom of vitamin B_6 deficiency. The deficiency can develop from either poor dietary intake or long-term use of medications that interfere with vitamin B_6 absorption or use, such as antituberculosis medications or oral contraceptives.

VITAMIN B_{12}. A deficiency of vitamin B_{12} causes reduced cell and tissue repair and results in dermatitis, changes in the lips and tongue, nerve damage, anemia, and intestinal upsets.

BIOTIN. A deficiency of biotin results in dermatitis, progressive hair loss and hair color, and other hair and skin disorders.

PANTOTHENIC ACID. Although a deficiency of pantothenic acid is rare, it has been induced in the laboratory and symptoms include dermatitis, burning sensations, and numbness and tingling in the hands and feet.

VITAMIN C. The primary symptoms of vitamin C deficiency result from the vitamin's function in the formation and maintenance of collagen. Small pinpoint hemorrhages under the skin, poor wound healing, the breakdown of old scars, dry and scaly skin, and swollen and bleeding gums are symptoms of inadequate vitamin C intake.

ESSENTIAL FATTY ACIDS. A deficiency of linoleic acid, a fatty acid found in nuts, wheat germ, and vegetable oils, produces a type of dermatitis characterized by red, dry, scaly skin that resembles eczema or dermatitis. The blotchy areas appear first on the face, clustered near the oil-secreting glands, and then in the folds of the nose and lips, the forehead, the eyes, and the cheeks. Dry, rough areas also appear on the forearms, thighs, and buttocks. Fish oils also show promise as an effective therapy in the treatment of psoriasis and other skin disorders.

Dietary Recommendations

A low-fat, high-fiber, nutrient-dense diet should be consumed, adequate in all vitamins and minerals and low in sugars and refined and convenience foods. The diet should contain a variety of fruits, vegetables, whole grain breads and cereals, cooked dried beans and peas, low-fat or non-fat dairy products, and lean meat, chicken, and fish. A tablespoon of safflower oil in salad dressing to supply linoleic acid and frequent servings of fish should be included in the diet. During times when the diet is inadequate, a multiple vitamin-mineral supplement should supply at least 100% of the USRDA for all vitamins including vitamin A, vitamin B_2, niacin, vitamin B_6, vitamin B_{12}, biotin, pantothenic acid, and vitamin C. In addition, regular exercise; effective stress management; avoidance of alcohol and tobacco; avoidance of cold, wind, harsh soaps, and detergents; frequent use of moisturizers, superfatted bath bars, and a humidifier; and showering after swimming in chlorinated waters are important for the prevention and treatment of dermatitis and dry skin.

DIABETES MELLITUS

Overview

Diabetes is characterized by a reduced ability to use and metabolize dietary carbohydrates, elevated blood sugar levels (hyperglycemia), and an abnormal amount of sugar in the urine. The two general types of diabetes are Type I, also called insulin dependent (IDDM) or juvenile-onset diabetes and Type II, also called noninsulin dependent (NIDDM) or adult-onset diabetes. IDDM usually begins in childhood. It begins suddenly, severe symptoms develop soon after onset, and control of the disorder requires insulin. NIDDM begins in the adult years, the progression of the disease is slow, and symptoms are mild in the beginning. Although genetics contribute to a person's risk for developing NIDDM, lifestyle factors such as being overweight, consuming a poor diet, and lack of exercise are important contributors to the development of this type of diabetes (Table 31).

Table 31.
DIFFERENCES BETWEEN TYPE I AND TYPE II DIABETES

Characteristics	Type I	Type II
Age at onset	Under age 40	Over age 40
% of all diabetics	< 10%	>90%
Inherited	Sometimes	Common
Appearance of symptoms	Sudden/severe	Slow
Obesity	Uncommon	Common
Beta cells of pancreas	Reduced	Normal or reduced
Insulin secretion	Reduced	Normal or reduced
Insulin receptors on cells	Normal	Reduced or normal
Remission	Rare	Common with weight reduction, diet, exercise

Individuals with IDDM usually have reduced numbers of active beta cells in the pancreas, the cells responsible for the production and secretion of insulin. The person with IDDM must inject insulin and balance the entry of insulin into the blood with food intake to maintain normal use of sugar. In contrast, individuals with NIDDM can have reduced beta cells in the pancreas or, more often, show adequate production and secretion of insulin, but the cells of the body are insensitive to the hormone. The insensitivity is often related to obesity. Consequently, excess sugar does not flow into the cells and blood sugar levels remain high. Oral hypoglycemic medications or injected insulin are sometimes used to overcome the insensitivity, although insulin insensitivity often is reversible with weight loss.

Nutrition and Diabetes

The goals of a diet program for the treatment of diabetes include improvement of overall health by achieving and maintaining optimal nutritional status and ideal body weight, stabilization of blood sugar levels within the normal range, and prevention or delay of the development of cardiovascular disease, kidney disease, and eye or nerve disorders. The most important aspect of the diet is the control of carbohydrate, protein, fat, and calories; however, vitamin and mineral intakes contribute to the prevention and treatment of the disease.

VITAMIN C. Adequate intake of vitamin C might help regulate blood sugar levels and aid in the prevention of diabetes. Vitamin C metabolism might be altered and tissue levels of the vitamin are reduced in diabetes, which would help explain the suppression of the immune response characteristic of diabetes. Caution must be used when diabetics supplement with vitamin C, however, as supplemental vitamin C at doses that approach common intakes or above might interfere with the urinary test for glucose.

VITAMIN E. Poor dietary intake of vitamin E might alter blood sugar levels, whereas increased intake of the fat-soluble vitamin might help reduce elevated blood sugar levels. In addition, blood levels of vitamin E are low in diabetics and people at risk for developing diabetes, which suggests that the use of vitamin E is altered as a result of the disease. Limited evidence shows that the progression of atherosclerosis, a common complication of diabetes, might be slowed when vitamin E is increased in the diet.

CHROMIUM. Chromium is a component of Glucose Tolerance Factor that aids insulin in increasing the absorption of sugar into the cells. As chromium is important to the proper functioning of insulin, which in turn controls blood sugar, a deficiency of the trace mineral can result in insulin insensitivity and elevated blood sugar.

A chromium deficiency resembles diabetes. The first sign of a marginal deficiency is an elevated insulin level in the blood. The person experiences numbness in the toes and fingers, an increase in blood sugar, glucose intolerance, and reduced muscle strength and coordination. In some people, all of these symptoms disappear with chromium supplementation.

The effects of increased chromium intake depend on individual nutritional status; more chromium does not improve glucose tolerance in a person who is already adequately nourished in the mineral. However, increased long-term chromium intake does improve glucose intolerance in a person who is chromium deficient.

A diet high in fat and refined carbohydrates, such as enriched white breads, ready-to-eat cereals, and sugar could contribute to elevated blood sugar levels because of the marginal chromium content of these foods. Blood levels of sugar and fat decrease when people avoid these highly processed foods and increase their consumption of chromium-rich foods.

Dietary Recommendations

The primary goal in the dietary management of diabetes, both IDDM and NIDDM, is control of blood sugar levels within a narrow range at least 80% of the time. A person with diabetes should work closely with a physician and dietitian to establish a diet and exercise program that balances blood sugar and food intake with exercise, body weight, and medication use.

MAINTAIN IDEAL BODY WEIGHT. More than three out of four diabetics are overweight and, in many cases, blood sugar stabilizes or returns to normal with a reduction in body weight.

COMPLEX CARBOHYDRATES. A diet higher in complex carbohydrates, such as whole grain breads and cereals, vegetables, cooked dried beans and peas, potatoes, and other unrefined starches, than in protein and fat is beneficial in the control of diabetes. Complex carbohydrates enhance the cells' sensitivity to insulin and produce a gradual rise in blood sugar as opposed to refined carbohydrates and sugars that produce a rapid rise in blood sugar levels. The American Diabetes Association recommends the following percentages based on total calories:

50% to 60% carbohydrates
15% to 20% protein
25% to 30% fat

Fiber also slows the rise in blood sugar after a meal, aids in the maintenance of normal blood sugar levels, and reduces the amount of sugar excreted in the urine. Oat bran and the fiber in cooked dried beans and peas is especially effective in the control of blood sugar levels, but consumption of all fibers, including the fiber in whole grain breads and cereals, vegetables, and fruits, is encouraged.

VITAMINS AND MINERALS. Consumption of a nutritious diet that derives most of its calories from whole grain breads and cereals, fresh fruits and vegetables, and cooked dried beans and peas with small amounts of lean meats, chicken, fish, and non-fat or low-fat dairy products will provide adequate amounts of most vitamins and minerals. If the calorie intake is below 2,000 calories or the diet is not optimal, a multiple vitamin-mineral supplement that contains all the vitamins and most of the minerals, especially chromium and magnesium, in amounts approaching 100% of the USRDA should provide adequate intake of these nutrients.

REGULAR EXERCISE. Exercise improves how the body uses insulin and aids in the regulation of blood sugar levels. Aerobic exercise, such as brisk walking, swimming, jogging, or stationary or outdoor bicycling, performed 3 to 4 times a week, for 20 minutes or more will have an overall lowering effect on blood sugar. A diabetic's exercise program should be developed with the help of a physician and trained exercise physiologist.

ECZEMA

Overview

Eczema, also called atopic eczema, eczematous dermatitis, or atopic dermatitis, is a general term for any chronic skin inflammation or irritation. Eczema develops from allergic reactions to pollens, cosmetics, dust, or other environmental factors or is a result of dry air, chemical irritants, or excessive exposure to sunlight. The symptoms of this skin disorder are often increased by anxiety, lack of sleep, or other stresses.

Nutrition and Eczema

Numerous nutrient deficiencies will produce eczema-like symptoms, and increased dietary intake of these nutrients will help if the skin disorder is a result of a vitamin or mineral deficiency.

VITAMIN A. A long-term deficiency of vitamin A will produce some of the symptoms of eczema including dry, scaly, and rough skin. The most common locations for vitamin A-induced skin disorders are the shoulders, neck, back, forearms, thighs, and abdomen.

THE B VITAMINS. A deficiency of vitamin B_2 results in dermatitis or eczema-like symptoms, including dryness, scaling, or itching of the skin. Symptoms of niacin deficiency include skin eruptions, such as darkened skin that is scaly and dry. Eczema-like symptoms also develop during a deficiency of vitamin B_6, vitamin B_{12}, folic acid, biotin, and pantothenic acid.

OTHER NUTRIENTS. Deficiencies of either vitamin C or the essential fatty acid linoleic acid produce skin disorders, including eczema.

Dietary Recommendations

A low-fat, high-fiber, nutrient-dense diet should be consumed, adequate in all vitamins and minerals and low in sugars and refined and convenience foods. The diet should contain a variety of fruits, vegetables, whole grain breads and cereals, cooked dried beans and peas, low-fat or non-fat dairy products, and lean meats, chicken, and fish. A multiple vitamin-mineral supplement that contains adequate amounts of the B vitamins, vitamin C, and vitamin A should be considered if the diet is not optimal. Regular exercise, effective stress management, avoidance of alcohol and tobacco, and moderate exposure to sunshine also are important for the prevention and treatment of eczema.

When food allergies are the cause of eczema, appropriate steps should be taken to eliminate the offending foods. Foods most often associated with allergies include wheat, corn, milk, eggs, chocolate, oranges, nuts, strawberries, and shellfish. For example, one study showed when people who suffered from eczema and who had been treated with emollients, topical steroids, and oral antihistamines were placed on a nutritious diet that excluded milk and egg products and used soy-based milk as a substitute, their symptoms improved, including a reduction in itching and redness. The management of food allergies should be planned with the help of a physician or dietitian. (See pages 133–138 for additional information on food allergies.)

EMOTIONAL DISORDERS

Overview

Until recently, the brain was thought to be impermeable to the effects of nutrition. Although other organs such as the liver and the heart show profound changes as a result of poor dietary intake of vitamins and minerals, the brain was thought to be protected from fluctuations in nutrient intakes by a series of partitions, called the *blood-brain barrier*, which separated the brain from the rest of the body. This concept is now recognized as incomplete and inaccurate. Food and nutrient intake have a powerful effect on a person's mood, behavior, and ability to learn.

Nutrition and Emotional Disorders

Vitamin and mineral deficiencies can change the structure and function of the brain and nervous system and affect behavior, memory, mood, and learning. Even the nutrient content of a single meal or marginal deficiencies of a single vitamin or mineral can alter mood and behavior, and disorders once considered irreversible show improvement when vitamin and mineral intake is increased.

Nutrition affects the fundamental units of the brain called the *neurons* or nerve cells and the chemicals, called *neurotransmitters*, secreted by these cells. Neurotransmitters transmit messages from one nerve cell to another or from one nerve cell to its target organ, such as a muscle or a gland that releases hormones. These processes regulate all thoughts, behaviors, physical actions, and the ability to learn. A nutrient deficiency causes changes in the structure or function of nerve cells or decreases the production of neurotransmitters. The result is reduced ability to remember or learn, depression, anxiety, and other mood disorders.

Several vitamins and minerals also affect how a person feels mentally and physically by affecting the production and maintenance of red blood cells. A nutrient deficiency, such as iron or folic acid, that reduces the number of red blood cells or the capacity of these cells to carry oxygen would reduce the supply of oxygen to the brain and other tissues and could cause lethargy, mood disorders, learning disabilities, and depression. It should be noted, however, that treatment of these disorders with food or vitamin supplements should only be done with the supervision of a physician.

VITAMIN E. Symptoms of a vitamin E deficiency include nervous system disorders and anemia, characterized by lethargy and depression.

People with rare fat malabsorption syndromes, such as cystic fibrosis and celiac disease, are susceptible to nerve damage, poor coordination, and anemia, probably resulting from inadequate absorption of vitamin E. Increased intake of the fat-soluble vitamin improves or removes these symptoms.

VITAMIN B$_1$. Vitamin B$_1$ deficiency causes nerve and brain disorders, such as fatigue, loss of appetite, mental confusion, tingling of the hands and feet, numbness, memory loss, emotional instability, reduced attention span, irritability, confusion, and depression. Increased intake of the vitamin reverses these symptoms.

VITAMIN B$_2$. A severe deficiency of vitamin B$_2$ causes depression or hysteria and lethargy associated with anemia. A vitamin B$_2$ deficiency is often accompanied by deficiencies of other B vitamins also related to nerve and brain function, such as niacin, vitamin B$_1$, and vitamin B$_6$.

NIACIN. One of the classic symptoms of niacin deficiency is dementia or depression. Other nerve and brain disorders associated with inadequate niacin intake include disorientation, irritability, insomnia, loss of memory, delirium, and emotional instability. As with vitamin B$_2$ deficiency, these symptoms usually are accompanied by other nutrient deficiencies, such as protein, iron, vitamin B$_1$, or vitamin B$_6$.

Niacin supplements have been used in conjunction with antiepileptic medications, such as phenobarbital and primidone, with some success. Large doses of niacin have been used in the treatment of schizophrenia; however, the results are conflicting and recommendations for niacin's therapeutic effectiveness cannot be made at this time. Some psychiatric disorders have been attributed to abnormal absorption or use of niacin or its dietary building block tryptophan. A few reports show improvement in patients with depression, hyperactivity, and sleep disturbances when tryptophan or niacin are increased in the diet.

VITAMIN B$_6$. Vitamin B$_6$ is an important contributor to the formation of several neurotransmitters, the chemicals that regulate brain and nerve function and that are secreted by nerve cells. Inadequate intake of vitamin B$_6$ results in reduced production or activity of these chemicals and can cause depression, insomnia, irritability, and nervousness. Low blood levels of neurotransmitters are found in suicidal or depressed patients and supplementation with vitamin B$_6$ often helps stabilize mood.

One study reported vitamin B$_6$ and magnesium supplementation was successful in the treatment of autism, characterized by language retardation and social detachment, in an otherwise healthy 4-year-old boy. Autism is apparently a disorder that occurs when there is impairment in the formation of certain neurotransmitters. Vitamin B_6 might help normalize this impairment. However, more evidence is necessary before the effectiveness and role of vitamin B_6 and magnesium in the treatment of autism is clearly understood.

High doses of vitamin B_6 also cause changes in nerve function including numbness and tingling in the hands and feet, poor coordination, and a stumbling gait. Some of this nerve damage might be permanent if the dosage has been very high for long periods of time.

VITAMIN B_{12}. Vitamin B_{12} is essential for the formation and maintenance of the insulation around nerve cells, called the *myelin sheath*, that speeds the conduction of nerve impulses. A long-term deficiency of vitamin B_{12} results in nerve damage, tingling and numbness, moodiness, confusion, agitation, dimmed vision, delusions, dizziness, and disorientation. Mental illness in the elderly might be linked to a deficiency of vitamin B_{12} in those people with vitamin B_{12}-deficient anemia.

Vitamin B_{12} also is important in the formation of all body cells, and a deficiency results in poor formation of red blood cells and the characteristic lethargy, depression, and fatigue associated with anemia. Anemia can be treated, but the nerve damage that results from long-term vitamin B_{12} deficiency is permanent.

FOLIC ACID. Folic acid is important in the formation of all types of cells and is essential for the growth and development of the nervous system. Irritability, weakness, apathy, hostility, paranoid behavior, and anemia are some of the symptoms of folic acid deficiency and are responsive to an increased intake of the vitamin. Limited evidence shows folic acid supplementation in conjunction with a special diet might be useful in the treatment of violent outbursts, seizures, bouts of amnesia, and sleep disorders in children unresponsive to anticonvulsant medication therapy.

BIOTIN AND PANTOTHENIC ACID. Although a deficiency of either biotin or pantothenic acid is very rare, when it does occur symptoms include numbness in the hands and feet, nausea, lethargy, lack of coordination, staggering gait, restlessness, irritability, and depression. These symptoms disappear when these B vitamins are added back to the diet.

CALCIUM AND MAGNESIUM. Calcium and magnesium are important in the regulation of nerve impulses. The nerves become overly sensitive in the rare occurrence when blood calcium levels drop below normal. Both of these minerals also aid in the formation of certain neurotransmitters. It is unclear how or if a calcium deficiency would alter mood or behavior, but it is known that depression, confusion, personality changes, lack of coordination, and weakness result from poor intake of magnesium.

IRON. The classic symptom of poor iron intake is anemia, characterized by lethargy, depression, poor concentration, irritability, decreased attention span, apathy, and personality changes. An iron deficiency affects the ability to understand or learn new information. Iron-deficient children do not perform well in school, do poorly on intelligence tests, show impaired attention span, and have a more limited capacity to remember information than do well-nourished children. Iron deficiency, even in the absence of anemia, also can affect job performance, mood, and memory in the adult.

Other vitamins and minerals related to nerve and brain function include vitamin C, chromium, copper, and zinc. A deficiency of any of these nutrients might produce nervous system disorders, such as depression, poor coordination, numbness, and learning disabilities.

AMINO ACIDS—PHENYLALANINE AND TYROSINE. Both phenylalanine and tyrosine are converted in the body to a series of neurotransmitters: dopamine, norepinephrine, and epinephrine (adrenaline). These chemicals transmit messages from one nerve cell to another and aid in the regulation of mood, pain, and behavior. Phenylalanine and tyrosine might be effective in the treatment of depression. Levels of these amino acids are low in the blood of patients who are depressed and, in some cases, supplementation with either phenylalanine or tyrosine is an effective therapy.

AMINO ACIDS—TRYPTOPHAN. The amino acid tryptophan is converted in the body to a neurotransmitter called *serotonin*, which is important in the regulation of mood, pain, sleep, and behavior. The amount of serotonin in the brain depends on how much tryptophan is available in the blood. Adequate dietary intake of tryptophan, especially if consumed with a low-protein, high-carbohydrate snack, encourages the production of serotonin and improves pain tolerance, insomnia, and depression. In addition, limited information exists that tryptophan might be effective in the treatment of certain forms of mental illness. Some people with acute mania or schizophrenia improve when tryptophan supplements are included in the diet.

CHOLINE AND LECITHIN. Choline is a nonessential substance produced by the body and found in the diet or as a component of lecithin. Choline is incorporated into the neurotransmitter acetylcholine, which aids in the regulation of memory and other brain and nerve processes. Levels of this neurotransmitter are low in the brains of people with Alzheimer's disease and Huntington's disease and one theory for the development of these disorders blames these low levels as the cause of the related memory loss.

Blood choline levels increase when the choline content of a meal is increased. The rise in blood choline stimulates an increase in brain levels of choline and more acetylcholine is produced. However, choline or lecithin supplementation does not always improve memory, especially in advanced stages of memory loss or in people with degeneration of nerve cells such as Alzheimer's patients.

Dietary Recommendations

Depression, lethargy, and other emotional disorders can result from a variety of factors, including life problems and nervous system disorders that are unrelated to nutrition. In addition, over-consumption of certain metals, such as mercury or lead, affects nerve and brain tissue causing temporary, and sometimes permanent, damage. However, proper nutrition is safe and potentially helpful in all circumstances.

A low-fat, high-fiber, nutrient-dense diet should be consumed, adequate in all vitamins and minerals and low in sugars and refined and convenience foods. The diet should contain a variety of fruits, vegetables, whole grain breads and cereals, cooked dried beans and peas, low-fat or non-fat dairy products, and lean meats, chicken, and fish. Consumption of sugar, highly processed and refined foods, and caffeine from coffee and cola drinks should be limited. Regular meals, including a well-balanced breakfast, are important for the prevention and treatment of emotional and learning disorders.

When the diet is not optimal, a multiple vitamin-mineral supplement should be considered that supplies all the vitamins and minerals in approximately 100% to 300% of the USRDA. In addition, regular exercise, effective stress management, and avoidance of alcohol, chronic use of medications, and tobacco are important in the prevention and treatment of emotional disorders.

EPILEPSY

Overview

Epilepsy is one of the oldest human diseases and affects approximately 1% of the population in the United States. The seizures or attacks vary in severity, duration, and frequency and are basically of two types: generalized epilepsy, also known as grand mal or petite mal seizures, and focal epilepsy. Generalized epilepsy involves all parts of the brain while focal epilepsy involves only a portion of the brain.

Dietary Recommendations

Epilepsy is usually treated with anticonvulsant medications, such as phenytoin (Dilantin), phenobarbital, and primidone. In these cases, a low-fat, high-fiber, nutrient-dense diet should be consumed, adequate in all vitamins and minerals and low in sugars and refined and convenience foods. The diet should contain a variety of fruits, vegetables, whole grain breads and cereals, cooked dried beans and peas, low-fat or non-fat dairy products, and lean meats, chicken, and fish. A multiple vitamin-mineral supplement as well as regular exercise, effective stress management, avoidance of alcohol and tobacco, and moderate exposure to sunshine are important in the treatment of epilepsy.

Nutrition therapy consists primarily of a specialized diet called the "ketogenic diet" and is used for those people who do not tolerate or respond to medication. The diet is very high in fat and low in carbohydrates (starchy foods such as vegetables, grains, breads, and fruits) and must be monitored carefully by a physician and dietitian (Table 32).

Table 32.
FOODS TO AVOID ON THE KETOGENIC DIET
USED IN THE TREATMENT OF EPILEPSY

The following foods contain carbohydrates and might be restricted on a ketogenic diet for the treatment of epilepsy:

Cake	Pastries
Candy	Pies
Chewing gum	Sherbet
Cookies	Soft drinks
Cough drops and syrup containing	Sugar
Sugar	Sweet rolls
Fruit flavored drinks	Sweetened condensed milk
Honey	Syrup
Ice cream	All breads, bread products, and
Jam and jelly	cereals, unless they are planned in
Marmalade	the daily meal plan
Molasses	

Vitamins and minerals most likely to be low in the specialized ketogenic diet are calcium, iron, the B vitamins, vitamin C, and vitamin D. A multiple vitamin-mineral preparation that contains these nutrients in amounts between 100% and 300% of the USRDA should be consumed daily.

Long-term use of anticonvulsant medications can alter vitamin and mineral absorption and use. Vitamin D, vitamin B_{12}, and folic acid are likely to be affected by these medications and increased intake might be necessary. However, large doses of folic acid can interfere with the action of certain anticonvulsant medications, such as phenytoin, and supplements of this B vitamin should be taken only with the approval of a physician.

EYE DISORDERS

Overview

How well a person sees is often an indicator of the health of the eye. Although the eye works, becomes fatigued, and ages as does every organ, many disorders of the eye are preventable or treatable.

Nutrition and Eye Disorders

Deficiencies of fish oil and several vitamins might alter vision and the health of the eye.

VITAMIN A. Vitamin A is essential to the development and mainte- nance of normal eye tissue and vision. Vitamin A binds with a special protein in the eye that makes vision possible in dim light. A condition called night blindness or poor dark adaptation is an early sign of poor vitamin A intake. A person with night blindness is unable to see well in dim light, especially when entering darkness from a bright light as in entering a darkened room or driving at night where the eyes must adjust rapidly from bright headlights to darkness.

Vitamin A also is necessary for the development and maintenance of epithelial tissues that line the external and internal surfaces of the body including the eyes. An inadequate supply of this fat-soluble vitamin causes these tissues to shrink, harden, and deteriorate. If the deficiency continues, the changes can include irreversible loss of vi- sion. The first symptoms of vitamin A deficiency in the eye include over-sensitivity to bright light, itching, or burning. The eyes and eye lids become dry and inflamed.

In advanced stages of vitamin A deficiency, the cornea, the clear transparent portion at the front and center of the eyeball, becomes dry, inflamed, and swollen with water. Infection follows, accom- panied by cloudiness and blindness.

Severe vitamin A deficiency is rare in the United States. Infants and small children are most susceptible to vitamin A deficiency, but loss of vision from lack of vitamin A can occur in any age group. Increased intake of vitamin A and vitamin A-rich foods, such as dark green or orange vegetables, reverses the damage, unless it has progressed beyond repair.

VITAMIN E. As an antioxidant, vitamin E protects the eyes from damage caused by highly reactive compounds called free radicals. The antioxidant nutrients, including vitamin E, are thought to protect the eyes from "oxidative" or free radical damage and thus help prevent several eye disorders, including cataract formation. (See pages 126–128 for an explanation of free radicals.)

VITAMIN B_2. Some of the symptoms of a vitamin B_2 deficiency are damage to the eye tissue, poor vision, burning and itching of the eyes, and increased blood vessels in the eye. The outer lining of the eyes becomes inflamed and ulcers appear on the cornea. Poor dietary intake of this B vitamin must continue for several months before changes in the eyes and vision develop. Increased intake of vitamin B_2 and vitamin B_2-rich foods, such as milk and low-fat dairy products and dark green leafy vegetables, reverses the damage. Low vitamin B_2 intake is associated with cataract formation and blood levels of B_2 are low in as many as 80% of these patients.

VITAMIN B_{12}. A deficiency of vitamin B_{12} results in poor vision that disappears when intake of the vitamin is increased.

VITAMIN C. Vitamin C might inhibit the progression and encourage the regression of some forms of cataracts. A type of sugar in the diet called galactose can produce cataracts and this form of cataract is responsive to vitamin C therapy in some people. Another form of cataract, called cortical cataracts, also might be associated with vitamin C deficiency. Patients with cortical cataracts have low levels of the water-soluble vitamin in the fluid portion of the eye.

FISH OILS. The omega 3 fatty acids found in fish oils might be essential nutrients for the normal development and maintenance of good eyesight. Large amounts of these fats are found in eye tissues and a prolonged deficiency during the early stages of life results in a significant loss of vision that might be permanent.

Dietary Recommendations

For the development and maintenance of healthy eyes and vision, a low-fat, high-fiber, nutrient-dense diet should be consumed, adequate in all vitamins and minerals and low in sugars and refined and convenience foods. The diet should contain a variety of fruits, vegetables, whole grain breads and cereals, cooked dried beans and peas, low-fat or non-fat dairy products, and lean meats and chicken. Frequent servings of steamed, baked, or broiled fish should be included in the diet. At times when the diet is not optimal, a multiple vitamin-mineral preparation that contains between 100% and 300% of the USRDA of vitamin A, vitamin E, vitamin B_2, vitamin B_{12}, and vitamin C as well as the other vitamins and minerals can supplement the diet. Regular exercise, effective stress management, avoidance of tobacco and excessive exposure to sunlight, regular medical check-ups and eye exams, and moderate use of alcohol also are important for the prevention and treatment of eye disorders.

GUM AND TOOTH DISORDERS

Overview

A healthy smile is dependent on several factors including strong bones and teeth, adequate blood supply to the developing and mature gums and teeth, healthy gums, and a balance between acid and alkaline in the mouth.

Nutrition and Gum and Tooth Disorders

The cells that line the mouth have a short lifespan and require a constant supply of nutrients for normal repair and replacement. Consequently, symptoms of a vitamin or mineral deficiency often will develop more quickly in the mouth than in other tissues. The hard structures in the mouth, the bones and teeth, are blueprints for dietary intake of calcium and other minerals. Dietary habits and intake of other nutrients, such as starch and sugars, also are determining factors in the maintenance or loss of a healthy smile.

The incidence of tooth decay is strongly influenced by dietary intake during tooth development. Periodontal diseases—diseases of the gums—also have nutritional components.

Tooth decay is the most common long-term disease in the United States. People in primitive cultures living in remote areas of the world far from "civilized" cultures have little or no problem with tooth decay; however, the incidence of tooth decay increases upon exposure to modernized cultures and dietary habits. Tooth decay is most likely to develop with frequent consumption of sugary foods, especially if the food sticks to the teeth or if the sugary foods are eaten alone. The effects of sugar consumption on tooth decay are most pronounced during infancy and childhood when the teeth are developing. Certain vitamins and minerals, however, can help strengthen the tooth and gum structure and aid in the prevention of tooth decay or periodontal disease.

VITAMIN A. Vitamin A is important in tooth formation and in the proper spacing of teeth. However, no evidence exists that vitamin A functions in the prevention of tooth decay.

VITAMIN D. A major function of vitamin D is in the regulation and use of calcium and phosphorus. The vitamin also aids in the formation and maintenance of normal teeth and bones, including the bones of the jaw.

VITAMIN E. It has been proposed that the mercury in silver amalgam dental fillings leaches out of the tooth and poses a potential health hazard, including increased risk for nerve and brain damage. The amount of mercury lost from dental fillings is extremely small and probably is not a problem to health; however, if this source of mercury is a concern, adequate intake of vitamin E would help protect the body against the toxic effects of this metal.

VITAMIN B_2. Early symptoms of vitamin B_2 deficiency include burning and soreness of the mouth, lips, and tongue and cracks at the corners of the mouth. The lining of the mouth becomes inflamed in advanced stages of vitamin B_2 deficiency. These symptoms are reversed when intake of vitamin B_2 or vitamin B_2-rich foods is increased.

VITAMIN B_{12} AND FOLIC ACID. Vitamin B_{12} and folic acid are essential for the normal repair and replacement of cells. A deficiency of these B vitamins causes cells to form improperly. One of the first areas affected are the cells that line the mouth and tongue, causing soreness and deterioration of these surfaces. These symptoms are reversed with increased intakes of vitamin B_{12} and folic acid.

VITAMIN C. Vitamin C is required for the normal formation of the connective tissue that holds together the gums and other structures in the mouth. Some of the symptoms of scurvy or vitamin C deficiency are bleeding gums, deterioration of the gums, and loosening of the teeth caused by a deterioration of the connective tissue. Increased intake of vitamin C or vitamin C-rich foods cures the bleeding gums, but some damage caused by long-term vitamin C deficiency might be irreversible.

CALCIUM. One of the first bones affected by poor dietary intake of calcium is the alveolar bone, the portion of the jaw bone where the lower teeth are embedded or where dentures rest. Even the most expertly cared for or repaired teeth are useless unless they are supported by healthy bone. Loss of calcium from the alveolar bone can result in deterioration of the bone, periodontal disease, and problems with ill-fitting dentures.

Marginal calcium intake throughout life contributes to periodontal disease. As is seen in the bones affected by osteoporosis, the strength and hardness of the alveolar bone is related to how much calcium a person consumes. When calcium intake is adequate, periodontal disease is less likely to occur. One study showed alveolar bone loss was reversed when people increased their intake of dietary or supplemental calcium. When supplementation was stopped the bone began to deteriorate; this deterioration was halted and bone strength was increased when calcium supplementation was resumed.

Calcium functions in several ways to prevent or treat dental problems. Low intake of calcium hinders the production and alters the structure of the connective tissue that holds together the gums (periodontium) and bone. As a result, the bone and tissues dissolve and periodontal disease or poorly fitting dentures are likely to occur. In addition, calcium is important in the formation of strong, well-developed teeth because the mineral comprises a large part of both the enamel and the underlying dentin layer.

MAGNESIUM. The balance between magnesium and calcium is important in the formation and maintenance of healthy teeth and bones, such as the jaw and alveolar bones. In addition, a deficiency of magnesium produces swollen and sore gums, which is reversed when magnesium is added to the diet.

PHOSPHORUS. Phosphorus is a major component of the enamel and dentin of teeth. The balance between phosphorus and calcium is essential for the normal formation of bones and teeth. Because much of the calcification of these tissues occurs during the last 2 months in the uterus and during the first few months of life, it is important that the mother consume adequate amounts of both phosphorus and calcium during these periods. Otherwise, the developing infant will drain the mother's stores of these minerals.

SULFUR. Sulfur is a component of bones and teeth. A deficiency of this mineral is rare and usually is secondary to a protein deficiency.

COPPER. Copper works with vitamin C in the formation of connective tissue. A deficiency of this trace mineral could result in faulty development of gums, teeth, and the jaw and alveolar bones.

FLUORIDE. Adequate consumption of fluoride during the first 18 years of life could reduce the incidence of tooth decay by more than 50% and maintain an increased resistance to decay throughout life. The incidence of tooth decay is high in areas of the United States where the water is not fluoridated and fluoride intake is low. Fluoride is effective possibly because it discourages plaque accumulation on the tooth surface, discourages the activity of decay-causing bacteria, and encourages calcium deposition while discouraging calcium loss from teeth. The inclusion of fluoride into the calcium structure of teeth makes the teeth more resistant to decay caused by bacterial acids. In addition, fluoride strengthens the bones and reduces calcium loss from the jaw (alveolar) bone, characteristic of osteoporosis.

One milligram of fluoride for every liter of water (1 part fluoride for every million parts water or 1 ppm) is considered optimal for the prevention of tooth decay. Excessive intake of fluoride causes mottling and discoloration of teeth.

MANGANESE. Manganese is important in the formation of connective tissue and a deficiency of this trace mineral results in bone deformities, such as a misshapened jaw bone.

ZINC. In animals, a deficiency of zinc, combined with deficiencies of vitamin C and folic acid, results in increased risk for developing periodontal disease. Zinc apparently is important in the formation and maintenance of healthy gum tissue and maintenance of the immune system to prevent infection in humans as well.

Dietary Recommendations

A low-fat, high-fiber, nutrient-dense diet should be consumed, adequate in all vitamins and minerals and low in sugars and refined or sugary convenience foods. Sugary foods that stick to the teeth or frequent consumption of sugary foods, especially if consumed alone, are of particular concern. Jams, jellies, desserts, candies, caramels, dried fruit, sugar, heavily sugared beverages and soft drinks, and sugared ready-to-eat cereals should be avoided or consumed infrequently. Consumption of raw and rough foods, such as raw carrot sticks, apples, and green salads, scrape the teeth and help prevent accumulation of plaque and the development of tooth decay. The diet should contain a variety of fruits, vegetables, whole grain breads and cereals, cooked dried beans and peas, low-fat or non-fat dairy products, and lean meats, chicken, and fish.

Nursing bottle syndrome, a condition in infants and small children, is characterized by extensive decay and loss of the upper teeth. This condition can be prevented by not giving the child a bottle at bedtime filled with any beverage that contains sugar, including sugared fruit drinks, orange juice, milk, or other fruit or commercial drinks. Water or a pacifier can be given to the child if necessary.

Regular dental visits, daily brushing and flossing, and consumption of fluoridated water also aid in the prevention of tooth decay.

HAIR PROBLEMS

Overview

Skin and hair are composed of the same protein, called *keratin*; however, they differ in shape, texture, and function.

Nutrition and Hair Problems

Although baldness and other hair disorders can be natural results of aging or symptoms of disease, in some cases vitamin and mineral deficiencies result in hair loss that can be corrected when the deficiency is treated. For example, inadequate intake of protein results in brittle, sparse, lusterless hair. Severe protein deficiency in children causes the hair to turn orange as a result of alterations in the pigments embedded in the hair shaft. These symptoms of protein deficiency disappear when the diet is improved.

VITAMIN A. Hair loss and dandruff develop as a result of vitamin A deficiency. If poor vitamin A intake is not a cause or if these symptoms do not disappear when vitamin A-rich foods are added to the diet, then other causes of the disorder should be investigated. Vitamin A toxicity also causes hair loss and dryness and itching of the skin.

VITAMIN B_6, FOLIC ACID, AND VITAMIN B_{12}. The hair is dependent on a constant supply of blood and oxygen for normal growth and health. Any nutrient that reduces the blood's ability to transport oxygen to the hair will have an effect on the health and appearance of the hair. Vitamin B_6, folic acid, and vitamin B_{12} are essential for the normal formation of red blood cells, the portion of the blood that carries oxygen to the tissues. A deficiency of these B vitamins causes anemia and diminished blood supply to the hair and skin.

BIOTIN. A deficiency of the B vitamin biotin causes hair loss. A deficiency is rare, however, as bacteria in the intestine produce biotin that is absorbed.

VITAMIN C. Hair splits and breaks easily as a result of a vitamin C deficiency. When the hair breaks below the surface of the skin, the developing hair is cramped, coils into an abnormal circular pattern, and forms improperly. As a result, the hair is dry, kinky, and tangles. These symptoms occur only in a severe vitamin C deficiency and are reversible when vitamin C intake is increased.

COPPER. Copper is necessary for the formation of red blood cells and the maintenance of an adequate supply of blood to the hair shaft. In addition, copper functions in the formation and maintenance of hair pigments. A deficiency of this trace mineral is associated with color changes and loss of color from the hair. Excessive intake of the trace mineral molybdenum might interfere with the body's ability to use copper and produce symptoms of copper deficiency, such as hair loss.

IRON. Iron functions in the formation of red blood cells and the maintenance of the oxygen-carrying capacity of the blood. Therefore, this trace mineral is essential to the maintenance of an adequate blood supply to the hair. Iron deficiency is associated with hair loss, which is corrected when iron intake is increased.

ZINC. Symptoms of a zinc deficiency include hair loss and baldness. These symptoms are reversible if caused by a zinc deficiency. Zinc also functions in the maintenance of the oil-secreting glands attached to the hair follicle.

Dietary Recommendations

Most cases of balding result from hereditary influences; however, a good diet is safe and potentially beneficial. To maintain healthy scalp and hair, a low-fat, high-fiber, nutrient-dense diet should be consumed, adequate in all vitamins and minerals and low in sugars and refined and convenience foods. The diet should contain a variety of fruits, vegetables, whole grain breads and cereals, cooked dried beans and peas, low-fat or non-fat dairy products, and lean meat, chicken, and fish. Several glasses of water each day also are beneficial for healthy hair.

Regular exercise, effective stress management, avoidance of alcohol and tobacco, avoidance of severe cold and wind, and washing with a mild shampoo are helpful. Additionally, limited use of medications such as anticoagulents that produce hair loss, stimulation of the scalp, and moderate exposure to sunshine are important for the prevention and treatment of non-inherited hair and scalp disorders.

HEADACHES

Overview

Any pain in the head is called a headache. An intense, throbbing headache often accompanied by nausea, vomiting, or disturbances in sensation or muscle movement is called a migraine headache.

Nutrition and Headaches

Several dietary factors are associated with an increased risk for developing headaches or migraine headaches. In addition, migraine headaches are sometimes caused by sensitivity to specific food components and often are successfully treated by removing the offending food from the diet.

VITAMIN A. Consumption of large doses of vitamin A, between 60,000 IU and 341,000 IU can cause headaches in adults. Children develop toxicity symptoms such as headaches at small doses. Large doses of carotene appear to be harmless.

B VITAMINS. Symptoms of marginal and clinical deficiencies of several of the B vitamins, including niacin and folic acid, might induce headaches.

CHOLINE. Blood levels of choline are low in people with headaches and headache symptoms improve when blood levels of choline increase. Whether the changes in choline status are a cause or a result of the headache is unclear.

COPPER. Altered copper metabolism might be the underlying factor in the association between the intake of some foods, such as chocolate, and migraine headaches. Food factors known to trigger migraine headaches also might affect copper metabolism. Changes in the intake, absorption, or use of copper might increase the incidence of migraine because the mineral is important in the production, use, and breakdown of chemicals in the brain the cause blood vessels to constrict or relax. Migraine headaches apparently occur more often when blood levels of copper are low than when blood levels are normal.

IRON. Headaches are a symptom of a marginal or clinical iron deficiency.

FISH OILS. The severity and frequency of migraine headaches might be reduced when the omega 3 fatty acids found in fish oils are increased in the diet.

AMINO ACID—TYRAMINE. Tyramine is a compound similar to the amino acid tyrosine and is found naturally in foods. It is estimated that between 20% and 25% of people who suffer from migraine headaches can be successfully treated by tyramine-free diets. Tyramine-containing foods include aged cheeses, herring, organ meats, peanuts and peanut butter, chocolate, sauerkraut, fermented sausages such as bologna and pepperoni, and alcoholic beverages.

PHENYLETHYLAMINE (PEA). PEA is a compound found in chocolate and might be a cause or an aggravator of migraine headaches. PEA causes the blood vessels in the head to enlarge, which places pressure on the surrounding brain tissue and results in migraine headaches in some people.

FOOD ADDITIVES. Nitrites are found naturally in foods and are preservatives added to bacon, hot dogs, and other sandwich meats. Some individuals who suffer from migraine headaches are sensitive to nitrites and the severity, frequency, and duration of headache symptoms might be reduced if foods that contain these additives are removed from the diet.

Monosodium glutamate (MSG) is a common food additive used in Chinese and other ethnic foods. The "Chinese Restaurant Syndrome" includes headache, flushing, nausea, or vomiting within an hour after consuming food high in MSG. The non-nutritive sweetener aspartame (NutraSweet) also increases the frequency of headaches in some people.

Dietary Recommendations

The tyramine-free diet is effective in many cases of migraine headache. If headaches continue after following this diet, then an elimination diet where foods thought to trigger headaches are removed one by one from the diet can be retried with the supervision of a physician or dietitian. A regular schedule of meals and sleeping hours and a record of headaches should be maintained to detect any hidden relationships between headaches and diet or other lifestyle patterns.

In addition, a low-fat, high-fiber, nutrient-dense diet should be consumed, adequate in all vitamins and minerals and low in sugars and refined and convenience foods. The diet should contain a variety of fruits, vegetables, whole grain breads and cereals, cooked dried beans and peas, low-fat or non-fat dairy products, and lean meats, chicken, and fish. When the diet is inadequate, a multiple vitamin-mineral supplement might be considered. Regular exercise; effective stress management; and avoidance of alcohol, caffeine, and tobacco also are important in the prevention and treatment of headaches.

HEARING DISORDERS

Overview

Hearing is a complex process that begins with the gathering of sound at the outer ear and ends with the interpretation of sound in the higher centers of thought and reasoning in the brain (Figure 1, page 27).

Nutrition and Hearing Disorders

VITAMIN D. Inadequate amounts of vitamin D in the body might be associated with ear abnormalities and hearing loss in some people. A lack of vitamin D produces calcium loss from the bones and might cause the fragile bone of the inner ear, the *cochlea*, to become porous and unable to transmit messages to the nerves that lead to the brain. The association between vitamin D and hearing loss is supported by findings that people with other vitamin D-related disorders often have hearing loss. Deafness caused by changes in the cochlea might respond to vitamin D supplementation. It is unknown whether or not calcium is important in this form of hearing loss.

IODINE. Hearing improves in some people when they increase their consumption of dietary iodine. How iodine affects hearing is unclear; however, iodine therapy appears to be effective only in those few people deficient in the mineral.

Dietary Recommendations

Vitamin D cannot cure all types of hearing loss. Deafness as a result of nerve damage is not affected by vitamin D intake. If deafness is caused by changes in the boney structure of the inner ear and if dietary intake of vitamin D-fortified milk or exposure to sunshine has been minimal over a long period of time, then an increase in the consumption of vitamin D and calcium, and exposure to moderate sunshine might be useful in the treatment of hearing loss.

HERPES SIMPLEX

Overview

The severity, frequency, and duration of the viral infection called herpes varies between individuals and depends on other lifestyle factors such as stress and nutritional status. No cure exists for genital herpes, but the symptoms can be treated by soaking in salt solutions or sitz baths, use of pain-killers or soothing ointments, and possibly an antibiotic cream to prevent secondary infections.

Nutrition and Herpes Simplex

Nutrition functions directly and indirectly by stimulating the immune response to reduce the frequency, severity, and duration of recurrences of herpes infections.

AMINO ACIDS—L-LYSINE. Lysine might reduce the frequency and severity of symptoms of recurrent herpes infections. Doses that exceed 1 gram of lysine appear to be necessary to obtain satisfactory results. Blood levels of lysine also are related to risk for recurrence; when blood levels of lysine are high the incidence of recurrent infections is reduced as compared to when blood levels of lysine are low.

The herpes virus thrives in an environment where there are large amounts of the amino acid arginine and low amounts of lysine. If lysine supplementation is an effective treatment for herpes it is probably because increased intake of lysine upsets the ratio of arginine to lysine and slows viral growth. The evidence in support of lysine for the treatment of herpes infections is limited and controversial and some studies have found lysine is not beneficial in the treatment of herpes.

BIOFLAVONOIDS. A few reports state that bioflavonoids might be effective in reducing the severity of symptoms during recurrent herpes infections. More evidence is necessary, however, before dietary recommendations can be made.

VITAMINS AND MINERALS. A person's susceptibility to herpes infection depends on exposure to the virus and the strength of the immune system to fight the infection. All nutrients associated with a well-functioning immune system are important to build the body's defense against infection and reduce the likelihood of recurrence. These nutrients include beta carotene, vitamin E, the B vitamins, vitamin C, iron, copper, selenium, and zinc. (See pages 128–129 for more information on nutrition and immunity.)

Dietary Recommendations

Supplementation with L-lysine combined with limited intake of arginine-rich foods, such as nuts, seeds, and chocolate, might discourage the growth of the herpes virus and reduce the risk for recurrence.

In addition, a low-fat, high-fiber, nutrient-dense diet should be consumed, adequate in all vitamins and minerals and low in sugars and refined and convenience foods. The diet should contain a variety of fruits, vegetables, whole grain breads and cereals, cooked dried beans and peas, low-fat or non-fat dairy products, and lean meats, chicken, and fish. A multiple vitamin-mineral supplement that contains between 100% and 300% of the USRDA for all nutrients related to the immune system (see page 00 for more information on nutrition and immunity), as well as regular exercise, effective stress management, adequate sleep, avoidance of alcohol and tobacco, and limited use of caffeine are important for the prevention and treatment of viral infections, such as herpes simplex.

HYPERTENSION

Overview

Blood pressure is the blood's force against the walls of the arteries and heart as the blood is pumped from the heart to the tissues. Two pressures make up blood pressure: systolic blood pressure, or the maximum amount of pressure in the arteries when the heart contracts (heartbeat), and diastolic blood pressure, or the least amount of pressure in the arteries when the heart relaxes between beats.

Hypertension is blood pressure that remains above the normal range and signifies a constant, excessive pulsing of blood against the walls of the arteries and heart. Hypertension is not a disease, but a symptom of an underlying disease. It also is one of the three primary risk factors for the development of the cardiovascular diseases of heart attack and stroke. The best defense against hypertension is prevention; the second best defense is to control existing hypertension with diet, lifestyle habits, and medication.

Nutrition and Hypertension

Diet is strongly linked to the prevention and treatment of essential hypertension. For example, body weight is a prime risk factor for the development or prevention of this disorder; as weight increases above the ideal, the risk for hypertension increases. In contrast, weight loss and maintenance of ideal body weight is effective in the prevention and treatment of hypertension, and the maintenance of ideal body weight for people with borderline hypertension might eliminate the need for medications.

A high-fat, low-fiber diet is linked to an increased risk for developing hypertension and an increase in fiber and reduction in fat intake, especially saturated fats found in foods from animal origin, might reduce blood pressure. Blood pressure drops when the fat content is reduced from the typical 37% to 25% of total calories and more poly-unsaturated fats from vegetable oils than saturated fats from meat and dairy products are consumed. It is theorized that if fat was re-duced to less than 25%, salt intake was restricted, and ideal body weight was maintained, hypertension might be controlled or elimi-nated without the need for medication in more than 85% of all cases.

SODIUM. Excessive salt (sodium chloride) intake is linked to increased risk for developing hypertension. In contrast, as salt intake decreases, so does the risk for developing hypertension. The link between salt and hypertension is still controversial and it appears some people are more susceptible than others to salt intake. This sensitivity to salt might be inherited, in which case the consumption of a low-salt diet from childhood would aid in the prevention of this disorder. However, there is no method for determining who is and who isn't salt-sensitive. As the intake of salt is excessive in the United States and reduction of intake poses no harm, it has been recommended that all Americans reduce their intake of salt.

POTASSIUM. The ratio of potassium to sodium might be a factor in the development of hypertension. A high intake of sodium-rich foods such as convenience foods, snack foods, and canned soups, coupled with a reduction in intake of potassium-rich foods is associated with a high incidence of hypertension. In contrast, a diet high in potassium pro-tects against the development of this disorder by lowering systolic and diastolic blood pressures.

CHLORIDE. Chloride, the other compound in table salt (sodium chlo-ride), also is linked to hypertension. Sodium and chloride work to-gether in the regulation of fluid balance and blood pressure. Some evidence shows that dietary intake of sodium without chloride does not increase blood pressure in salt-sensitive people with hypertension and the intake of both sodium and chloride are necessary for the disorder to develop.

CALCIUM. Calcium might be as strongly linked as sodium to hyperten-sion. People who consume low amounts of calcium or calcium-rich dairy products are more likely to develop high blood pressure than are people who consume at least the RDA or more of calcium. Diastolic blood pressure drops when diets are supplemented daily with 1,000 mg of calcium. People with hypertension might have altered levels of calcium in their blood and these changes are related to dietary cal-cium intake. In animal studies, a high-calcium diet consumed during pregnancy and breastfeeding discourages the development of high blood pressure in the offspring; in contrast, a low-calcium diet increases the risk of high blood pressure in the offspring. A high-calcium diet might help counteract the harmful effects of a high-sodium diet. However, for maximum benefits, a low-sodium, high-potassium, high-calcium diet should be consumed.

MAGNESIUM. People with hypertension often have low levels of magnesium in their blood. In many cases, elevated blood pressure returns to normal when the intake of magnesium-rich foods is increased or if magnesium supplements are added to the daily diet.

Some anti-hypertension medications affect the amount of magnesium in the body. Diuretic medications, such as the thiazides, lower blood pressure by increasing urinary excretion of fluid and reducing blood volume. They also increase the excretion of magnesium and might increase the risk for magnesium deficiency. People with hypertension who take diuretic medications have low blood levels of magnesium and the combination of magnesium and hypertension medication might be more effective in lowering blood pressure than medication alone.

Magnesium might aid in the regulation of blood pressure by its effect on the blood vessel walls. Magnesium influences how the heart and the blood vessels contract and relax. Artery walls spasm and an irregular heartbeat develops when magnesium intake is low; artery walls relax and the heartbeat returns to normal when blood levels of the mineral are adequate. Constriction or spasms of the blood vessels are linked to hypertension, whereas relaxation of the blood vessels increases the size of the blood vessel, reduces resistance to blood flow, and lowers blood pressure.

FISH OILS. The omega 3 fatty acids found in fish oils might lower blood pressure. Blood pressure drops as much as 24% when a person includes frequent servings of fish in the weekly diet or includes fish oil supplements in the daily menu. Evidence is limited, however, and recommendations cannot be made at this time.

Dietary Recommendations

Maintenance of ideal body weight is important for the prevention and treatment of essential hypertension. Also, a low-fat, high-fiber, nutrient-dense diet should be consumed, adequate in all vitamins and minerals and low in sugar, salty foods, and refined and convenience foods. The diet should contain a variety of fruits, vegetables, whole grain breads and cereals, cooked dried beans and peas, low-fat or non-fat dairy products, and lean meats, fish, and chicken. Foods should be baked, steamed, and broiled, rather than fried or sauteed. A multiple vitamin-mineral supplement and a calcium and magnesium supplement should be consumed if the diet does not supply at least the RDA for these nutrients.

Regular aerobic exercise, such as walking, jogging, swimming, or jumping rope, is also necessary for weight and blood pressure maintenance. Effective stress management, frequent blood pressure checkups, compliance with medications, moderate use or avoidance of alcohol and caffeine, and avoidance of tobacco are important for the prevention and treatment of hypertension.

INFECTION

Overview

Infection is any invasion of the body by disease-causing microorganisms (germs), such as bacteria or viruses, that results in a reaction of the tissues, inflammation, and a response from the immune system. Many areas of the body are normally inhabited by microorganisms, but disease develops when the body's defense system is faulty or the microorganisms migrate from their natural spot to another area in the body. Other disease-causing microorganisms are transmitted through food, air, contact with other people and the environment, contact with insects and animals that transmit disease, or water. Microorganisms find entry into the body through the skin, nose, mouth, ears, the intestinal or urinary tracts, and other body openings.

In addition to common infections, several diseases are attributed to exposure and susceptibility to specific microorganisms, such as the diseases caused by bacterial infection including scarlet fever, rheumatic fever, meningitis, measles, tuberculosis, whooping cough, and food poisoning. Also included are the diseases caused by viral infections including rabies, mumps, influenza, acquired immunodeficiency syndrome (AIDS), hepatitis, herpes, chickenpox, infectious mononucleosis, and smallpox.

The strength of the immune system is an important factor in the prevention or development and treatment of infection. (See pages 128–129 for more information on the immune system.)

Nutrition and Infection

Nutrition is a major contributor to the functioning of the immune system. All organs and cells of the immune system are affected by a person's nutritional status. General poor nutrition, including inadequate intake of protein and calories, suppresses the immune response and increases the risk for developing infection and disease; however, even single vitamin or mineral deficiencies in the presence of otherwise adequate nutrition can reduces a person's ability to fight infection. On the other hand, optimal intake of all vitamins and minerals and consumption of a diet low in fat and high in fiber enhances the immune response and reduces a person's risk for developing infection.

The vitamins and trace minerals associated with the immune response include vitamin A, beta carotene, vitamin E, the B vitamins, vitamin C, copper, iron, selenium, and zinc. Inadequate intake of any of these nutrients results in reduced activity of the immune system and increased susceptibility to colds and infection. In addition, infection drains essential nutrients from the body and increases the daily requirement in order to fight the infection and repair the damaged tissues. Marginal nutrient deficiencies have a harmful effect on the immune system long before obvious signs of more severe deficiencies and malnutrition develop.

Dietary Recommendations

To maintain a healthy immune system and prevent infections, a low-fat, high-fiber, nutrient-dense diet should be consumed, adequate in all vitamins and minerals and low in sugars and refined and convenience foods. The diet should contain a variety of fruits, vegetables, whole grain breads and cereals, cooked dried beans and peas, low-fat or non-fat dairy products, and lean meats, chicken, and fish. A multiple vitamin-mineral supplement that supplies between 100% and 300% of the USRDA for all vitamins and minerals should be chosen when the diet is not optimal. Regular exercise, effective stress management, avoidance of alcohol and tobacco, compliance with antibiotic medications, daily consumption of several glasses of water, adequate amounts of sleep, and good sanitation are also important for the prevention and treatment of infection. (For additional information on specific infections see the sections on The Immune System, Acne, AIDS, the Common Cold, Dermatitis, and Herpes.)

INSOMNIA

Overview

The most common sleep disorder is insomnia. Insomnia can be a result of difficulty falling asleep, difficulty staying asleep during the night, or waking too early in the morning. The relative decrease in the need for sleep that is the normal accompaniment of aging is not included in this category. Insomnia results from numerous disorders such as depression, chronic physical pain, stress, and many medications.

Nutrition and Insomnia

Deficiencies of niacin and vitamin B_6 are related to insomnia; however, supplementation with these nutrients is only effective if a nutrient deficiency is the cause of the sleep disorder. One of the symptoms of a niacin deficiency is insomnia, and increased niacin intake is an effective cure for this form of the disorder. Vitamin B_6 is an important contributor to the formation of serotonin, a neurotransmitter that aids in the regulation of sleep. A diet low in vitamin B_6 is associated with increased risk for developing insomnia, irritability, and depression, and increased intake of the vitamin reverses these symptoms.

AMINO ACIDS—TRYPTOPHAN. The dietary amino acid tryptophan is converted to the neurotransmitter serotonin in the body. Serotonin is one of the chemicals that regulates sleep. Tryptophan supplementation increases serotonin levels, reduces the time required to fall asleep by as much as 50%, and can improve the quality and length of sleep. Tryptophan supplements or foods rich in tryptophan must be taken at night for the amino acid to be an effective inducer of sleep. The effects of tryptophan are most pronounced if the amino acid is taken with a carbohydrate (starch)-rich, low-protein snack, such as toast and jam. The effects of tryptophan are short-term and the amino acid might be most effective in inducing sleep, rather than in preventing night awakenings or sleepiness the next morning. In the fall of 1989, the Food and Drug Administration removed tryptophan supplements from the marketplace because of reports of a rare blood disorder associated with their use.

Dietary Recommendations

Short-term insomnia might be treatable with tryptophan-rich foods, such as milk, cheese, turkey, or bananas. Tryptophan entry into the brain is increased if a meal or snack high in starchy foods and low in protein is consumed. Tryptophan supplements currently are under investigation for their potential association with a rare blood disorder. Long-term insomnia should be treated with the help of a physician and may require medication and stress reduction or psychological counseling. Stress reduction techniques such as regular exercise and good diet might aid in the treatment of insomnia. Avoidance of caffeine, tobacco, and other stimulants or drugs is also beneficial.

JET LAG

Overview

Jet lag is a physiological and psychological syndrome experienced by many people when they travel by air across three or more time zones; symptoms are most severe in flights traveling west to east. People do not develop jet lag when traveling north and south. Within the first day at the destination, a person might feel tired, experience poor concentration, have memory lapses, or perform poorly on normal tasks. Later symptoms include increasing weariness, gastrointestinal disturbances such as constipation or diarrhea, insomnia, loss of appetite, headaches, reduced ability to see at night, and limited peripheral vision. The symptoms last from a day to 2 weeks, depending on individual variation and the number of time zones crossed. In general, it takes the body 1 day to adjust for each time zone crossed.

Nutrition and Jet Lag

THE AMINO ACIDS—TRYPTOPHAN. Tryptophan-rich foods, such as milk, cheese, turkey, or bananas, have a sedative effect that might be useful in the treatment of jet lag without the adverse side effects of other sedatives, such as drowsiness. Tryptophan absorption and effectiveness is most pronounced when the amino acid is consumed as a part of a high-carbohydrate, low-protein meal.

Dietary Recommendations

A jet lag diet program has been developed that might aid in the prevention of weariness and related symptoms associated with long-distance air travel. Four days prior to the estimated breakfast time at the destination the meals should be hearty, high in protein at breakfast and lunch, and high in carbohydrates at dinner. Coffee and tea are allowed only between 3 P.M. and 5 P.M. The second day of the program, the meals are light, such as salads, simple soups, fruits and fruit juices, and vegetables. This "fast" day is designed to deplete the body's stores of carbohydrates and help "reset" the internal time clock. The last 2 days of the diet the feast and fast cycle is repeated, except on the fourth day people flying westbound drink a caffeinated beverage in the morning, while people flying eastbound drink a caffeinated beverage between 6 P.M. and 11 P.M. The feast-fast cycle is broken at what should be breakfast time at the destination by consuming a high-protein breakfast. The person should eat this meal regardless of when the breakfast hour occurs, even if he/she must get up in the middle of the night or eat at 2 A.M. on the plane.

In addition, sleep and meal times should be shifted 1 hour each day prior to the trip to prepare the body for the time change. The traveler should begin the trip well rested and not plan activities for the first day after arrival. Fluids should be consumed before and during the flight to replace body water lost due to low humidity in the pressurized airplane cabin.

KIDNEY DISORDERS

Overview

The kidneys and urinary system maintain the chemical balance of all body fluids. They filter out and remove waste products from the blood; maintain the normal ranges of nutrients in the blood by removing and excreting excess amounts of minerals, vitamins, and other compounds; and regulate the normal acid-base (pH) balance of the body. Kidney and urinary disorders include the following:

Acute glomerulonephritis. Temporary inflammation of the portion of the kidneys that filters waste products from the blood.

Chronic glomerulonephritis. Long-term inflammation that sometimes develops from the acute form of the same disorder.

Nephrotic syndrome or nephrosis. A disease characterized by water retention, protein loss in the urine, tissue deterioration, and malnutrition.

Uremia. A toxic condition caused by the accumulation of waste products in the blood that is a symptom of kidney failure.

Acute and chronic kidney failure. The inability of the kidneys to remove waste products characterized by the accumulation of toxic chemicals and acids in the blood.

Kidney stones. Kidney stones are crystals of calcium oxalate, calcium phosphate, uric acid, or a mixture of these or other substances. The urinary concentration of calcium, oxalate, and other substances, and the presence (or absence) of factors in the urine that promote or inhibit stone formation, called crystallization, determine whether a stone will develop.

Urinary tract infections. Infections such as a bladder infection result from bacteria in the urethra, bladder, or ureters.

Nutrition and Kidney Disorders

Dietary management for all kidney disorders except kidney stones includes consideration for the intake of protein, fluid, salt, potassium, calcium, phosphorus, vitamin D, fluoride, and all vitamins. Dietary control of these kidney disorders must be monitored closely by a physician and a dietitian.

VITAMIN A. Vitamin A is essential for the development and maintenance of the lining of the urinary system.

VITAMIN D. Excessive intake of vitamin D can result in calcium deposits in the kidneys and irreversible kidney damage. Vitamin D, however, also improves zinc status in kidney patients on dialysis.

VITAMIN E. A deficiency of vitamin E produces a form of anemia called *hemolytic anemia* where red blood cells are fragile and break easily. This form of anemia is common in patients on dialysis for the treatment of advanced kidney disease, and supplementation with the vitamin might help prevent or correct this secondary disorder.

Kidney stones are comprised of several different substances including calcium and uric acid. Dietary management of kidney stones should be designed and monitored by a physician and a dietitian and depends on the type of stone. Treatments attempt to reduce these substances in the urine or keep them in solution rather than allowing them to solidify into stones. The use of acid-ash or alkaline-ash diets in the treatment of kidney stones refers to the products the foods will eventually yield after use in the body. The acids in fruits or milk are used in the body and the remaining products for excretion include alkaline substances such as potassium or calcium. In contrast, the waste products of a diet high in meat are acidic and produce an acid ash, such as uric acid and phosphoric acid, that is excreted by the kidneys. The most common form of kidney stones are calcium-containing stones that are caused by abnormal absorption of calcium from the intestine, abnormal filtering of calcium from the kidneys, or abnormal activity of hormones that regulate calcium use in the body. A high dietary intake of calcium does not cause kidney stones except in those people who are prone to kidney stone formation. Foods that produce an acid ash, such as meat, starchy foods, cranberries, and prunes, help keep calcium from crystallizing into a stone. Other techniques for the control of calcium stones include the use of diuretic medications that reduce the amount of calcium in the urine and gel medications that reduce the absorption of calcium from the intestine. A low-calcium diet is often prescribed, but increases the risk for developing osteoporosis and other bone diseases. In contrast, uric acid stones require an increased intake of alkaline ash foods, such as milk, vegetables, and fruits and a reduced intake of meats and other acid ash foods.

VITAMIN B_6. A vitamin B_6 deficiency might increase the risk for developing oxalate-containing kidney stones. Supplementation with the vitamin reduces the amount of oxalate in the urine and reduces a person's risk for developing kidney stones or kidney damage.

VITAMIN C. Large doses of vitamin C might encourage the formation of oxalate-containing kidney stones in people prone to stone formation. In addition, evidence shows that vitamin C intake should be limited to the RDA in people with kidney disorders because large doses of the vitamin raise blood and urinary levels of oxalic acid, a compound that aggravates kidney disease.

MAGNESIUM. Magnesium inhibits the formation of crystals in the urine, possibly as a result of the ratio of magnesium to calcium in the urine. The magnesium content of the urine of stone formers and stone nonformers is similar; however, stone formers excrete large amounts of calcium, making their urinary ratio of magnesium to calcium very low. Increased intake of magnesium raises the magnesium concentration in the urine, alters the ratio of magnesium to calcium to resemble the urinary magnesium concentration of stone nonformers, and reduces the formation of kidney stones.

Kidney stones are most common in affluent nations where typical diets are high in protein, refined carbohydrates, fat, alcohol, and phosphorus. These dietary factors also increase the daily need for magnesium.

Dietary Recommendations

For the prevention of kidney disorders, a person should consume a low-fat, high-fiber, nutrient-dense diet, adequate in all vitamins and minerals and low in sugars and refined and convenience foods. The diet should contain a variety of fruits, vegetables, whole grain breads and cereals, cooked dried beans and peas, low-fat or non-fat dairy products, and lean meats, chicken, and fish. A multiple vitamin-mineral supplement as well as several glasses of water daily, limited use of bubble baths and hygiene sprays, regular physical examinations that include a urine culture, regular exercise, effective stress management, avoidance of alcohol and tobacco, and daily bathing are important.

Urinary tract infections have been treated with mixed results by drinking large amounts of cranberry juice or consuming large doses of vitamin C to acidify the urine. The best treatment after a diagnosis, based on an analysis and culture of the urine, is the use of prescribed medications such as antibiotics or sulfa drugs combined with increased water intake. Coffee, tea, alcohol, and spicy foods should be avoided during the period of infection.

The treatment of kidney diseases should be designed and monitored by a physician and dietitian, and includes dietary, medication or medical, and lifestyle components.

LIVER DISORDERS

Overview

The liver is the largest and one of the most important organs in the body and has the greatest variety of functions. Most of the nutrients absorbed from the diet are transported directly to the liver for storage, repackaging, or combining with other compounds. Poisons that enter or are produced in the body are detoxified in the liver. Many compounds essential to growth and development are produced in the liver, such as fat, proteins, sugar, cholesterol, and the blood carriers of fat called *lipoproteins*. The liver serves as a storehouse for nutrients, such as the fat-soluble vitamins, vitamin B_{12}, vitamin C, copper, and iron, and the storage form of energy called *glycogen*. The liver also releases substances into the blood when levels are low, such as sugar to maintain blood sugar levels and a special protein called *albumin* that maintains fluid balance in the blood. The liver packages other compounds for excretion, such as converting cholesterol to bile for excretion into the intestine. The liver converts vitamins to their active forms, such as carotene into vitamin A.

Damage to the liver has profound effects on numerous body processses, including digestion, absorption, storage, and use of vitamins and minerals. In addition, the manufacture of proteins decreases, fat production is altered and results in fat accumulation in the liver, and the manufacture of enzymes necessary for the detoxification of alcohol and other poisons is reduced so that these substances accumulate in the body.

Diseases of the liver include the following:

Hepatitis. Inflammation of the liver caused by a virus, toxin or drug, or blockage of the duct leading from the liver to the gallbladder.
Cirrhosis. A replacement of healthy liver tissue with tough, fibrous tissue resulting in a reduction in liver function,
Jaundice. The symptom of an underlying liver disorder, which is characterized by a yellowish discoloration of the skin and eyes caused by accumulation of bile in the body.
Hemochromatosis. A rare, excessive accumulation of iron in the liver.

Nutrition and Liver Disorders

Liver disease causes malnutrition for three reasons: it hinders the digestion and absorption of food, it affects the utilization of nutrients in the body, and it reduces food intake because of nausea, loss of appetite, and vomiting. The manufacture, use, and excretion of protein, carbohydrate, and fat are altered and the absorption and use of numerous vitamins and minerals are reduced.

VITAMIN A. Adequate intake of vitamin A might help prevent the accumulation of tough, fibrous tissue in the liver characteristic of disease. Animals with liver disease show reduced damage to the tissue when the diet is high in vitamin A as compared to when vitamin A intake is poor. Long-term and excessive intake of the fat-soluble vitamin might cause liver enlargement and disease.

VITAMIN E. A vitamin E deficiency produces liver damage, but no evidence exists that increased vitamin E intake will reverse liver disorders unless the damage is a result of a deficiency.

VITAMIN K. Large doses of vitamin K produce jaundice and damage to brain tissue in infants.

BIOTIN. Large doses of biotin over long periods of time might cause abnormal enlargement of the liver.

COPPER. An inherited disorder in the use of copper called Wilson's disease is characterized by excessive accumulation of copper in tissues and results in reduced liver function. Treatment of Wilson's disease includes a diet low in copper and the medication penicillamine that binds to copper and increases its excretion in the intestine.

Nutritional consequences of liver disease might include reduced formation of vitamin D, which contributes to osteoporosis, increased loss of vitamin B_6 and possible deficiency, and reduced formation of the protein that transports vitamin A in the blood that will cause night blindness. Additionally, increased loss and possible deficiencies of folic acid, calcium, magnesium, and zinc might occur.

Dietary Recommendations

The dietary management of all liver disorders should be designed and monitored by a physician and dietitian. Protein, carbohydrates, fat, and calories must be balanced, and vitamin and mineral intake should be optimal to reduce nutritional stress on the liver and provide all the nutrients necessary for repair of the damaged tissue. Vitamins should be consumed in their active forms, especially vitamin A and the B vitamins, as the liver, which is responsible for producing the active forms of vitamins from dietary building blocks, is unable to function normally. Water-soluble forms of vitamins A, D, E, and possibly K might be necessary if the person is unable to absorb fats. In addition, a person should avoid alcohol, environmental and dietary toxins, and substances that stress the body, such as tobacco. Use of medications known to cause liver damage should be monitored closely by a physician.

To prevent liver disease, avoid alcohol, and consume a low-fat, high-fiber, nutrient-dense diet, adequate in all vitamins and minerals and low in sugars and refined and convenience foods. The diet should contain a variety of fruits, vegetables, whole grain breads and cereals, cooked dried beans and peas, low-fat or non-fat dairy products, and lean meats, chicken, and fish. A multiple vitamin-mineral supplement as well as regular exercise, effective stress management, avoidance of tobacco, removal of all environmental and dietary toxins, and regular physical examinations are important.

LUNG DISORDERS

Overview

The main function of the lungs is to supply the bloodstream with oxygen and remove unwanted gases, such as carbon dioxide, from the system. Carbon dioxide is removed with each exhalation and oxygen is absorbed into the blood with each inhalation. This exchange of gases is called *respiration* and is essential to life.

The lungs are exposed to numerous environmental substances that could cause infection, including molds, bacteria, viruses, and pollens. The barriers to infection in the respiratory tract include enzymes that destroy foreign substances, a strong lining (epithelial lining) that forms a physical barrier to contaminants, a mucous coating that covers the lining of the lungs and further prevents invasion by harmful germs and substances, and a layer of minute hair-like structures (cilia) on the lining of the respiratory tract that sweep inhaled debris into the stomach for excretion. In addition, white blood cells and the other factors of the immune system constantly monitor the respiratory tract and prevent establishment of infectious bacteria and other germs. Tobacco smoke, alcohol, and air pollution deteriorate the lining of the lungs and reduce the strength of the immune system, increasing the lungs' susceptibility to disease and infection.

Lung disorders associated with environmental conditions or tobacco use include bronchitis, emphysema, and lung cancer. A healthy immune system combined with an active antioxidant system is important for the prevention and treatment of these lung disorders; however, tobacco use and secondhand smoke are the greatest contributors to these lung diseases. Allergies and asthma, two disorders that involve the respiratory tract, are discussed in detail on pages 133–138 and 146–147.

Nutrition and Lung Disorders

Vitamins and minerals function to maintain healthy lung tissue by strengthening the immune system and increasing the body's resistance to infection, maintaining lining of the lungs, and deactivating highly reactive compounds called *free radicals* that cause lung damage and possibly cancer.

VITAMIN A AND BETA CAROTENE. Vitamin A and beta carotene are necessary for the development and maintenance of healthy epithelial tissue and mucous membranes, such as the lining of the lungs, bronchi, and other respiratory tissues. Epithelial tissue forms a barrier to bacteria and other foreign substances and directly aids in the prevention of infection and disease. Beta carotene also strengthens the immune system and provides resistance to infection.

An adequate intake of foods high in beta carotene reduces a person's risk for developing lung cancer. In contrast, the lung tissues of people who smoke or who develop cancer are lower in vitamin A and beta carotene than the lung tissues of healthy people. Beta carotene is especially effective as an anti-cancer nutrient in the prevention of lung cancer. Vitamin A or beta carotene might reduce cancer risk by strengthening the epithelial lining of the lungs and discouraging the formation of abnormal cells.

VITAMIN D. If vitamin D is important to the maintenance of healthy lung tissue it is because this fat-soluble vitamin aids in the regulation of the immune system and improves the lungs' resistance to infection.

VITAMIN E. As an antioxidant, vitamin E protects the membranes in the lungs from damage by free radicals found in air pollution and tobacco smoke and aids in the prevention of tumor growth that develops from free radical destruction of tissue. People with lung cancer, compared to healthy people, show low levels of vitamin E in their tissues. (See pages 126–128 for more information on antioxidants and free radicals.)

THE B VITAMINS. Adequate intake of vitamin B_6 is necessary for optimal functioning of the immune system; however, large doses of this B vitamin do not provide added benefits. Vitamin B_{12} is important in the formation and maintenance of white blood cells, necessary components of the immune system and essential to the body's resistance to infection and disease. A deficiency of the B vitamin pantothenic acid results in increased risk for developing respiratory tract infections.

VITAMIN C. Adequate intake of vitamin C might increase a person's resistance to colds and other infections. Optimal dietary intake of vitamin C reduces the severity and duration of the common cold, while poor dietary intake increases a person's risk for developing lung infections and the common cold. Excessive intake of vitamin C might lower the body's resistance to lung infections. Vitamin C used in conjunction with the medication indomethacin might improve the symptoms, such as easier breathing, of bronchoconstriction (constriction of the bronchial tubes or air passages in the lungs).

COPPER. Inadequate intake of copper, especially during the formative years when the respiratory tract is developing, might be linked to later development of lung damage similar to emphysema. Copper deficiency is associated with reduced resistance to disease and increased likelihood of developing colds and infection.

IRON. Iron contributes to a healthy immune system and increases a person's resistance to colds, infection, and disease.

MAGNESIUM. One of the symptoms of magnesium toxicity is difficulty breathing.

MANGANESE. Manganese functions as an antioxidant to protect lung tissue from damage by free radicals in air pollution and tobacco smoke.

SELENIUM. A deficiency of the antioxidant selenium is associated with increased risk for developing lung cancer. Lung cancer is more prevalent in people with low levels of selenium in their lung tissues than in people with moderate to high selenium concentrations. The anticancer effects of selenium are enhanced if the mineral is consumed in conjunction with vitamin E. Limited evidence shows that selenium also is important in the maintenance of the immune system and the body's resistance to infection.

ZINC. Zinc stimulates the immune response and aids in the prevention of colds and infection. In addition, zinc appears to have a direct effect on slowing the growth of infectious organisms, especially viruses that invade the lungs and increase risk for developing colds or lung infections. Excessive intake of zinc reduces resistance to infection.

Dietary Recommendations

There is no specific diet that will prevent all types of lung disorders, although the dietary guidelines for the prevention of cancer apply to lung cancer. In general, a low-fat, high-fiber, nutrient-dense diet should be consumed, adequate in all vitamins and minerals and low in sugars and refined and convenience foods. The diet should contain a variety of fruits, vegetables, whole grain breads and cereals, cooked dried beans and peas, low-fat or non-fat dairy products, and lean meats, chicken, and fish.

A multiple vitamin-mineral supplement that provides between 100% and 300% of the USRDA for all vitamins and minerals, especially vitamin A and the antioxidant nutrients, as well as regular exercise, effective stress management, avoidance of alcohol, and limited exposure to air pollution and other toxic environmental gases are important considerations. Avoidance of tobacco and secondhand smoke is one of the most important contributors to the prevention and treatment of lung and respiratory disorders.

LUPUS ERYTHEMATOSUS

Overview

Lupus erythematosus or lupus is one of a number of autoimmune diseases (auto = self) characterized by a defect in the immune system and an accumulation of white blood cells that attack the body, rather than attacking foreign invaders such as a virus or bacteria.

Nutrition and Lupus Erythematosus

VITAMIN E. Tissue destruction in lupus results from free radical damage to cell membranes and might be a result of an actual or relative deficiency of the antioxidant vitamin E. Improvement in symptoms, including reduced inflammation of the skin and sensitivity to sunlight, are reported when people with lupus consume between 800 IU and 2,000 IU of natural vitamin E (d-alpha tocopheryl acetate or d-alpha tocopheryl succinate) daily. Doses of 300 IU or below appear to have no effect on immune function and the treatment of lupus.

Supplemental iron and estrogen therapy reduce vitamin E's effectiveness. Vitamin E should not be taken in large doses for the treatment of lupus without the supervision of a physician.

VITAMIN A. Vitamin A supplementation might improve the immune response and resistance to colds and infection in patients with lupus.

Dietary Recommendations

A low-fat, high-fiber, nutrient-dense diet should be consumed, adequate in all vitamins and minerals and low in sugars and refined and convenience foods. The diet should contain a variety of fruits, vegetables, whole grain breads and cereals, cooked dried beans and peas, low-fat or non-fat dairy products, and lean meats, chicken, and fish.

A multiple vitamin-mineral supplement and a vitamin E supplement, as well as regular exercise, effective stress management, avoidance of alcohol and tobacco, and frequent monitoring of the disease by a physician are important in the treatment of lupus.

OSTEOMALACIA

Overview

Osteomalacia or adult rickets is a bone disorder characterized by softening and deformities of the bones of the legs and arms, spine, thorax, and pelvis and caused by inadequate intake of calcium or vitamin D. The condition results from loss of minerals from the bones called *demineralization*. Rickets is the childhood form of osteomalacia. It is characterized by severely bowed legs or knock knees, malformed rib cage called pigeon breast, delayed growth, delayed eruption of and malformed teeth, and in infants, an enlarged head.

Osteomalacia is most common in women with multiple pregnancies and chronic calcium and vitamin D deficiency or in women who avoid sunlight or are heavily clothed. Elderly people living alone are at risk for developing osteomalacia because of poor diet, inadequate exposure to sunlight, limited ability to produce vitamin D, and limited intake of vitamin D-rich foods.

Osteomalacia is often confused with osteoporosis, but there are distinct differences between these two bone disorders. In osteomalacia, people complain of chronic pain and muscle weakness, whereas pain is usually associated only with bone fractures, while muscle weakness is uncommon in osteoporosis. Bone fractures are uncommon, but deformities of the bones are very common in osteomalacia; the opposite is true in osteoporosis. Finally, people with osteomalacia respond quickly to vitamin D therapy, while the vitamin produces little response in people with osteoporosis (Table 33).

Table 33.
SYMPTOMS AND DIAGNOSIS OF OSTEOPOROSIS AND OSTEOMALACIA

Symptoms	Osteoporosis	Osteomalacia
Skeletal pain	Periodic, usually associated with a fracture	Chronic, major complaint
Muscle weakness	Uncommon	Usually present, often produces disability or unusual gait
Fractures	Common	Uncommon
Skeletal deformity	Occurs with fractures	Common
Loss of bone density	Occurs in most bones	Infrequent or only in spine
Blood levels of calcium/phosphorus	Normal	Low
Blood levels of alkaline phosphatase	Normal	High
Urinary excretion of calcium	Normal or high	Low

Nutrition and Osteomalacia

A poor diet that contains marginal amounts of calcium and vitamin D over long periods of time is usually the cause of osteomalacia. In some cases, poor absorption or use of these two nutrients increases the daily requirement above the recommended dietary allowances. Osteomalacia is rare in people who are physically active, spend time in the sunlight, and eat a well-balanced diet. One dietary survey found that older adults consume daily only 88 IU of vitamin D, or less than half the RDA. Those who supplemented their diet had higher blood levels of vitamin D and a reduced rate of bone loss than did those who did not take a vitamin D supplement.

Dietary Recommendations

A low-fat, high-fiber, nutrient-dense diet should be consumed, adequate in all vitamins and minerals and low in sugars and refined and convenience foods. The diet should contain a variety of fruits, vegetables, whole grain breads and cereals, cooked dried beans and peas, calcium and vitamin D-rich dairy products, such as milk and lean meats, chicken, and fish.

A multiple vitamin-mineral supplement that contains vitamin D and a calcium supplement might be necessary if dietary intake is not optimal. Regular exercise, effective stress management, avoidance of alcohol and tobacco, and moderate exposure to sunshine are important for the prevention and treatment of osteomalacia.

OSTEOPOROSIS

Overview

Osteoporosis is a degenerative bone disease characterized by long-term loss of calcium from the bones, especially the bones of the jaw, spine, pelvis, and the long bones of legs. The bones gradually become porous, brittle, and break easily. The humped posture common in people with osteoporosis is called dowager's hump and also results from changes in the spine as the bones deteriorate and compress. The brittle bones in the legs, pelvis, or arms are susceptible to fracture and seemingly harmless movements, such as coughing, walking down stairs, or receiving a strong hug, can cause them to break. In some cases, the first sign of osteoporosis is a bone fracture. Loss of bone tissue in the jaw causes problems with teeth and dentures and can result in limited food intake and malnutrition (see Table 33).

Nutrition and Osteoporosis

For every man who develops osteoporosis, eight women develop the bone disease. Women are at particular risk for developing osteoporosis because of their lifestyle and dietary habits as well as their small body size relative to men. Women are more likely than men to follow calorie-restricted weight loss diets that contain inadequate amounts of nutrients, especially calcium and vitamin D. A diet of less than 1,600 calories, the average calorie intake of women in the United States, is likely to be low in several vitamins and minerals associated with the development and maintenance of bone density. For example, loss of bone density in women is associated with a calcium intake 50% below the RDA of 800 mg/day. Frequent consumption of diet soft drinks that contain phosphoric acid and avoidance of dairy products that contain calcium and vitamin D upsets the ratio of calcium to phosphorus intake and contributes to calcium loss from bones. High intakes of caffeinated beverages, such as coffee and cola drinks, increase the loss of calcium in the urine and might contribute to bone loss. Regular exercise that places pressure on the bones, such as walking, jogging, or jumping rope, increases bone density and discourages bone loss; whereas inactivity results in calcium loss from bones and an increased risk for developing osteoporosis. Finally, women's bones, in general, are smaller than men's bones and less calcium loss is required before signs of osteoporosis develop.

VITAMIN D. Vitamin D is essential to the absorption of dietary calcium from the intestine and deposition of calcium into bone. A long-term deficiency of this fat-soluble vitamin is associated with calcium loss and bone deterioration. However, reports are mixed on whether vitamin D supplementation is effective in the treatment of osteoporosis. Blood levels of vitamin D are low in people with osteoporosis, suggesting a reduced production of the vitamin. The ability to manufacture vitamin D in the skin when exposed to sunlight might be reduced as a person ages and the need to depend on dietary sources of the vitamin is even more important than in previous years.

VITAMIN B$_6$. Vitamin B$_6$ might aid in the healing of bones after a fracture. A deficiency of this B vitamin results in reduced bone density and width.

CALCIUM. Osteoporosis might be a preventable disease, if adequate calcium intake is maintained throughout life. Calcium intake is important during childhood and adolescence to develop strong, dense bones. Calcium intake during the middle years, when calcium loss from bones exceeds calcium gain, is important to slow the rate of bone loss. Calcium intake during and after menopause is essential to prevent the development of rapid bone loss associated with the advanced stages of osteoporosis.

The adult Recommended Dietary Allowance (RDA) for calcium of 800 mg/day might not be adequate to prevent osteoporosis and it is recommended that premenopausal women consume 1,000 mg daily. Postmenopausal women who are not on estrogen therapy might require as much as 1,500 mg to 1,700 mg of calcium daily. Estrogen therapy aids in the prevention of bone loss in postmenopausal women and 1,000 mg to 1,500 mg of calcium combined with estrogen replacement therapy has been shown effective in the prevention of osteoporosis. However, the use of estrogen is controversial as some studies show no benefits to its use in the treatment of osteoporosis and the hormone is linked to an increased risk for cancer. Currently, a combination of progesterone and estrogen with calcium supplementation is used to treat osteoporosis, while minimizing the estrogen-induced risk for cancer.

Adequate calcium intake might help regenerate bone tissue in people with osteoporosis. Restoration and maintenance of bone tissue is observed in people who consume, over several years, a high-calcium diet plus 750 mg of calcium/day from calcium supplements and 375 IU/day of vitamin D.

COPPER. A long-term copper deficiency results in reduced bone formation and bone deformities, possibly from the trace mineral's effect on the protein webbing that forms the matrix for calcium and other minerals in bone tissue. Calcium loss from the bones also is associated with a copper deficiency.

FLUORIDE. People who live in areas of the country where the water contains fluoride have a lower incidence of osteoporosis than people who do not consume a regular source of fluoride. However, other studies show that fluoride consumption at the level of 80 mg of sodium fluoride each day might increase the risk for hairline fractures in the bones of postmenopausal women with osteoporosis.

MAGNESIUM. Magnesium is important in the development and maintenance of strong bones. Pregnant animals who consume a magnesium-deficient diet give birth to offspring with bone deformities. The magnesium content of osteoporotic bone is altered from that of healthy bones. Bone formation also depends on the ratio of calcium and magnesium and a deficiency of either mineral could result in reduced deposition of calcium into bones and poor formation of bones. How a magnesium deficiency affects bone loss and the effectiveness of magnesium supplementation in the prevention and treatment of osteoporosis is unclear.

MANGANESE. A long term deficiency of manganese is associated with calcium loss from bone, possibly because of the trace mineral's role in bone metabolism. Manganese might be essential for skeletal growth and maintenance.

Dietary Recommendations

Calcium intake should meet or exceed the RDAs throughout life. At least three servings a day of calcium-rich dairy products, such as non-fat or low-fat milk, low-fat cheese, or low-fat yogurt, plus a variety of nutrient-rich foods, such as dark green leafy vegetables, cooked dried beans and peas, and whole grain breads and cereals, should be consumed daily to supply the 1,000 mg to 1,500 mg of calcium recommended to prevent osteoporosis. Fortified non-fat or low-fat milk is the only reliable source of vitamin D; one quart provides 400 IU, the RDA for children and adolescents and three cups provides 300 IU, the RDA for adults. A calcium supplement should be used if calorie restriction or aversion to milk products prevents adequate consumption of calcium from the diet. A well-chosen multiple vitamin-mineral supplement provides adequate amounts of most nutrients, including vitamin D, but does not supply the RDA for magnesium or calcium. Separate mineral preparations might be required to meet the daily need for these nutrients if the diet is poor (Table 34).

Table 34.
HOW TO INCREASE CALCIUM IN THE DIET

- Add non-fat milk powder to casseroles, soups, meatloaf, cheese sauces, or milkshakes.
- Add non-fat milk powder to recipes for French toast, muffins, dips, puddings, pie fillings, homemade breads, mashed potatoes, creamy salad dressings, or creamed soups.
- Cook rice, hot cereals, or other grains in milk.
- Use non-fat or low-fat yogurt as a partial substitute for sour cream in recipes.
- Combine non-fat or low-fat milk with non-fat milk powder in recipes.
- Use low-fat cheeses with fruit and crackers for snacks.
- Increase the daily consumption of calcium-rich foods of plant origin (broccoli, dark green leafy vegetables, or soy products).

In addition, regular weight-bearing exercise, avoidance of alcohol and tobacco, effective coping skills for stress, limited intake of caffeine-containing beverages, and moderate but not excessive intake of protein are important in the prevention and treatment of osteoporosis.

PREMENSTRUAL SYNDROME (PMS)

Overview

Premenstrual syndrome (PMS) is a variety of physical and psychological changes that develop before the beginning of menstruation. More than 150 symptoms, including mood disturbances, water retention, breast soreness, and changes in eating patterns, are attributed to this disorder.

The causes of PMS are unclear; however, the disorder probably results from a complex interaction between hormones, chemicals called *neurotransmitters* that regulate nerves, stress, and dietary factors. Several lifestyle factors, such as a sedentary lifestyle, a diet high in sugar and fat, consumption of alcohol and caffeine, and stress might increase the severity of PMS symptoms.

Nutrition and Premenstrual Syndrome

Generally poor dietary intake is associated with an increased risk for developing symptoms of PMS. Women with PMS tend to have poor dietary habits; they consume more refined sugars and starch and consequently less B vitamins and trace minerals, such as iron, manganese, and zinc, than do women who are symptom-free. The cravings for sweets characteristic of PMS might result from fluctuations in blood sugar and insulin levels common during menstruation.

A possible link between specific vitamin-mineral deficiencies and PMS might exist. For example, vitamin A and zinc show promise in reducing the symptoms of PMS. Dietary treatment of PMS has not produced consistent results, however, and many times, regardless of the nutrient, both the group on the supplement and the group on a placebo (a pill that contains no active ingredient) report improvements in symptoms. This suggests that psychological factors might have a greater effect on the development and treatment of PMS than does diet.

VITAMIN B$_6$. A deficiency of vitamin B$_6$ appears to be a contributing factor in the development of PMS. Vitamin B$_6$ is a necessary nutrient in the manufacture of certain chemicals called neurotransmitters that regulate nerve function. These neurotransmitters, in particular serotonin and dopamine, direct mood, water balance, memory, and sleep. It has been speculated, but not proven, that the fluctuations in the female hormones progesterone and estrogen prior to the onset of menstruation cause a temporary deficiency of vitamin B$_6$. This deficiency reduces the manufacture and activity of the neurotransmitters and results in some of the symptoms of PMS. In support of this theory, symptoms such as headaches, water retention, bloating, depression, and irritability are reduced when vitamin B$_6$ is increased in the diets of some PMS patients.

Limited evidence shows that consumption of 50 mg of vitamin B$_6$ throughout the month and increased doses prior to menstruation cause estrogen levels in the blood to drop, progesterone levels to rise, and symptoms of PMS to vanish. Symptoms responsive to vitamin B$_6$ supplementation include depression, irritability, tension, breast tenderness, water retention, bloating, headaches, and acne. Vitamin B$_6$ also aids in the regulation of magnesium levels in the blood and a deficiency of the vitamin might alter magnesium status and result in temporary symptoms of deficiency that resemble PMS symptoms. The evidence linking a deficiency of vitamin B_6 with PMS is preliminary and limited and some studies have found no association between the vitamin and the disorder.

VITAMIN E. Breast tenderness during PMS might be reduced with vitamin E supplementation; however, the evidence is limited and inconclusive.

MAGNESIUM. Low blood levels of magnesium are found in women during PMS. Headache, dizziness, and craving for sweets sometimes respond to an increased dietary intake of magnesium. Whether this change in blood levels of magnesium is a result of a magnesium deficiency, changes in hormones, or a temporary deficiency of vitamin B_6 is unclear.

Dietary Recommendations

No specific dietary recommendations have been established. In general, a low-fat, high-fiber, nutrient-dense diet should be consumed, adequate in all vitamins and minerals and low in sugars and refined and convenience foods. The daily diet should contain a variety of fruits; vegetables; whole grain breads and cereals; cooked dried beans and peas; low-fat or non-fat dairy products; lean meats, chicken, and fish; several glasses of water; and one to two tablespoons of safflower oil. Caffeine should be avoided by people who experience anxiety and breast tenderness. Salt and salty foods should be limited for people who experience fluid retention.

A multiple vitamin-mineral supplement that contains vitamin B_6 as well as other vitamins and minerals, regular exercise, effective stress management, avoidance of alcohol and tobacco, and an adequate amount of sleep are important in the prevention and treatment of PMS.

PSORIASIS

Overview

Psoriasis is an inflammatory skin disorder characterized by dry, red skin patches covered with silvery white scales. Small spots of bleeding appear under the sores. Psoriasis can be a chronic or sporadic condition.

Nutrition and Psoriasis

A very low-fat, moderately low-protein diet is effective for the treatment of psoriasis in some people. The diet is difficult to follow, however, and long-term compliance is poor; psoriatic symptoms reappear upon return of normal eating habits. Dr. Kempner's Rice Diet, developed in the 1940s and used as a therapeutic diet for patients with certain degenerative diseases, also might be effective in the treatment of psoriasis. People with psoriasis who are unresponsive to medication or ointments report improvement in symptoms when they consume the Rice Diet.

VITAMIN D. Vitamin D might be helpful in the treatment of psoriasis. Three in four people reported improvements within 3 months after taking a daily vitamin D supplement or using a lotion that contained vitamin D.

LINOLEIC ACID. Inadequate dietary intake or poor absorption of the essential fatty acid called linoleic acid, found in vegetable oils, nuts, and seeds, might contribute to the outbreak and severity of psoriasis. Increased intake of this nutrient might improve symptoms. Safflower oil is high in linoleic acid.

ZINC. Zinc losses through the skin might be higher in people with psoriasis than in healthy people. Zinc is necessary for the absorption of linoleic acid, a nutrient suspected to cause or worsen the symptoms of psoriasis when deficient in the diet. It is speculated that a zinc deficiency might increase the likelihood of a linoleic acid deficiency and subsequent outbreaks of psoriasis.

FISH OILS. Fish oils have been used with some success in the treatment of psoriasis. The signs and symptoms of psoriasis improve when patients with active outbreaks of psoriasis are placed on a daily supplement of fish oil for several months. The reason for the improvement in psoriasis symptoms is probably because of the effect fish oils have on the production of chemicals called *leukotrienes* that regulate inflammation. Leukotrienes affect the development and progression of psoriasis and reducing their production might be beneficial in the treatment of this skin disorder. The omega 3 fatty acids found in fish oils lower blood levels of leukotrienes, which slows or stops the process of inflammation.

Dietary Recommendations

Kempner's Rice Diet consists of 10 ounces of dry rice cooked, small amounts of sugar, and fresh or preserved fruit, supplemented with a multiple vitamin-mineral preparation. Use of this diet should be monitored by a physician or dietitian as the diet is extremely imbalanced; lacks adequate amounts of numerous nutrients, such as protein, vitamin A, vitamin C, the B vitamins, and trace minerals; and cannot be expected to sustain life for long-periods of time.

No specific diet has been developed to prevent or treat psoriasis. In general, a nutritious diet such as a low-fat, high-fiber, nutrient-dense diet should be consumed, adequate in all vitamins and minerals and low in sugars, refined and convenience foods, and fats, especially saturated fats. The diet should contain a variety of fruits, vegetables, whole grain breads and cereals, cooked dried beans and peas, low-fat or non-fat dairy products, frequent servings of water, one to two tablespoons of safflower oil, and lean meats, chicken, and fish.

A multiple vitamin-mineral supplement that contains vitamin D and zinc, as well as regular exercise; effective stress management; avoidance of alcohol, caffeine, and tobacco; and compliance with prescribed medications or ointments might be important for the prevention and treatment of psoriasis.

SICKLE CELL ANEMIA

Sickle cell anemia is an inherited disorder characterized by crescent-shaped rather than the normal kidney-shaped red blood cells. The abnormal cells block the flow of blood to tissues and cause severe pain, growth retardation, liver damage, hepatitis, jaundice, gallstones, and kidney failure.

The treatment for sickle cell anemia centers around reducing the symptoms of pain. The excess accumulation of iron characteristic of this disorder requires a reduction in iron intake and avoidance of iron-rich foods for some people; however, some sickle cell patients are iron-deficient. The diet should be high in folic acid, zinc, vitamin B_2, and possibly vitamin E. Improvements in growth rate, pain, and frequency of infections are noted when children with sickle cell anemia are given a multiple vitamin-mineral preparation that contains zinc, iron, folic acid, and vitamin E. Blood levels of vitamin C are low in people with sickle cell anemia and supplementation with the vitamin might protect red blood cells from free radical damage and prolong red blood cell lifespan.

STRESS

Overview

Stress is the body's response to any demand, such as hunger, a telephone ringing, an unexpected tap on the shoulder, a death in the family, divorce, or a car accident. Stress cannot be avoided and positive stress can encourage a person to strive and achieve goals. Harmful stress is called *distress* and can cause anxiety, nutrient deficiencies, and emotional or physical disease. Diseases related to stress include atherosclerosis and heart disease, high blood pressure, obesity, peptic ulcer, and asthma. In many cases, these diseases are preventable when effective coping skills and guidelines for a well-balanced diet are followed.

Nutrition and Stress

Stress and nutrition are related. First, a nutrient deficiency is a stress in itself. Second, how well stress is handled is related to how well the body is nourished. Stress and its widespread effects on body chemistry and functions can interfere with digestion and reduce nutrient absorption and retention. A well-nourished individual is better equipped to cope with stress than is a poorly-nourished individual. Even a diet that contains marginal amounts of one or more nutrients can produce a deficiency when the compounding burden of stress is present. Third, adequate intake of vitamins and minerals is important in preventing the loss of nutrient stores within the body. A tension-filled day increases losses of several nutrients in the urine, and blood levels of many vitamins and minerals are also low during times of stress.

Finally, vitamins and minerals are important contributors to the immune response, the system that defends the body against infection and disease. The body's response to stress includes release of several hormones that suppress the immune response and increase the body's susceptibility to infection. Adequate intake of the vitamins and minerals, such as vitamin A, the B vitamins, vitamin C, and the trace minerals, that maintain a strong defense system stimulates the formation and activity of antibodies, white blood cells, and other aspects of the immune system. Body stores of these nutrients are less likely to be depleted and the immune system is less likely to be jeopardized if nutrient intake is adequate prior to and during times of stress.

Diet appears to make a difference in the body's ability to handle stress. People who consume a diet low in refined carbohydrates, sugar, and caffeine and high in whole grain breads and cereals and other nutritious foods showed greater improvement in their ability to cope with stress as compared to individuals who consume their normal diets with sugar or caffeine.

B VITAMINS. The B complex vitamins are needed for the maintenance of the nervous system. Diets high in sugars and other refined carbohydrates require B vitamins to adequately process these foods for energy. These foods do not supply ample amounts of these nutrients, however, and can cause a relative deficiency. A low intake of the B vitamins or the relative deficiency caused by consuming a nutrient-poor diet can alter nerve function and increase the symptoms of stress, such as depression and irritability.

VITAMIN C. The vitamin C content of stress-related tissues, such as the pituitary and adrenal glands, is reduced during stress. The reduced body stores are a result of either poor dietary intake or increased daily need for vitamin C during times of stress. During physical stress and heart attack vitamin C levels drop in the blood. Increased intake of vitamin C during times of stress might reduce the harmful effects of the stress hormones, such as adrenaline, and improve the body's ability to cope with the stress response.

MAGNESIUM. Magnesium stores are depleted and large amounts of the mineral are lost in the urine during times of stress. Some of the symptoms of stress, including stimulation of the nervous system, are reduced when blood levels of this mineral are normal to high and are accented in the presence of a magnesium deficiency. Animals fed a magnesium-deficient diet react violently to previously well-tolerated noise; consuming adequate amounts of magnesium prior to and during the stressful noise reduces the stress reaction. Hospitalized patients who experience physical and emotional stress are often low in magnesium, which might contribute to the stress reaction and interfere with optimal recovery.

ZINC. People in physical stress, such as hospitalized patients, often are deficient in zinc. The zinc deficiency interferes with the body's ability to recuperate from illness and might contribute to chronic leg ulcers, infection, and secondary diseases. The physical stress of strenuous exercise might increase urinary loss of zinc and other trace minerals, such as chromium and copper, and alter blood levels of these minerals. Whether these changes increase the daily requirement for the trace minerals is unknown.

Dietary Recommendations

No specific dietary recommendations have been established for people during stress. In general, a low-fat, high-fiber, nutrient-dense diet should be consumed, adequate in all vitamins and minerals and low in sugars and refined and convenience foods. The diet should contain a variety of fruits, vegetables, whole grain breads and cereals, cooked dried beans and peas, low-fat or non-fat dairy products, several glasses of water, and lean meats, chicken, and fish.

A multiple vitamin-mineral supplement that contains between 100% and 300% of the USRDA for the B vitamins, vitamin C, magnesium, and the trace minerals, as well as regular exercise, effective stress management, avoidance of alcohol and tobacco, and avoidance of caffeine-containing beverages, such as coffee and cola drinks, are important practices prior to and during times of stress.

THYROID DISORDERS

Overview

The most pronounced symptom of thyroid malfunction is enlargement of the thyroid gland or goiter, also called *endemic goiter*. The thyroid gland enlarges in an attempt to maintain normal function despite an insufficient supply of iodine necessary for thyroxine production.

Nutrition and Thyroid Disorders

Poor dietary intake of iodine results in goiter in adults and if the diet is low in iodine during pregnancy, the baby will be born with a condition called *cretinism*. In addition, excessive consumption of foods containing goitrogens, such as cabbage, soybeans, and turnips, reduces the absorption of iodine and increases the risk of developing goiter.

ZINC. Significant changes in how the body uses and stores zinc are present in patients with thyroid disease. It is unknown whether these imbalances are caused by dietary deficiency or result from the disease.

Dietary Recommendations

Daily consumption of iodine-containing foods or iodized salt, especially if a person lives in the goiter belt (the northern states, the states bordering on the Great Lakes, the New England states, and portions of the central-western states, such as Nevada, Colorado, and Arizona) where the iodine in foods and water is low, will prevent goiter and cretinism. People who live in coastal regions obtain iodine from fresh fish and shellfish and produce grown locally.

CHAPTER 6

How Medications, Alcohol, and Tobacco Affect Vitamin and Mineral Status

OVERVIEW

From the superstitions of primitive cultures to the high technology of today's medical system, medication has had a primary role in the patient's care. More than 1.51 billion prescription drugs are dispensed each year and more than 100,000 different medications are available in the United States. The widespread use of prescription and non-prescription medications, also called over-the-counter or OTC drugs, coupled with the increasing interest in nutrition and diet, has encouraged research into the interactions between diet and drugs.

Prescription and nonprescription medications can alter vitamin and mineral status in four ways: 1) medications can increase or decrease appetite and alter the amount of vitamins and minerals consumed, 2) reduce vitamin and mineral absorption even with adequate intake, 3) alter how a nutrient is used by the body, and 4) increase vitamin and mineral excretion so even if dietary intake and absorption is adequate the nutrient is not retained in the body. The result is possible marginal, and sometimes clinical, vitamin and mineral deficiencies.

Some medications increase and other medications decrease appetite and food intake. Examples of appetite-stimulating medications are some antidepressants and certain antihistamines. Many of these drugs stimulate appetite by improving a person's mental status or emotional stability. Other medications reduce appetite by their effects on the central nervous system; by direct irritant action on the stomach and small intestine causing nausea, discomfort, constipation or diarrhea, and vomiting; or by altering taste. Amphetamines act on the central nervous system and reduce the desire to eat. Some medications reduce appetite by altering the sense of taste and smell, reduce saliva and cause a dry mouth, cause stomach or intestinal irritation, produce nausea and vomiting, or reduce the desire to eat. The reduced desire to eat increases the likelihood of poor food and nutrient intake and vitamin or mineral deficiencies. Medications also reduce food and nutrient intake by altering mood or behavior. In other cases it is not the medication, but the underlying disease or a combination of disease and medication that upsets this balance and causes a loss of appetite.

Medications, vitamins, and minerals are absorbed in the small intestine and can interact to alter the absorption of one another. Some medications bind to a vitamin or mineral in the small intestine and interfere with the nutrient's absorption. For example, mineral oil binds to the fat-soluble vitamins and hinders their absorption. A medication also can alter the shape or function of a vitamin, making it less likely to be absorbed. Other medications increase the speed with which nutrients pass through the small intestine; the reduced contact time vitamins and minerals have with the intestinal wall results in decreased absorption. Some medications physically or chemically block the absorption sites on the wall of the small intestine or alter the absorption sites so the vitamins or minerals cannot pass through. Finally, medications can interfere with the digestive juices required for normal absorption of vitamins and minerals. Medications that change the acidity or pH of the stomach and small intestine will reduce the absorption of vitamins and minerals dependent on normal acidity for absorption. For example, antacids increase the pH to a more alkaline environment in the small intestine and reduce the absorption of iron and calcium. Other medications inhibit the activity of bile salts, digestive juices necessary for normal digestion of the fat-soluble vitamins. Other medications alter the digestive juices produced by the pancreas.

Prescription and nonprescription medications alter how the body uses vitamins or minerals in a variety of ways. Certain medications change specific requirements for vitamins and minerals by altering absorption, availability, storage, and use of the nutrient. Some

226 THE ESSENTIAL GUIDE TO VITAMINS AND MINERALS

medications are shaped chemically similar to a vitamin, but have no vitamin activity. In the body, these medications are mistaken for the vitamin and block the real vitamin from entering into normal body processes. The vitamin is available but inaccessible, and symptoms of a marginal deficiency develop. Other medications alter the storage sites for vitamins and minerals. For example, oral contraceptives affect the distribution or possibly decrease blood levels of vitamin B_{12} in the body. Other medications bind to the biologically active portion of an enzyme where a vitamin normally would attach. The body mistakes the unattached vitamin for an excess of the nutrient and excretes it in the urine, the medication-bound enzyme cannot function, and all body processes depending on the enzyme are stopped. An example of this medication-nutrient interaction is vitamin B_6 and oral contraceptives. The effects of this medication-induced vitamin deficiency are subtle and can cause emotional disturbances, altered sleep, irritability, lethargy, and reduced resistance to infection and disease.

Diuretics, laxatives, and cathartics are examples of medications that increase the excretion of vitamins and minerals and if used in excess could result in nutrient deficiencies. Minerals are most susceptible to this form of medication-nutrient interaction. The absorption, use, and excretion of minerals in the body depend on a delicate balance; a medication that interferes with one mineral will probably upset the status of other minerals. It is common for an individual to take more than one medication at a time and the combined effects of these medications might result in numerous changes in mineral status.

Medication-nutrient interactions might result in, or increase, a vitamin deficiency. This interaction occurs at a time when optimal nutritional status is important to a person's health and recovery from disease. In addition, these marginal nutrient deficiencies produce subtle symptoms, such as depression or reduced resistance to infection, that proceed unnoticed or are excused as a side-effect of the disease or medication.

Note: Eating patterns and nutrients also can decrease or increase the therapeutic effectiveness of many prescription or nonprescription medication. These nutrient-drug interactions are usually listed with the medication's accompanying literature or are explained by your physician or pharmacist.

WHO IS AT RISK FOR DEVELOPING MEDICATION-INDUCED VITAMIN AND MINERAL DEFICIENCIES?

A person who is well-nourished, with optimal amounts of vitamin and minerals stored in the body, who has no problems with digestion and absorption of food, who has consumed a nutritious diet prior to and during illness, and who must take a prescription or nonprescription medication for only a short time is at low risk for developing medication-induced nutrient deficiencies. In contrast, malnutrition and marginal vitamin and mineral deficiencies are most likely to develop in people on long-term medication therapy, especially if they consume a nutrient-poor diet. In particular, the elderly, children, alcoholics, and people who are chronically ill are the most vulnerable to medication-induced nutrient deficiencies. Poor vitamin and mineral status, however, can result from a variety of factors, including poor dietary intake of nutrients prior to the onset of disease and medication therapy. Malnutrition is less likely to develop if the long-term diet contains a variety of fresh and nutritious foods. Everyone, however, should begin preventive and rehabilitative dietary measures and should monitor nutritional status while taking prescription and nonprescription medications.

Seniors

Seniors account for the highest sales of prescription and nonprescription medications; more than 80% of these older adults use more than two medications daily and 61% take nonprescription medications. Many older people are at risk for vitamin and mineral deficiencies, even if they are not taking medications. The added stress of long-term use of one or more medications, coupled with poor dietary habits, chronic disease, and reduced ability to absorb and use vitamins and minerals places this segment of the population at high risk for drug-induced nutrient deficiencies. In addition, limited income, reduce mobility or access to nutritious foods and food preparation, special diets, reduced appetite, disinterest in food, and oral and dental problems also contribute to poor dietary intake and increase risk for developing vitamin and mineral deficiencies. Finally, living alone, loneliness, and social isolation can jeopardize nutritional status.

Problem Drinkers

Alcohol is the number one cause of malnutrition in people who are otherwise disease-free. Abuse of alcohol results in loss of appetite and reduced food and nutrient intake, especially the B vitamins, the trace mineral zinc, and protein. Alcohol damages the lining of the small intestine and reduces the absorption of nutrients. Deficiencies of several vitamins and minerals are common in people who abuse alcohol. Vitamin and mineral deficiencies also develop secondary to alcohol-induced disorders, including inflammation of the stomach, intestine, pancreas, or liver; lactose intolerance; and cirrhosis of the liver.

People with Long-Term Illness

Medication-induced vitamin and mineral deficiencies might develop in people with long-term diseases, such as cancer, diabetes, epilepsy, disorders of the gastrointestinal tract, behavioral or emotional disorders, or heart and blood vessel diseases. Nutrient deficiencies are possible because of long-term exposure to medication and the likelihood of multiple medication therapy. Dosage also contributes to the potential for nutrient deficiencies; a high-dose medication taken over long periods is more likely to cause vitamin and mineral deficiencies than a low-dose over a short time. This dose effect also holds true for nonprescription medications, such as laxatives and aspirin.

Nutrient depletion of tissues, as a result of the disease or the medication, is gradual and often goes undetected until nutrient stores are exhausted. Preventive measures to maintain or replenish nutrient stores are essential as long-term medication therapy might threaten nutritional health.

People with Increased Vitamin and Mineral Needs or Decreased Vitamin and Mineral Intakes

People on weight reduction diets or calorie/food restricted diets; adolescents who eat sporadically, but have high vitamin and mineral requirements; and pregnant and breastfeeding women are at risk for medication-induced vitamin and mineral deficiencies. People in these groups often are marginally nourished because of restricted food intake, reliance on high calorie-low nutrient foods, or increased need for vitamins and minerals. The poor dietary intake coupled with long-term use of medications increases the possibility of malnutrition.

SPECIFIC MEDICATIONS AND OTHER SUBSTANCES: EFFECTS ON VITAMIN AND MINERAL STATUS

Alcohol

Chronic or abusive alcohol consumption predisposes the drinker to malnutrition in several ways. First, alcohol supplies between 10% and 20% of the calories in the diet of the average person, but provides little or no other nutrients and requires additional vitamins, such as vitamin B_1, vitamin B_6, biotin, and niacin, for its detoxification in the liver. For example, vitamin E and other antioxidant nutrients are needed to repair the tissue damage from alcohol, and vitamin C, folic acid, vitamin B_{12}, and vitamin B_6 are needed to build new tissue. The body functions in a deficit without adequate amounts of these nutrients. Although beer and wine contain some vitamins and minerals, the amounts are minute (i.e., the nutrient content of 1 ounce of bread exceeds the nutrient content of 12 ounces of beer). The calories from alcohol either replace more nutritious foods or are supplied in addition to a day's allotment of calories. Whether it is nutrient deficiencies or obesity, malnutrition can result.

Second, alcohol irritates the stomach, pancreas, and intestine, and inhibits absorption of vitamin C, vitamin B_1, vitamin B_{12}, folic acid, the fat-soluble vitamins, calcium, and other nutrients. A cycle might develop where poor absorption of nutrients results in malnutrition, which further limits absorption of vitamins and minerals and encourages the development of alcohol-related diseases, such as liver disease.

Third, alcohol and its by-products can inhibit the body's ability to use vitamins. Many dietary vitamins must be altered by the liver before they are of use in metabolic reactions. In the presence of excess alcohol, vitamins D, B_1, B_6, and folic acid are not converted to their active forms and deficiency symptoms might develop even if dietary intake is adequate.

Fourth, alcohol sabotages vitamin stores in the body. For example, liver stores of vitamin A are decreased with long-term alcohol intake. Alcoholism also depletes the body's store and blood levels of antioxidant nutrients, such as selenium and vitamin E. Selenium deficiency can cause liver damage similar to that seen in alcoholism. This effect on antioxidant nutrients might leave the body defenseless against damage from highly reactive substances called *free radicals* that are linked to the development of cancer and premature aging. Low blood selenium levels are found in alcoholics despite adequate selenium intake, which suggests an increased requirement for the trace mineral when alcohol is consumed. However, it is not known whether supplementation with these nutrients would halt or retard the damage induced by alcohol. (See pages 126–128 for more information on antioxidants and free radicals.)

Fifth, alcohol increases urinary loss of some nutrients, such as magnesium, potassium and zinc, and is associated with reduced tissue levels of several vitamins and minerals. In particular, a zinc deficiency might initiate a cycle where the alcohol-induced zinc deficiency then encourages excessive consumption of alcohol. In studies on animals, excessive alcohol consumption stops when animals are fed a diet high in zinc.

The best treatment for malnutrition caused by abuse of alcohol is to stop drinking and consume a diet rich in vitamins and minerals and low in fat. Supplements cannot protect the body from the toxic effects of alcohol and cannot prevent the formation of scar tissue or fatty infiltration of the liver. However, they might help minimize the long-term nutritional consequences. The vitamins and minerals most likely to be depleted with alcohol abuse are folic acid, vitamin B_1, vitamin B_6, vitamin C, vitamin A, vitamin D, vitamin B_{12}, calcium, iron, magnesium, potassium, and zinc.

Antacids

Antacids are sometimes used in excess to minimize the discomfort experienced from the misuse of other dietary substances, such as alcohol or coffee, excessive eating, or to curb the stomach pain from high levels of stomach acid secreted during times of stress. This overuse of antacids might result in vitamin or mineral deficiencies.

Large doses of magnesium and aluminum hydroxides in antacids interfere with the absorption of phosphorus and calcium and might upset the delicate balance between these minerals. The result is that calcium and phosphorus are not deposited properly into bones and there is an increased risk for bone disorders. The risk of antacid-induced bone disease is higher in older people than in other segments of the population because the ability to absorb calcium decreases with age, and older people often do not consume adequate amounts of calcium-rich foods, such as milk, yogurt, cheese, and dark green leafy vegetables. However, they rely heavily on antacids.

Antacids can affect calcium and bone health. Sodium bicarbonate (baking soda) used to buffer stomach acid might increase the risk for calcium deficiency. This possible effect on calcium and bone status is only a concern if sodium bicarbonate is consumed daily and the diet is low in calcium. Aluminum absorption from antacids might be increased when they are consumed with citrus fruits and juices. Aluminum toxicity is associated with damage to the nervous system and bones. However, more information is needed before dietary or medication recommendations can be made.

Mineral and vitamin deficiencies and anemia might develop with overconsumption of antacids. These nonprescription drugs neutralize stomach acid and alter the acidity or pH of the stomach. Nutrients, such as iron, calcium, and vitamin B_{12} are not absorbed well in the more alkaline environment created by antacids. The absorption of folic acid and vitamin A also is reduced with abuse of antacids. Iron, vitamin B_{12}, and folic acid are essential to the formation of red blood cells and reduced dietary intake or excessive or long-term antacid use could result in anemia. Another medication that inhibits the secretion of stomach acid and is used in the treatment of ulcers or "nervous stomach," cimetidine (Tagamet), also reduces the absorption of vitamin B_{12}.

The potential for vitamin or mineral deficiencies varies depending on when the antacids are taken. Aluminum hydroxide antacids should be taken 1 to 2 hours before a meal or before bed to maximize their buffering action on stomach acid in the treatment of ulcers. A larger quantity of antacids is sometimes required in the treatment of duodenal ulcer than is required in stomach ulcers because the patient with duodenal ulcer usually also has excessive secretion of stomach acid. In this case, the antacid is taken when no food is present in the stomach, so the antacid will not interfere with nutrient absorption and is not likely to produce vitamin or mineral deficiencies. When the same medication is taken with meals, the likelihood increases for reduced absorption of calcium, iron, vitamin B_{12}, and folic acid (Table 35). Aluminum hydroxide is particularly effective in neutralizing stomach acid and is often the preferred antacid for the treatment of ulcer; however, it also is most likely to reduce the absorption of phosphorus and other minerals and vitamins. This type of antacid should be consumed between meals if it is taken for long periods of time.

Table 35.
THE EFFECTS OF ANTACIDS ON VITAMINS AND MINERALS

Type Of Antacid	Nutritional Effects
Aluminum hydroxide	Aluminum toxicity, reduced absorption of calcium, iron, and vitamin B_{12}
Aluminum or Magnesium hydroxide	Phosphate depletion, reduced absorption of calcium, iron, and vitamin B_{12}
Magnesium hydroxide	Magnesium overload
Sodium bicarbonate	Sodium overload, Milk-alkali syndrome

Antibiotics

Antibiotics are important in the treatment of infections but might have nutritional side effects. Antibiotics are effective because they interfere with the growth of disease-causing bacteria; however, antibiotics also interfere with bacteria that promote health. Some essential nutrients are produced by bacteria living in the large intestine, and this source of a vitamin or mineral contributes an important proportion of the daily recommended allowance. Antibiotics disturb the normal intestinal bacterial growth and limit or destroy the vitamin-producing bacteria. For example, a deficiency of vitamin K or biotin might result with long-term use of antibiotics.

Long-term use of the antibiotic tetracycline, especially in conjunction with a poor diet, has produced deficiencies of vitamin K and might reduce vitamin C stores in the body. Tetracycline interacts with dietary minerals, such as calcium, iron, and magnesium, and absorption and use of both the medication and the minerals are reduced when these minerals and the medication are consumed at the same meal. Neomycin causes malabsorption of vitamin B_{12}, calcium, iron, and potassium, which is reversed when the medication is discontinued.

Para-aminosalicylic acid (PAS), an antibacterial prescription medication used in the treatment of tuberculosis, alters the absorption of several nutrients, including vitamin B_{12} and folic acid. In some cases, the reduction in vitamin B_{12} absorption results in anemia. The malabsorption of vitamin B_{12} and folic acid is reversible with discontinuation of the medication or with physician-supervised injections of folic acid and vitamin B_{12}.

Antibiotic-induced vitamin and mineral deficiencies are not likely to develop if the diet contains a variety of fresh and nutritious foods prior to and during medication therapy and if the use of antibiotics is temporary.

Anticonvulsants

Anticonvulsant medications are used in the treatment of epileptic seizures and to prevent or treat seizures resulting from head injuries or surgery on the nervous system. Long-term use of the anticonvulsant medications phenytoin (Dilantin), phenobarbital, primidone, or carbamazepine might cause bone disorders, such as rickets in children or osteomalacia in adults. These medications interfere with the manufacture of vitamin D in the body. A person taking anticonvulsants cannot synthesize adequate amounts of this fat-soluble vitamin even with adequate exposure to sunlight. As vitamin D acts as a hormone in the regulation of calcium absorption and use, a deficiency of this vitamin, even with adequate calcium intake, might cause calcium loss from bones and bone deterioration. The severity of these bone changes increases with long-term treatment and large doses of the medication.

More than 15% of people on long-term use of anticonvulsant medications show reduced blood levels of vitamin D and skeletal disease. Because of the high incidence of drug-induced vitamin D deficiency, it is recommended that everyone on long-term anticonvulsant medication therapy take a vitamin D supplement that contains 400 IU to 800 IU of the vitamin or consume 1 quart or more of vitamin D-fortified milk each day.

Long-term use of anticonvulsant medications also might cause deficiencies of the vitamins associated with red blood cell formation and maintenance, which would result in anemia. Phenytoin, phenobarbital, and primidone induce a folic acid deficiency and birth defects in infants born of women on anticonvulsant therapy might be a result of the drug's effect on folic acid. Consumption of large doses of folic acid in an attempt to counteract this deficiency might upset vitamin B_{12} metabolism. Vitamin B_{12} is usually unaffected by anticonvulsant medications, but the increase in red blood cell production stimulated by increased intake of folic acid increases the demand for vitamin B_{12}. The combined deficiency and altered metabolism of these two vitamins results in reduced production of red blood cells and anemia. Vitamin K levels might drop on long-term anticonvulsant therapy, resulting in hemorrhage and blood loss. It is important for a physician to monitor folic acid, vitamin B_{12}, and vitamin K status in patients on anticonvulsant therapy and to prescribe supplements of these nutrients where necessary. Supplements of folic acid should not be taken without the supervision of a physician as large doses of this vitamin might interfere with the effectiveness of the anticonvulsant medication and increase the likelihood of convulsions. Long-term use of anticonvulsants also lowers blood and tissue levels of copper and zinc.

Antidepressants

Long-term use of antidepressant medications and tranquilizers might alter nutrient status because these prescription drugs influence the desire to eat, reduce or increase food intake, and increase vitamin or mineral excretion. Some of the side effects of the antianxiety medications meprobamate, lorazepam, oxazepam, alprazolam, chlordiazepoxide (Librium), and diazepam (Valium) include nausea, vomiting, dry mouth, loss of appetite (anorexia), diarrhea, reduced salivation, and stomach upsets. Any one of these symptoms might reduce appetite or the desire to eat.

The tricyclic antidepressants amitriptyline, imipramine, doxepin, amoxapine, protriptyline, or lithium carbonate and the tranquilizer chlorpromazine increase or decrease appetite and might cause weight gain or weight loss. These drugs also might cause nausea, vomiting, diarrhea, flatulence, peculiar taste sensations, sore mouth, and abdominal cramps; all symptoms that could impair optimal food and nutrient intake. In addition, these medications increase urinary excretion of the B vitamins and vitamin C and alter the body's use of magnesium. For example, diazepam might alter magnesium status and increase the urinary excretion of calcium. Urinary loss of calcium during long-term antidepressant therapy coupled with medication-induced loss of calcium from the bones increase risk for developing bone disorders when taking these medications over long periods of time.

Patients on antidepressants also might need to supplement with B vitamins. One study showed patients on lithium therapy have low blood levels of folic acid, and supplementation in moderate doses (approximately 200 mcg) reduces behavioral problems in these people. However, more information is necessary before dietary recommendations can be made. In one study, patients on the antidepressant phenelzine (Nardil) showed symptoms of vitamin B_6 deficiency, including depression and hyperirritability, that responded to vitamin supplementation. Vitamin B_6 deficiency also might contribute to the pre-existing depression.

The sedative-hypnotic medication glutethimide (Doriden) increases the daily requirement for vitamin D and might cause loss of calcium from the bones and bone disease if large doses are taken over an extended period of time.

The monoamine oxidase inhibitors (MAOI) are used in the treatment of depression, usually for adult patients unresponsive to other antidepressant medication therapies. Acute hypertension (high blood pressure) might occur in people taking MAOIs when foods high in a nonnutritive substance called *tyramine* are consumed. Tyramine-containing foods include aged and fermented foods, such as cheese, yogurt, sour cream, tenderized meats, fermented sausages, pickled herring, beer, red wine, yeast, and soy sauce. Alcohol and caffeine also should be avoided when taking MAOI medications as these substances could cause headaches and other unusual symptoms.

In general, vitamin and mineral deficiencies are unlikely if the diet is adequate in vitamins and minerals prior to and during medication. However, poor diet coupled with long-term or high dosage antidepressant medication therapy might encourage deficiencies.

Arthritis Medications

D-penicillamine (Cuprimine) is used in the treatment of rheumatoid arthritis. Possible side effects resulting from D-penicillamine use that might affect food and nutrient intake include sores and inflammation of the mouth and tongue, loss of appetite, stomach pain, nausea, vomiting, occasional diarrhea, altered taste sensation, ulcer, disorders of the pancreas and liver affecting the release of digestive juices, and inflammation of the large intestine. Loss of appetite might result in weight loss, muscle wastage, and general malnutrition.

D-penicillamine binds to iron, zinc, and other essential dietary minerals. For this reason, this anti-arthritis medication should be taken on an empty stomach, 1 hour before or 2 hours after a meal and at least 1 hour apart from any other medication, food, or beverage other than water. The loss of appetite, hair loss, and skin changes associated with D-penicillamine use might be partially a result of a drug-induced zinc deficiency, as the medication has been shown to reduce absorption of zinc and clinical symptoms of zinc deficiency include these signs. The potential for iron deficiency is also possible, especially in children and in menstruating women. Supplements of iron should be taken in small doses, 2 hours before or after the medication as iron interferes with the effectiveness of the medication.

Long-term use of D-penicillamine increases the daily requirement of vitamin B_6 and supplementation during periods of medication prevents the development of a vitamin deficiency. It is recommended that patients take a supplement containing 25 mg of this B vitamin each day. In Wilson's disease, the supplement must be free of copper as supplemental copper intake could block the action of the medication. Anyone taking D-penicillamine should consult a physician or pharmacist before taking a daily vitamin and mineral supplement.

Aspirin, Pain-Killers, and Anti-Inflammatory Medications

Moderate to excessive use of aspirin causes bleeding in the stomach or intestines in many people. The loss of blood means a loss of iron and iron deficiency can result. People with pre-existing stomach disorders, such as ulcer, are especially susceptible to aspirin-induced blood and iron loss. Deficiencies of folic acid, vitamin C, and potassium and malabsorption of vitamin B_{12} also have been reported in people on long-term large doses of aspirin.

Vitamin A might help prevent stomach ulcers and bleeding in people on long-term medication with aspirin. Moderate intake of vitamin A within the recommended dietary allowance of 4,000 IU to 5,000 IU might be sufficient to prevent stomach disorders induced by low intake of aspirin (325 mg/day). However, more information is necessary before dietary recommendations can be made.

Ibuprofen is both a nonprescription medication (Advil and Nuprin) and a prescription medication (Motrin and Rufen) for the treatment of minor pains and aches. The possible side effects associated with ibuprofen that affect food and nutrient intake include stomach irritation, heartburn, vomiting, nausea, cramps, diarrhea, flatulence, and ulcers. However, these side effects are not common.

The anti-inflammatory medication colchicine is used in the treatment of gout because it reduces the inflammation and pain associated with this joint disorder. Colchicine reduces the absorption of vitamin B_{12}, increases the excretion and tissue loss of calcium and potassium, and reduces the absorption of folic acid. Other side effects that influence the intake of food and nutrients include nausea, vomiting, diarrhea, and abdominal pain, especially when large doses are taken.

The anti-inflammatory medication salicylazosulfapyridine (Azulfidine) decreases the absorption of folic acid and the inclusion of several servings each day of folic-acid rich foods might be necessary to counteract the effects of anti-inflammatory medications on folic acid status.

Cancer Medications

Chemotherapy is the treatment of a disease with chemicals or medication. The term is most commonly used in reference to cancer. Although chemotherapy is an effective therapeutic effort, it has numerous side effects, one of which is nutritional consequences.

The effects of chemotherapeutic agents are not limited to the growth or function of cancer cells, but extend to healthy tissues as well. These toxic effects influence dietary intake and vitamin-mineral status. For example, many chemotherapeutic drugs produce sore or dry mouth, inflammation of the mouth and throat, and altered taste sensation. Nausea and vomiting are common for most chemotherapies. Loss of appetite results from this drug-induced damage to tissues of the mouth, throat, and stomach and the variety and quantity of appealing food choices decreases. The medication 5-fluorouracil alters taste sensations, affects appetite, and produces nutrient deficiencies, including vitamin B_1. The results of these conditions are malnutrition, tissue wastage, and weight loss.

The lining of the intestine is also harmed by some chemotherapies and diarrhea, constipation, or reduced absorption of vitamins and minerals might result. The toxic effects on the stomach and intestine are usually short-term and subside within a few days after each chemotherapy treatment; however, in some cases the damage is severe and prolonged. Some chemotherapies, such as the corticosteroids, damage tissues and cause excessive loss of potassium, calcium, and other minerals in the urine. The vitamin and mineral deficiencies that might result from these medications reduce the effectiveness of the immune system to fight disease, alter mood and behavior resulting in a greater likelihood of depression and sleep abnormalities, and generally are counterproductive to regaining health.

Some chemotherapeutic medications interfere with the use of vitamins within the cells and tissues. For example, methotrexate alters folic acid metabolism. Cells cannot divide and multiply without an available supply of folic acid and they die. Cancer cells multiply more rapidly than healthy cells and are more dependent on the folic acid levels in the body; therefore, a deficiency of this B vitamin affects them most severely. However, all cells in the body are affected by a folic acid deficiency including red blood cells. People on methotrexate therapy should not self-medicate with folic acid supplements without the prior approval of a physician as large doses of this vitamin could alter the effectiveness of the medication therapy.

It is difficult, but possible to maintain adequate vitamin and mineral status during chemotherapy and it is vitally important to the outcome of the treatment. Chemotherapy is most effective when a person is adequately nourished. An adequate supply of all nutrients, including vitamins and minerals, lessens the harmful effects of chemotherapy on healthy tissue and enhances the destruction of cancer cells. Optimal supplies of all vitamins and minerals improves the sense of well-being, preserves healthy tissue function, repairs tissue damage caused by the disease and the chemotherapy, and strengthens the body's natural defense system to fight infection and disease.

In contrast, poor nutrition and inadequate intake of vitamins and minerals are harmful to the outcome of the therapy because a malnourished person has a narrow margin of tolerance to chemotherapy as compared to a well-nourished person. Poor dietary intake of vitamins and minerals and the resultant malnutrition can be the most disabling aspect of cancer. Malnutrition reduces the person's quality of life and contributes to an increased risk for continuation of the disease.

The two goals of nutrition therapy during treatment for cancer are to maintain optimal nutritional status or correct pre-existing deficiencies of vitamins, minerals, and other nutrients and to minimize weight loss resulting from the disease or the medication. The guidelines for meeting these goals must be individualized to the person and should be designed and monitored by a physician and registered dietitian (Table 36, page 238).

Table 36.
NUTRITIONAL GUIDELINES DURING CHEMOTHERAPY

Problem	Diet	Foods To Avoid
Nausea	Choose small, frequent meals. Eat slowly. Chew food well. Eat dry foods (crackers). Drink cold liquids.	Liquids at mealtimes, sweets and fatty foods
Acute stomach or intestine toxicity/pain	Drink clear, cold liquids.	Milk, milk products, soups, cereals, sandwiches
Post-treatment stomach or intestine pain	Choose liquid and soft foods, carbonated beverages, frozen fruit.	Citrus juice, milk, milk products, meat, raw foods
Dry mouth	Choose high-fluid foods: gravies, sauces, soups, casseroles. Drink beverages with meals. Include citrus fruits.	Dry foods, meat, bread products
Reduced taste	Choose a regular diet. Season foods. Choose spicey foods and textured foods with aroma.	Bland foods
No taste	Choose a regular diet of cold foods: milk, milk products. Experiment with different foods and textures.	Red meats, chocolate, coffee
Diarrhea	Choose liquid or soft foods, high-protein and high-calorie foods.	Raw fruits, vegetables, milk, spicy foods
Fullness/Bloating	Take meals with no fluids. Eat slowly Choose easily digested foods and small meals.	Gas-forming foods, fatty foods
Heartburn	Choose small, frequent meals.	Pureed foods, alcohol, coffee, tea, spicy foods, fatty foods

Medications for Cardiovascular Disease and Elevated Blood Cholesterol Levels

Some of the medications used to lower blood cholesterol in the treatment of atherosclerosis and cardiovascular disease (CVD) include cholestyramine, clofibrate, and colestipol. These medications are called cholesterol-lowering agents. Lovastatin, a medication that reduces cholesterol synthesis in the liver, is a new medication for the treatment of CVD. Its nutritional side effects, if any, are unknown.

The cholesterol-lowering medications reduce the absorption of the fat-soluble nutrients, such as the fat-soluble vitamins A, D, E, and K, and the essential fatty acid called linoleic acid. The risk for nutrient deficiencies is high because cholesterol-lowering medications are used for chronic diseases and long-term drug therapy is common. Gradual depletion of body stores of the fat-soluble vitamins resulting from long-term poor absorption of these dietary nutrients could produce night-blindness and increased risk for some forms of cancer in the case of vitamin A, osteomalacia and related bone disorders in the case of vitamin D, and susceptibility to hemorrhage in a vitamin K deficiency. A linoleic acid deficiency produces skin disorders, such as eczema. It is advised that people on long-term medication with lipid-lowering medications take a supplement of vitamins A, D, E, and K in water-soluble form.

Cholestyramine (Questran) also interferes with the absorption of vitamin B_{12}, folic acid, and iron, and chronic use of this cholesterol-lowering medication is associated with low blood levels of folic acid and other nutrients. Long-term medication therapy might result in anemia unless supplementation with these vitamins and iron is combined with the medication therapy. Cholestyramine increases the urinary excretion of calcium, increases blood levels of other fats, called *triglycerides*, and reduces body stores of iron when taken over a long period of time or at high doses. Other possible side effects from long-term use of cholesterol-lowering agents include constipation, abdominal pain, bleeding in the stomach or intestine, belching, flatulence, nausea, vomiting, diarrhea, heartburn, loss of appetite, and steatorrhea (loss of excessive amounts of fat and fatty substances in the stool). Clofibrate causes changes in taste sensation and might reduce the desire to eat.

Colestipol is another medication used in the treatment of elevated blood cholesterol and heart disease. Deficiencies of the fat-soluble vitamins A, D, and E and the B vitamin folic acid are possible when this medication is taken over long periods of time. Vitamin K supplementation also is required, but only in the presence of poor blood clotting and episodes of prolonged bleeding. The effectiveness of colestipol might be increased when it is combined with the B vitamin nicotinic acid (niacin).

Medications classified as calcium-channel blockers (slow channel blockers or calcium antagonists) are popular treatment for cardio-vascular disease. Nifedipine (Procardia), diltiazem (Cardizem), and verapamil (Calan, Isoptin) are examples of calcium-channel blocking agents. The terms used for these medications falsely suggest a possible danger in taking calcium supplements or eating calcium-rich foods during medication therapy. The assumption is dietary intake of calcium should be reduced, because these drugs reduce heart disease and hypertension by blocking calcium and calcium therefore must be the "bad guy." This assumption is wrong. A high-calcium diet in conjunction with a reduced intake of sodium (salt) lowers blood pressure and reduces the risk for developing cardiovascular disease. Any dietary advice for people with cardiovascular disease who are on calcium-channel blockers should include a recommendation to maintain adequate calcium intake and blood levels.

Another class of medications used in the treatment of cardiovascular disease and hypertension is the beta blocking agents propranolol, metoprolol, acebutolol, and timolol. Possible side effects that might affect vitamin and mineral intake include stomach pain, flatulence, constipation, nausea, diarrhea, dry mouth, vomiting, loss of appetite, bloating, abdominal cramping, and inflammation of the pancreas or liver. No vitamin or mineral deficiencies have yet been identified with long-term use.

Oral Contraceptives

Oral contraceptives affect the absorption and use of several nutrients within the body. They increase appetite and encourage weight gain, reduce the absorption of folic acid and other vitamins, and redistribute nutrients within tissues. Oral contraceptives are associated with several vitamin and mineral deficiencies or alterations in nutrient metabolism. Some women who take oral contraceptives have high blood levels of vitamin A and copper and low blood levels of vitamin E, vitamin C, vitamin B_6, folic acid, vitamin B_1, vitamin B_2, vitamin B_{12}, iron, and zinc. Limited evidence shows oral contraceptives also might increase the absorption of calcium. These nutritional effects are moderate to mild, vary between individuals, and might be related to other physical disorders or poor dietary intake of nutrients.

Although low blood levels of iron have been reported in users of oral contraceptives, other studies show blood levels of this mineral are increased. The low blood levels of iron in some studies might be a result of poor dietary intake of iron-rich foods of the subjects rather than a medication-induced nutrient deficiency. Menstrual flow is reduced in women on oral contraceptives, which reduces loss of blood and iron and should help prevent iron deficiency.

The effects of oral contraceptives on vitamin B_6 status are of particular interest because the behavioral changes, such as depression, irritability, and insomnia, that are common side effects of these medications might be at least partially a result of the medication's effect on vitamin B_6 status. Vitamin B_6 is an essential component in the body's production of several chemicals responsible for nerve transmission, behavior, and body processes, called neurotransmitters and hormones. For example, serotonin is a neurotransmitter found in the brain and is responsible for regulating sleep, several emotions, and mood. Low levels of serotonin are associated with depression, irritability, and insomnia. The amount of serotonin available and its activity depends on the dietary intake and availability in the body of the building blocks for this neurotransmitter, tryptophan and vitamin B_6. Inadequate intake or reduced availability of either of these nutrients can result in limited production of serotonin and mood and sleep disorders. Medications, such as oral contraceptives, interfere with vitamin B_6 metabolism and might suppress the production of serotonin. In some cases, the mood swings and depression accompanying these medications are reduced or eliminated when vitamin B_6 intake is increased.

Some people are more sensitive than other people to medication-induced vitamin and mineral deficiencies. Nutrient deficiencies also might be dependent on the particular oral contraceptive used, the length of time it is used, and the nutritional status of the woman prior to and during the use of the medication.

Medications for Hyperactivity

Amphetamines, such as dextroamphetamine (dexedrine), and psychotherapeutic agents, such as methylphenidate (Ritalin) are examples of drugs used in the treatment of hyperactive children. Long-term use of these medications is associated with reduced growth, specifically in suppressed gains in height and weight. This medication-induced effect on growth is possibly a result of the loss of appetite and subsequent food and nutrient intake that often accompanies amphetamine use. Amphetamines are appetite suppressants, so much so that similar compounds are used in weight loss or "diet" pills. Evidence shows children on methylphenidate (30 to 40 mg/day) or dextroamphetamine (10 to 15 mg/day) consume less food and gain weight at a much slower rate than do children who discontinue these medications. The growth retardation stops and catch-up growth occurs when children discontinue amphetamine use. Other possible side effects of long-term amphetamine use that might influence food and nutrient intake include nausea and abdominal pain.

Vitamin and mineral deficiencies are possible during "growth spurts" when the child's nutrient needs are high, but the appetite is low because of amphetamine therapy. Every attempt should be made to encourage a child to eat a variety of fresh and wholesome foods, such as fresh fruits and vegetables, low-fat dairy products, whole grain breads and cereals, and lean meats or cooked dried beans and peas and to avoid nutrient-poor foods such as fatty convenience or fast foods, commercial snack foods such as potato chips and corn chips, and sugary foods. A multiple vitamin-mineral preparation containing approximately 100% of the fat-soluble and water-soluble vitamins, calcium, magnesium, and the trace minerals also is recommended.

Hypertensive Medications

The diuretic medications (water pills) used in the treatment of high blood pressure (hypertension) and congestive heart failure include ethacrynic acid, furosemide, mercurials, spironolactone, thiazides, and triamterene. These diuretics increase the urinary excretion of sodium and chloride (salt) and probably are effective in the treatment of hypertension because of this influence on sodium and fluid balance; however, other nutrients are lost in the urine as well. Many of the diuretics, unless they are called potassium-sparing diuretics such as amiloride HCL, triamterene, or spironolactone, increase urinary excretion of potassium and can precipitate symptoms of a potassium deficiency, including irregular heartbeat. It is recommended that an individual include several servings each day of potassium-rich foods or take a potassium supplement when using these medications. A person might experience bone disorders, paralysis, temporary sterility, muscle weakness, nerve disorders, and kidney damage if severe potassium deficiency is allowed to progress. A physician or pharmacist should be consulted about whether or not a diuretic requires potassium supplementation before self-medicating with the nutrient. Other medications that deplete the body of potassium include:

- L-DOPA
- Salicylates
- Senna (Senokot)
- Phenolphthalein (Ex-Lax, Feen-A-Mint)
- Gentamicin
- Corticosteroids
- Amphotericin B
- Bisacodyl (Dulcolax)

Magnesium is another mineral that can be depleted when diuretics, such as thiazides, are used. Magnesium deficiency is observed in people on long-term diuretic therapy for cardiac (heart) failure or hypertension. This diuretic-induced marginal magnesium deficiency might be a result of the loss of appetite experienced by some people on these medications and subsequent poor dietary and nutrient intake and the increased urinary excretion of the mineral.

Magnesium is important for normal heartbeat and the regulation of blood pressure. Artery walls spasm and an irregular heartbeat develops when magnesium intake is low; artery walls relax and the heartbeat returns to normal when blood levels of the mineral are adequate. Constrictions or spasms of blood vessels are linked to hypertension, whereas relaxation of the blood vessels increases the size of the blood vessel, reduces resistance to blood flow, and lowers blood pressure. Magnesium deficiency also is associated with heart failure, atherosclerosis, and destruction of the heart muscle. People with hypertension, especially those who take diuretic medications, often have low levels of magnesium in their blood. Elevated blood pressure returns to normal in many cases when the intake of magnesium-rich foods is increased or if magnesium supplements are included in the daily diet. Increased loss of other minerals, including calcium, iodine, and zinc, and low blood levels of folic acid are associated with long-term use of diuretics and might result in marginal mineral and vitamin deficiencies unless the dietary intake of these nutrients is adequate. (See pages 239–240 for information of the beta-blocking agents and calcium channel-blocking medications in the treatment of hypertension.)

Laxatives

Laxatives interfere with the absorption of nutrients by reducing the amount of time vitamins and mineral are in contact with the intestine. The laxatives phenolphthalein (Alophen, Ex-Lax, Feen-A-Mint), senna (Senokot), and bisacodyl (Dulcolax) alter the intestinal lining so nutrients might not be optimally absorbed. As a result, several vitamins and minerals, including calcium, potassium, and vitamin D, are excreted rather than absorbed and deficiencies could result if laxatives are used frequently or over a long period of time.

Mineral oil is another laxative that binds to the fat-soluble vitamins A, D, E, and K and the essential fatty acid linoleic acid. These nutrients are then lost because mineral oil is not absorbed and the complex of oil and nutrients is excreted. Long-term use of mineral oil could produce deficiencies of these nutrients, and cause conditions such as night blindness and increased risk for developing cancer in the case of vitamin A, bone disorders with vitamin D deficiency, and frequent hemorrhage with vitamin K deficiency.

Steroid Medications

The nutritional side effects of using steroid hormones include nausea, vomiting, diarrhea, abdominal pain, loss of appetite, and burning of the tongue. Steroid medications should only be used with the consent of a physician.

Estrogen therapy for the treatment of menopause symptoms might cause abdominal pain, loss of appetite, diarrhea, and nausea in some women. These side effects reduce food and nutrient intake or increase nutrient losses. Salt and fluid retention and weight gain also are possible on estrogen therapy.

Tobacco

Cigarette smoke affects the smoker's and nonsmoker's nutritional status. Inhalation of cigarette smoke depletes the tissues of vitamin C and increases the daily need for this water-soluble vitamin. Vitamin A and beta carotene levels in lung and mouth tissues exposed to cigarette or cigar smoke or chewing tobacco are low; tissues that contain adequate amounts of vitamin A are less likely to become cancerous. In addition, vitamin E might reduce the damage to lung tissue from outside air pollution. It is unclear whether this fat-soluble vitamin reduces lung tissue damaged by indoor air pollution, such as cigarette smoke. Women who smoke during pregnancy have low zinc levels in their blood and are more likely than are non-smokers to give birth to zinc deficient babies. These babies are at an increased risk for birth defects and disease.

Nonsmokers are a growing majority. More than 30 million people have kicked the tobacco habit and only one in every four people smokes cigarettes. Nonsmokers are passive smokers. They inhale both the mainstream smoke (the exhaled cigarette smoke from the smoker) and the sidestream smoke (the smoke from the end of the burning cigarette). Sidestream smoke contains greater amounts of dangerous gases than the smoke filtered through the cigarette before entering the smoker's lungs; it contains twice as much tar and nicotine, 3 times as much benzo(a)pyrene (a cancer-causing substance), 3 times as much poisonous carbon monoxide, and 73 times as much ammonia. These toxic gases enter the lungs and bloodstream of the smoker and surrounding nonsmokers and remain for hours after the person leaves the smoke-filled room or puts aside the cigarette.

Inhalation of carbon monoxide reduces the oxygen supply to the heart, brain, and other tissues. The nonsmoker or smoker might experience headaches, and the risk for developing lung cancer and heart disease increases in both groups. Nonsmokers, including the children of smokers, also experience a higher incidence of breathing difficulties, bronchitis, pneumonia, eye irritations, and tonsil operations. The smoke also increases the symptoms of asthma and allergies. Stillbirths and deaths in infants up to 1 year old are more common when the mother smokes.

The best prevention of lung cancer and respiratory disease, such as emphysema and bronchitis, is to not smoke or quit smoking and avoid other's cigarette, pipe, and cigar smoke. In addition, adequate intake of some vitamins might help prevent the harmful effects of other's smoke.

Tuberculosis Medications

Isoniazid (isonicotinic acid hydrazide or INH) kills actively growing tuberculosis bacteria and is used in the long-term treatment of this disease. It is usually recommended that the medication be taken between meals, but isoniazid can be consumed with food to reduce stomach upset. Alcohol should be avoided while taking this antituberculosis medication. Certain foods, such as tyramine-containing foods and tuna, also should be avoided. The medication can produce toxic symptoms in the liver and symptoms of nausea, headache, fatigue, loss of appetite, vomiting, or numbness of the hands and feet should be reported immediately to a physician or pharmacist. The potential nutritional side effects include a possible vitamin B_6 deficiency. Isoniazid binds to the vitamin and the two are excreted, and the medication interferes with normal use of vitamin B_6 in the body. Supplementing the diet with 50 mg of vitamin B_6 each day might be sufficient to prevent the nerve damage observed in patients on isoniazid (16 mg/2.2 pounds of body weight). However, this vitamin therapy should be followed only with the consent and supervision of a physician as moderate to large doses of vitamin B_6 has reduced the effectiveness of isoniazid in animals with tuberculosis.

Niacin deficiency has been reported in people taking isoniazid. The symptoms disappeared with a combination of niacin and vitamin B_6 therapy. However, the niacin deficiency is probably a result of vitamin B_6's role in converting the amino acid tryptophan to niacin rather than poor dietary intake of niacin. In addition, patients with tuberculosis often do not feel like eating and food and nutrient intake might be poor. The poor diet and niacin intake prior to and during medication therapy coupled with the medication-induced effects on vitamin B_6 and the manufacture of niacin from tryptophan might encourage a previous marginal vitamin deficiency to develop into a clinical vitamin deficiency.

Weight Control "Diet" Medications

The quick and easy weight loss promised by "diet" pills has not been substantiated. The active ingredient often used in these nonprescription medications is phenylpropanolamine (PPA). PPA is chemically similar to ephedrine, a common decongestant and appetite suppressant. The long-term effects on weight loss are minimal with this medication, but there is a risk for developing elevated blood pressure, and damage to the heart. Other side effects include nervousness, irritability, insomnia, restlessness, headache, dizziness, and serious central nervous system effects, such as seizures, hallucinations, agitation, and stroke. People with a history of heart disease, diabetes, moderate to severe high blood pressure, kidney disease, hyperthyroidism, depression, or glaucoma should not take PPA. In addition, more than 10,000 cases of toxic effects attributed to PPA have been reported to FDA's Poison Control Center.

The only effective "diet" for long-term weight loss and weight maintenance is one that contains a variety of low-calorie, nutrient-dense foods combined with frequent aerobic exercise. This diet and exercise program must be followed for life if weight loss is to be maintained.

SECTION 3

THE VITAMIN/MINERAL-RICH DIET

CHAPTER 7

Vitamins, Minerals, and Food

Most people equate nutrition with the "balanced diet." When people ask what they should eat, it is common to hear, "a balanced diet." Nutritionists recommend the balanced diet rather than vitamin-mineral supplements to meet most people's daily nutrient needs. Parents are told their children should eat a balanced diet. Teenagers are scolded about their unbalanced diets, and the family meal planner worries about preparing at least one balanced meal for the family each day. The term "balanced diet" is used loosely and the vagueness of the term often leaves people confused. What is a "balanced diet?"

Only a few years ago a Sunday meal of baked ham, candied yams, buttered beans, and gravy was considered a balanced and wholesome meal. Scientific research now states a diet that contains large amounts of fat and cholesterol, as found in baked ham, buttered beans, and gravy, elevates blood cholesterol levels and increases the risk for developing heart disease and cancer. The salt in the processed ham and the salt added during cooking and at the table contributes to the development of hypertension. Although the evidence on sugar, as found in candied yams, is controversial, the extra calories with no additional nutrients contribute to either obesity or malnutrition, not to mention dental caries. In addition, even marginal deficiencies of vitamin C, vitamin A, magnesium, chromium, zinc, calcium, or other vitamins and minerals have been linked to suppressed immune function and increased risk for infection and disease, osteoporosis, arthritis, depression, and numerous other emotional and physiological disorders. It appears the "balanced" diet of years past can no longer be considered healthful.

What can a person eat and how much is enough? First, it is important to recognize the benefits of good nutrition. Healthy dietary habits and proper food and meal selections improve resistance to colds and infections, reduce the risk for developing acute or chronic disease, increase resistance to stress and stress-related disorders, maintain a feeling of "well-being," aid in the prevention of premature aging, aid in the maintenance of a healthy appearance, help maintain each individual's maximum energy level to enjoy life and perform necessary work, improve the outcome of pregnancy and the health and well-being of the infant, and aid in the regulation of a stable emotional and social life. Nutrition is one of the most important factors in a long and healthy life.

The good news is that the guidelines for good nutrition and a "balanced" diet are simple and require, in most cases, only moderate changes in current eating habits.

1. Base the day's food intake on the modified Four Food Group plan.
2. Limit the fat in the diet to no more than 30% of total calories and limit cholesterol to 300 mg/day or less.
3. Increase the fiber in the diet. Limit processed, refined, or commercial convenience foods that are often high in fat, sugar, salt, cholesterol, or highly processed ingredients.
4. Choose a variety of wholesome, nutritious foods every day.
5. Be moderate in food selection, portion size, and all other dietary habits.
6. Be patient. Gradually make dietary changes.

The above six guidelines combined with careful selection of fresh and wholesome food and proper food preparation methods will help guarantee consumption of a balanced, nutritious diet that aids in the prevention of disease and premature aging and helps maintain optimal health.

The Four Food Group Plan

There are numerous ways to design a balanced diet today; however, the most common in the United States is the Four Food Groups Plan.

This plan consists of four basic categories of foods to be included in the daily menu:

- the fruit and vegetable group
- the whole grain breads and cereals group
- the low-fat milk group
- the lean meat-legume group

The foods are categorized according to their specific nutrient contributions. For example, foods in the low-fat milk group are good sources of calcium, protein, and vitamin B_2, while foods in the fruit and vegetable group are reliable sources of fiber, vitamin C, vitamin A, and folic acid. Food selections in the lean meat-legume group are good sources of iron, protein, zinc, B vitamins, and phosphorus, and foods in the whole grain breads and cereals group are high in B vitamins, iron and other trace minerals, and fiber.

Exclusion of a food group would place a person at increased risk for a deficiency of the nutrients supplied by that food group. For example, the low-fat milk group supplies more than 40% of a person's need for vitamin B_2 and calcium and it is the only dietary source of vitamin D. Avoidance of low-fat milk and low-fat milk products would require careful menu planning to ensure these nutrients were supplied in adequate amounts. Vegetarians are at increased risk for developing a zinc deficiency as lean meats, chicken, or fish, the best dietary sources of this trace mineral, are avoided in the vegetarian diet.

The Four Food Groups Plan includes recommendations for the minimum number of servings for each group. The size of each serving also is important because neither a tablespoon of peas in a chicken pot pie nor a 16 ounce steak are correct serving sizes (Table 37).

Table 37.
GUIDELINES FOR PROPER SERVING SIZES

VEGETABLES AND FRUITS (4+ servings/day)

(at least 1 serving dark green or orange and at least 1 serving citrus or other vitamin C-rich selection)

1 serving   one piece of fruit or vegetable, such as a medium apple, orange, carrot, or tomato; or 1 cup raw, such as lettuce salad, cole slaw, or carrot sticks; or ½ cup cooked, such as spinach, broccoli, or lima beans

WHOLE GRAIN BREADS AND CEREALS (4+ servings/day)

1 serving   1 slice of bread; or ½ English muffin, hamburger bun, bagel; or ½ cup cooked grain, such as cooked oatmeal, brown rice, whole wheat noodles, wheat berries, barley, or millet

Table 37. (*continued*)
GUIDELINES FOR PROPER SERVING SIZES

MEATS AND LEGUMES (4+ servings/day)

(*2 servings lean meat, chicken, or fish and 2 servings of cooked legumes or peanut butter*)

1 serving   2 to 3 ounces of lean meat, chicken, or fish; or ½ cup cooked legumes, such as kidney beans, black beans, split peas, lentils, soybeans, or garbanzo beans; or 4 Tbsp peanut or nut butter; or 2 eggs

LOW-FAT DAIRY PRODUCTS (2 servings/day)

1 serving   1 cup (8 ounces) non-fat or low-fat milk/yogurt; or 1½ ounces hard, low-fat cheese; or 2 cups low-fat cottage cheese

OTHER FOODS

1 serving   1 Tbsp safflower, corn, or other vegetable oil (excluding palm or coconut oils)

A minimum of four servings each day are recommended for fruits and vegetables, including at least one vitamin C-rich selection, such as an orange, grapefruit, or tangerine, and one dark green or orange vegetable such as broccoli, chard, or yams. A serving size is equivalent to ½ cup cooked produce, 1 cup raw, or 1 piece, such as 1 carrot or one apple.

At least four servings of whole grain breads and cereals should be consumed daily, such as whole wheat bread, oatmeal, brown rice, noodles, or bagels. A serving size is 1 slice of bread, ½ cup cooked cereal or other grain, or 1 ounce ready-to-eat cereal.

Two servings of lean meat, chicken, and fish, and two servings of cooked dried beans and peas for a total of four servings are recommended. A serving size is 3 ounces of lean meat, chicken or fish or ½ cup cooked dried beans and peas. Three ounces of meat is approximately 3 inches in diameter and ½ inch thick.

Two servings of low-fat or non-fat milk and milk products, such as low-fat yogurt or low-fat cheese are recommended. A serving size is 1 cup (8 ounces) of milk or yogurt, 1 ½ ounces of low-fat cheese, or 2 cups cottage cheese.

The diet also should include one serving of oil, such as a tablespoon of salad dressing, mayonnaise, or vegetable oil. The plan basically states that approximately two-thirds of the servings in the daily diet should come from fresh fruits and vegetables and whole grain breads and cereals. The other one-third of daily food selections should come from lean meats, chicken (without the skin), fish, cooked dried beans and peas, peanut butter, nuts and seeds, and low-fat dairy products such as low-fat milk or yogurt. If only the minimum number of servings from the Four Food Group Plan is chosen each day, a person would consume approximately 2,000 to 2,200 calories and at least 75% of the Recommended Dietary Allowance for all vitamins and minerals.

Limit Dietary Fat

The Four Food Group plan is not foolproof. Poor choices can be made within each group that can result in a nutritionally-lacking diet. One way to avoid this and to reduce the risk for developing cardiovascular disease, cancer, obesity, and other disorders is to limit the daily intake of fats, fatty foods, and fatty methods of food preparation.

Fat is a general term for triglycerides (also known as unsaturated and saturated fats) and cholesterol. Triglycerides are the fats found in vegetable oils, beef, butter, and all fatty foods. Triglycerides are also found in the blood and are the storage form of fat in the body. When the scale reads a gain or loss of 2 pounds, that fluctuation in weight is probably a result of changes in triglycerides. Triglycerides, whether saturated as in beef fat or unsaturated as in vegetable oil, contain 9 calories for every gram of fat. An ounce of dietary fat (triglycerides) contains 252 calories and a pound of body fat, i.e., triglycerides, is equivalent to 3,500 calories. A diet high in fat, as saturated or unsaturated triglycerides, is associated with an increased risk for developing cardiovascular disease, hypertension, cancer, and other degenerative disorders (Table 38).

Table 38.
THE FAT CONTENT OF SELECTED FOODS

FOODS THAT CONTAIN MORE THAN 75% FAT CALORIES*

Avocado	Luncheon meats (bologna)
Bacon	Nuts
Beef (sirloin, hamburger)	Olives
Coconut	Peanut Butter
Coleslaw	Pork (sausage, spareribs, loin,
Cream	untrimmed ham)
Cream cheese	Seeds (sesame, sunflower)

FOODS THAT CONTAIN 50% TO 75% FAT CALORIES**

Beef (rump, corned)	Fish, fried
Cake, pound	Ice cream
Cheese (blue, cheddar, Swiss)	Lamb (chops, rib)
Chicken, with skin	Pork (Ham loin, shoulder)
Chocolate	Tuna, packed in oil
Creamed soups	Veal
Eggs	

Table 38. (*continued*)
THE FAT CONTENT OF SELECTED FOODS

FOODS THAT CONTAIN 30% TO 50% FAT CALORIES†

Beef (lean, flank steak, chuck roast)	Milk, low-fat (2%)
Cake, no icing	Pumpkin pie
Chicken, roasted no skin	Salmon, canned
Cheese, cottage	Soup, bean with pork
Fish, halibut broiled	Turkey, roasted dark skin
Ice milk	Yogurt, low-fat (2%)

FOODS THAT CONTAIN 30% OR LESS FAT CALORIES

Beef (sirloin, lean only)	Milk, non-fat
Beans, peas, lentils	Pancakes
Bread	Seafood (scallops, shrimp)
Cake, angel food, sponge	Soups, split pea or vegetable
Cereal	Tuna, packed in water
Cheese, cottage uncreamed	Turkey, roasted white meat
Fish, broiled	Wheatgerm
Fruits	Vegetables
Grains	

* More than 8 grams of fat for every 100 calories.

** Between 5 grams and 8 grams of fat for every 100 calories.

† Between 3 grams and 5 grams of fat for every 100 calories.

A second type of fat is cholesterol. Cholesterol is found only in foods of animal origin, such as liver, heart, kidneys, eggs, muscle meats, chicken, fish, milk, cheese, butter, and other fatty dairy products. Cholesterol is not found in peanut butter, vegetable oils, potato chips, avocados, or any other plant. Cholesterol is a fat, but it does not supply calories, so it cannot be walked off, burned off, sweated out, or exercised away. It is also manufactured by the body and is not needed in the diet. A diet high in cholesterol is associated with an increased risk for developing cardiovascular disease (Table 39).

Table 39.
CHOLESTEROL IN FOODS

Food	Amount	Cholesterol (mg)
Brains	3 ounces	1,700
Liver	3 ounces	370
Kidney	3½ ounces	375
Egg, yolk	1	250–300
Pie, lemon chiffon	1 piece	181

Table 39. (*continued*)
CHOLESTEROL IN FOODS

Food	Amount	Cholesterol (mg)
Custard, homemade	³/₅ cup	165
Beef, lean	3 ounces	80
Pork, lean	3 ounces	76
Chicken, with skin	¹/₂ breast	63
Ice cream	¹/₂ cup	53–84
Waffles	1 medium	45–64
Sweet roll	1	39
Cake, devil's food	1 piece	38
Butter	1 Tbsp	35
Milk, whole	1 cup	34
Cheese, cheddar	1 ounce	28
Doughnut, cake	1	27
Biscuits, cornbread, or muffins (made with eggs)	1 or 1 piece	16–31
Milk, low-fat	1 cup	20
Pie, apple	1 piece	16
Cheese, part skim	1 ounce	15
Milk, non-fat	1 cup	5
Egg substitute	¹/₄ cup	1

Dietary fats come in a variety of forms including visible fats, such as butter, sour cream, cream cheese, margarine, vegetable shortening, vegetable oils, and the visible fat surrounding meat or in chicken skin. Invisible fats are found in pie crust and other desserts, the marbled fat in meats, the hidden fats in fatty fish, doughnuts, croissants, many frozen entrees and other convenience foods, commercial snack foods such as potato chips and corn chips, and gravies and sauces. Limiting fatty foods also includes fatty food-preparation methods, such as frying and sauteeing; foods served in cream sauces and gravies; and curtailing the use of salad dressings, mayonnaise, shortening, and other added fats and fatty spreads.

Limiting fat does not mean reducing the quantity of food intake. It does mean reducing calorie intake. For example, a medium baked potato contains approximately 100 calories and is a rich source of vitamin C, protein, fiber, and several minerals. The addition of butter and sour cream can more than triple the calorie intake without changing the portion size. A 3 ¹/₂ ounce breast of fried chicken contains twice the calories of the same piece baked or broiled. Two tablespoons of dressing contain more calories than 2 cups of lettuce and assorted salad vegetables.

Increase Dietary Fiber

A high-fiber diet is associated with a reduced risk for colon cancer, cardiovascular disease, diabetes, hypertension, and several intestinal disorders. Fiber is a general term for a variety of compounds, including the bran in whole wheat and oats, pectin in apples and other fruits, guar gum, locust bean gum, and the fiber in whole grain breads and cereals and vegetables and fruits. Cooked dried beans and peas also are excellent sources of fiber. The insoluble fibers, such as wheat bran, are associated with a reduced risk for colon cancer and intestinal diseases, whereas the soluble fibers, such as pectin and oat bran, reduce blood cholesterol and sugar levels and risk for cardiovascular disease and diabetes. Both types of fibers are essential to health and work together to prevent disease. The best source of fibers is whole, unprocessed foods, rather than refined and processed bran cereals, or powdered fiber products.

A recommendation for the optimal quantity of fiber in the daily diet has not been established. In general, an adequate intake of fiber is likely if the Four Food Group plan is followed. More than 50 grams of fiber each day is not recommended as excessive intake (remember the moderation guideline) can cause intestinal upset and might reduce the absorption of certain trace minerals, such as iron and zinc. The following daily inclusions in the diet would provide approximately 37 to 45 grams of natural fibers.

6 servings of whole grain breads and cereals .... 13 grams
4 servings of fresh fruits and vegetables .... 15–23 grams
1 serving of cooked dried beans and peas .... 9 grams
Total .... 37–45 grams

Choose a Variety of Foods

Variety in the diet is important in guaranteeing adequate intake of the more than 45 essential nutrients (and possibly as yet unrecognized nutrients) and to avoid excessive consumption of potentially toxic compounds found naturally in some foods or unintentionally added during processing or storing. Many people repeatedly consume the same foods and often choose from less than 50 foods for their weekly diet. In these cases, many highly nutritious foods—low in fat and high in fiber, vitamins, and minerals—are ignored. Individuals should try to include at least three new foods in the diet each week.

Moderation

Good nutrition and choosing a healthful diet is not an "all-or-nothing" decree. It is a process of emphasizing wholesome, low-fat foods and limiting intake of highly processed, refined, and fatty foods. There are no perfect foods and no one food needs to be included in a diet in order for the diet to be nutritious. In contrast, the occasional addition of one fatty or processed food to an otherwise nutritious diet will not reduce the diet's nutritional quality. Bacon and eggs for breakfast every day is not advised because of the high amount of fat, cholesterol, nitrites (cancer-causing substances), and low fiber provided by this meal. However, a breakfast of bacon and eggs once a month is harmless. The diet should be reviewed according to the daily or weekly food intake, not according to each food. Moderation also applies to serving size. Remember, each of the Four Food Groups supplies specific nutrients necessary for optimal health. Overemphasis of one group to the exclusion or limitation of another group increases a person's risk for developing deficiencies of vitamins or minerals.

Be Patient

Making dietary changes can be difficult. Success is more likely and discomfort is minimal if changes are made gradually; failure, resentment, frustration, and loss of motivation are more likely if too many difficult changes are undertaken at one time. A person must recognize that lasting change occurs slowly, even if major adjustments in dietary intake are needed.

A nutritious diet is based on a few, simple guidelines. A low-fat, high-fiber diet based on the modified Four Food Groups, that includes a variety of wholesome foods, that limits consumption of highly refined and processed foods, and that maintains ideal body weight is most likely to supply the more than 45 essential vitamins, minerals, and nutrients in the proper ratio and combination to maintain optimal health. Limiting salt and alcohol and drinking at least 6 glasses of water each day are also recommended. Fresh foods should be selected and should be prepared to retain the most vitamins and minerals. How those foods are consumed, whether it be in three square meals a day or six small meals throughout the day, does not matter and depends more on an individual's preference and time schedule than on biological needs. A person should take time, however, to relax while eating so that the stomach and intestine can function optimally in digesting and absorbing nutrients. It should never be forgotten that food is more than nutrients; it is a source of pleasure, socialization, and enjoyment.

MEAL-PLANNING GUIDELINES

Guidelines for a nutritious diet are only as effective as the understanding of how to apply them. Reducing dietary fat sounds simple, but often fats are hidden in foods and a diet can remain high in fat or other unwanted substances without the person knowing it. In contrast, preparing vitamin and mineral-rich meals does not have to be time-consuming or complicated. Simple adjustments to favorite recipes and a few additions to the menu might be all that is needed.

Shopping for Nutritious Foods

Most of the foods included in the modified Four Food Groups plan are found around the periphery of the grocery store. The produce section, the dairy section, the meat section, and the bread section or bakery usually line the side walls and back of the grocery store. The other foods, such as whole grain cereals, noodles, canned and frozen vegetables, and legumes are located on a few aisles, while the greatest percentage of the aisle shelves are devoted to foods that are often highly processed and convenience foods (Table 40).

Table 40.
The Grocery List For Low-Fat, Nutritious Foods

DAIRY
Non-fat (skim) milk or yogurt (less than 1% fat, by weight)
Low-fat milk or yogurt (less than 2% fat, by weight)
Buttermilk (less than 2% fat, by weight)
Low-fat cheeses
  Pot cheese
  Dry curd cottage cheese
  Low-fat cottage cheese (1% fat, by weight)
  Hoop cheese
  Sap sago cheese
  Partially-skimmed mozzarella cheese
  Partially-skimmed ricotta cheese

EGGS
Use only the whites

BREAD
Whole wheat, rye, pumpernickle, multi-grain, or sourdough bread
Corn tortillas
Whole wheat pita bread

Table 40. (*continued*)
THE GROCERY LIST FOR LOW-FAT, NUTRITIOUS FOODS

CRACKERS
Rye crisp
Wasa crackers
Rice cakes

HOT CEREALS
Oat bran
Wheatena
Orowheat hot cereal
Rolled oats

Cornmeal
Cracked wheat
4-grain and 7-grain hot cereals

COLD CEREALS
Shredded Wheat
Puffed wheat, rice, millet, or corn
Grape-Nuts
NutriGrain, wheat, barley, rye, corn cereals

GRAINS
Bran
Brown rice
Millet
Kasha
Barley
Rye
Triticale
Whole wheat flour, graham, and
   pastry flour

Whole wheat berries
Rye flour
Oat flour
Cornmeal
Tabouli mix, rice pilaf, wheat pilaf,
   Spanish rice
Popcorn (dry pop)
Wild rice

PASTAS
All pastas, limit egg noodles
Whole wheat pasta
Spinach pasta
Buckwheat pasta
Rice noodles

FRUITS AND VEGETABLES AND JUICES
All fresh fruit
All fresh vegetables (olives and avacados are high in fat)
Fresh and canned 100% vegetable or fruit juices
Tomato products: paste, sauce, enchilada sauce, picante sauce, tomato
   juice, V-8 juice, whole tomatoes, plum tomatoes, crushed tomatoes, green
   chili salsa
Raisins, apricots, prunes, and other dried fruits (no added sugar)

OTHER CANNED ITEMS
Canned pumpkin, water chestnuts,
   bamboo shoots, green chilis
Canned artichoke hearts (canned in
   water)

Unsweetened apple juice
Water-packed tuna
Water-packed salmon
Beets

Table 40. (*continued*)
THE GROCERY LIST FOR LOW-FAT, NUTRITIOUS FOODS

OTHER CANNED ITEMS
Canned corn   Evaporated non-fat milk
Unsweetened pineapple juice   Canned beans, rinsed

FROZEN VEGETABLES AND FRUITS AND THEIR JUICES
Unsweetened concentrated apple, grapefruit, orange, or pineapple juice
All frozen vegetables without sauces
Frozen strawberries, blueberries, boysenberries (unsweetened)

BEVERAGES
Mineral water   Caffix
Spring water   Celestial Seasoning teas
Seltzer water   Postum

CONDIMENTS
Tamari   Wines (white or red burgandy),
Soy sauce   sherry, sauternes, dry vermouth,
Mustard   port
Miso   Picante sauce
Tabasco sauce   Horseradish
Vinegar   All spices, herbs, and seasonings
Dry mustard   (check for added salt)

LEGUMES
All beans, including soybeans, kidney, black, garbanzo, dried limas, navy,
   white, and mung
Tofu
Soybean cheese
Tempeh (fermented soybean curd)

MISCELLANEOUS STOCK ITEMS
Non-fat dry milk   Pearl tapioca
Cornstarch   Matzo meal
Arrowroot   Whey powder
Unflavored gelatin   Lemon juice (unsweetened)
Active dry yeast   Lime juice (unsweetened)
Baking powder   No-fat salad dressings
Baking soda

READ LABELS. In the "good ol' days" there was no reason for the warning "consumer beware." Everyone knew what was in mother's cookies, bread, cakes, and pancakes or grandmother's pickles, preserves, and canned goods. Vegetables were grown on the farm and the pork and beef came from the livestock raised by the family. Today, food is grown far from the family home and processed in factories far from the family kitchen. Many foods are fabricated or engineered in laboratories far removed from the conventional kitchen.

The shopper can learn much about a food by reading the label. The calorie and fat gram content can help compare one similar food item with another or can be used to determine the percentage of calories that come from fat (i.e., multiply the grams of fat by 9, divide by the total number of calories, and multiply by 100 to obtain percentage of fat calories). The grams of sugar can be equated with the number of teaspoons of sugar in the product (eg, 4 grams = 1 teaspoon). Often labels contain cholesterol content information and the USRDAs per serving for several vitamins and minerals (Figure 3).

THE USRDAs. The United States Recommended Daily Allowances (USRDAs) were developed by the Food and Drug Administration (FDA) and are condensed lists of nutrient requirements derived from the RDA charts. They are used in labeling foods and nutrient supplements (Table 41).

Table 41.
THE UNITED STATES RECOMMENDED DAILY ALLOWANCES (US RDAs)

Nutrients That Must Appear On The Label	US RDA
Vitamin A	5,000 IU
Vitamin C	65 mg
Vitamin B_1	1.5 mg
Vitamin B_2	1.7 mg
Niacin	20 mg
Calcium	1,000 mg
Iron	18 mg

Nutrients That May Appear On The Label	US RDA
Vitamin D	400 IU
Vitamin E	30 IU
Vitamin B_6	2.0 mg
Folic Acid	400 mcg
Vitamin B_{12}	6 mcg
Phosphorus	1,000 mg
Iodine	150 mg
Magnesium	400 mg
Zinc	15 mg
Copper	2 mg
Biotin	300 mcg
Pantothenic Acid	10mg

Figure 3

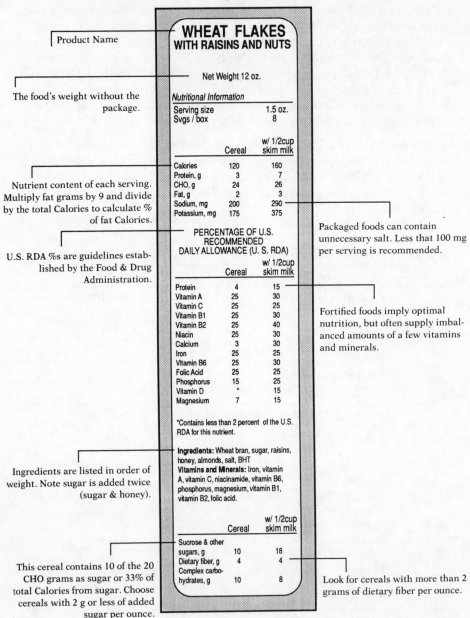

Product Name

The food's weight without the package.

Nutrient content of each serving. Multiply fat grams by 9 and divide by the total Calories to calculate % of fat Calories.

U.S. RDA %s are guidelines established by the Food & Drug Administration.

Ingredients are listed in order of weight. Note sugar is added twice (sugar & honey).

This cereal contains 10 of the 20 CHO grams as sugar or 33% of total Calories from sugar. Choose cereals with 2 g or less of added sugar per ounce.

Packaged foods can contain unnecessary salt. Less that 100 mg per serving is recommended.

Fortified foods imply optimal nutrition, but often supply imbalanced amounts of a few vitamins and minerals.

Look for cereals with more than 2 grams of dietary fiber per ounce.

WHEAT FLAKES
WITH RAISINS AND NUTS

Net Weight 12 oz.

Nutritional Information

Serving size		1.5 oz.
Svgs / box		8

	Cereal	w/ 1/2cup skim milk
Calories	120	160
Protein, g	3	7
CHO, g	24	26
Fat, g	2	3
Sodium, mg	200	290
Potassium, mg	175	375

PERCENTAGE OF U.S.
RECOMMENDED
DAILY ALLOWANCE (U. S. RDA)

	Cereal	w/ 1/2cup skim milk
Protein	4	15
Vitamin A	25	30
Vitamin C	25	25
Vitamin B1	25	30
Vitamin B2	25	40
Niacin	25	30
Calcium	3	30
Iron	25	25
Vitamin B6	25	30
Folic Acid	25	25
Phosphorus	15	25
Vitamin D	*	15
Magnesium	7	15

*Contains less than 2 percent of the U.S. RDA for this nutrient.

Ingredients: Wheat bran, sugar, raisins, honey, almonds, salt, BHT
Vitamins and Minerals: Iron, vitamin A, vitamin C, niacinamide, vitamin B6, phosphorus, magnesium, vitamin B1, vitamin B2, folic acid.

	Cereal	w/ 1/2cup skim milk
Sucrose & other sugars, g	10	18
Dietary fiber, g	4	4
Complex carbo-hydrates, g	10	8

The nutritional content of a food as listed on the label is a valuable resource for the consumer. For example, a person is guaranteed that he or she will meet at least a quarter of the calcium daily recommendation if a label states a food contains 25% of the USRDA for calcium. To determine the exact amount of calcium in each serving, multiply the percentage listed on the label with the USRDA for that nutrient, ie, $0.25 \times 1,000$ mg of calcium = 250 mg of calcium per serving.

FORTIFIED AND ENRICHED. The term "enriched" traditionally refers to the addition of three vitamins (vitamin B_1, vitamin B_2, and niacin) and one mineral (iron) to processed grain. Breads and rice that have been processed and then "enriched" contain the same amount of these four nutrients as did the original whole wheat or brown rice. The term is deceiving, however, as it implies added nutrition when in reality the other nutrients and fiber lost in processing have not been replaced. These "enriched" products are poor substitutes for the original whole grain items, which are also better sources of fiber, pantothenic acid, folic acid, vitamin B_6, chromium, selenium, magnesium, zinc, and other nutrients.

The term "fortified" refers to the addition of a vitamin or mineral to levels not naturally found in the food. For example, milk is fortified

---

The Vitamin And Mineral Content Of White Bread Compared To Whole Wheat Bread

White bread contains . . . . 22% of the magnesium in whole wheat bread

. . . . 38% of the zinc

. . . . 28% of the chromium

. . . . 42% of the copper

. . . . 12% of the manganese

. . . . 4% of the vitamin E

. . . . 18% of the vitamin B_6

. . . . 63% of the folic acid

. . . . 56% of the pantothenic acid

with larger amounts of vitamin D than is usually found in nature. This is beneficial as there is no other reliable source of vitamin D in the diet, and the fat-soluble vitamin is essential for calcium absorption and use in the body. The fortification of salt with iodine resulted in a marked reduction in the incidence of goiter and cretinism.

Fortification can be misused to sell otherwise nutrient-poor foods. Vitamins and minerals may be added in arbitrary amounts and combinations to breakfast cereals, protein powders, breakfast drinks, fruit-flavored or sugary beverages, or even candy bars. Fortification with a few nutrients gives an otherwise poor product the facade of being nutritious. These processed foods are never fortified with all the essential vitamins and minerals in balanced amounts that promote optimal nutrition. The natural product, such as orange juice, is always more nutritious and less expensive than a processed product, such as an orange-flavored, vitamin C-fortified fruit drink.

INGREDIENTS LIST. The ingredients in packaged food must be listed in descending order according to weight. For example, a loaf of bread labeled "whole wheat" that lists enriched wheat flour as its first ingredient is made primarily from white flour. A product will be primarily sweet and nutrient-poor if the first or second ingredient listed is sugar. Sweeteners come in a variety of names and their total contribution to the product should be considered. For example, if sugar is listed second on the list of ingredients, honey listed fourth, and dextrose or "natural sweeteners" listed sixth, a product should be considered high in sugar (Figure 3, page 262).

The ingredient list also provides information on the types of fat in a product. Corn oil, vegetable oil, and partially hydrogenated vegetable oil are very different forms of fat. Corn oil is a high polyunsaturated fat. Vegetable oil may or may not be polyunsaturated depending on whether it is safflower oil or corn oil or a highly saturated vegetable fat such as palm oil or coconut oil. Partially hydrogenated vegetable oil contains both saturated and polyunsaturated fats. People who are concerned about saturated fats and their influence on the development of cardiovascular disease will want to avoid products that contain saturated fats or that list vegetable oil, but fail to mention the type of oil. Sometimes a label will state "vegetable oil (may contain one or more of the following: soybean, coconut oil, or palm oil)." This wording allows the manufacturer to use whichever oil was cheapest at the time of processing and provides no guarantee to the consumer of nutritional quality. It is important to remember, however, that the intake of all fats—saturated and unsaturated—is associated with the development of cancer, and all fats should be reduced in the diet.

STANDARDS OF IDENTITY. The Food and Drug Administration (FDA) has developed Standards of Identity for 350 common foods. Ingredient standards for foods such as bread, meat products, margarine, mayonnaise, ketchup, flour, salad dressing, jam, and peanut butter were determined, and these manufactured foods must contain the ingredients established by the FDA. For example, commercial mayonnaise must contain not less than 65% vegetable oil by weight, vinegar or lemon juice (not less than 2.5% by weight of mayonnaise), and egg or egg yolk (frozen, liquid, or dried). One problem with the Standards of Identity is that the ingredients and additives in foods on this list do not have to be printed on the label. The label on salad dressing does not have to list the use of stabilizers, emulsifiers, flavorings, colorings, or other additives. The consumer must write the FDA in Washington, DC to obtain the Standard of Identity list on these products, and then will only be told what is allowed in the product, not what actually is included. It is hoped that future legislation will require nutritional labeling on all food products, regardless of the presence or absence of a Standard of Identity.

Food Storage

To maximize the vitamin and mineral content of foods:

- Purchase only the amount of fresh fruits and vegetables that will be eaten within a few days.
- Store refrigerated foods at less than 40°F, frozen foods below 0°F, and canned and dry goods in a cool, dry place. Even small fluctuations in temperature can result in considerable loss of vitamin C in frozen foods.
- Store canned or frozen foods for no more than 3 to 5 months as the vitamin content can decline as much as 75% or more with longer storage times.
- Store bulk dried beans and peas, noodles, rice, and flour in dark containers or in the refrigerator to reduce their exposure to ultraviolet light, which destroys vitamin B_2.

Food Preparation

The three most important considerations in cooking are the preservation of the vitamin and mineral content of the food, the maintenance of an overall low-fat menu, and the preservation of the taste, texture, color, smell, and appearance of the food.

Preserving Vitamins and Minerals. In general, vitamins and minerals are best preserved by cooking in a minimal amount of water, for a minimal amount of time, with a minimal amount of chopping or dicing of the food, and by keeping the cooked food for a minimal amount of time prior to serving and eating (Table 42 and Table 43).

Table 42.
Preservation Of Vitamins And Minerals During Food Preparation

- Cook food in a minimal amount of water for a short amount of time.
- Cook food to a temperature above 140°F to destroy harmful bacteria.
- Carefully read cooking instructions on packages.
- Use low to moderate heat for cooking meats.
- Thaw frozen meat, poultry, and fish in refrigerator before cooking.
- Cook frozen vegetables without thawing.
- Add shredded or grated cheese at the end of the cooking time.
- Cook eggs and milk mixtures over low heat.
- Use a vegetable peeler to remove only the outer layer of skin on produce.
- Cook produce in covered pan for a short amount of time.
- Cook vegetables just until crisp-tender.
- Peel, cut, chop vegetables just before eating or cooking.
- Prepare salads just before serving.
- Immediately refrigerate or freeze leftovers.
- Use leftover liquids for sauces, soups, stews, or cooking water for cereals, rice, or noodles.
- Save celery leaves, parsley, and other leftover vegetables for soup stock.

Table 43.
Vitamin And Mineral Losses During Food Handling

Light
Vitamin B_2
Vitamin A and beta carotene
Vitamin D
Vitamin E
Vitamin K

Heat	
Vitamin C	Folic acid
Vitamin B_1	Vitamin B_{12}
Pantothenic acid	Vitamin A

Exposure to Air	
Vitamin C	
Folic acid	Vitamin A
Vitamin B_{12}	Vitamin D
Biotin	Vitamin E
	Vitamin K

Table 43. (*continued*)
VITAMIN AND MINERAL LOSSES DURING FOOD HANDLING

LEACHING INTO COOKING WATER

Vitamin C	Vitamin B_6
Vitamin B_1	Selenium
Vitamin B_2	Potassium
Niacin	Magnesium
Pantothenic acid	Phosphorus

ACID/ALKALINE pH

Vitamin C (alkaline)	Folic acid (alkaline or acid)
Vitamin B_1 (alkaline)	Vitamin B_{12} (alkaline)
Vitamin B_2 (alkaline)	Biotin (alkaline)
Pantothenic acid (alkaline or acid)	

THE LOW-FAT MENU. The lower the fat content of the diet the more foods rich in vitamins, minerals, and fiber can be included in the daily fare and the less risk for developing marginal vitamin or mineral deficiencies, disease, or obesity. The common recommendation is to reduce dietary fat to no more than 30% of total calories.

A reduction in dietary fat and cholesterol is accomplished by following a few simple guidelines.

1. Emphasize low-fat and non-fat milk and milk products.
2. Use only lean meat, chicken without the skin, and fish, and only consume the amount recommended by the modified Four Food Group Plan.
3. Limit or avoid cooking with fats (butter, margarine, vegetable oil, or animal fats, such as bacon fat or lard). Limit total daily intake to less than 2 tablespoons.
4. Emphasize whole grain breads and cereals, fresh fruits and vegetables, cooked dried beans and peas, and nuts (Table 44).

Table 44.
REDUCING FAT IN THE DIET: MEAT AND GENERAL GUIDELINES

RATHER THAN . . .	CHOOSE TO . . .
1. using gourmet recipes as is	1. eliminate egg yolks (use egg substitute or two egg whites for every whole egg), butter, cream, salt, and substitute spices, wine, and other seasonings.
2. making fatty homemade soup	2. refrigerate stock and skim fat before preparing soup, stews, gravies, or sauces.

Table 44. (*continued*)
REDUCING FAT IN THE DIET: MEAT AND GENERAL GUIDELINES

RATHER THAN . . .	CHOOSE TO . . .
3. basting in oil	3. baste with wine, fat-free liquids, and spices
4. using mayonnaise	4. mix imitation or low-calorie mayonnaise with non-fat yogurt. Use for tuna or chicken salad.
5. preparing grilled sandwiches in butter	5. use a non-stick pan or PAM
6. preparing 4-8 oz servings of meat	6. prepare 2-3 oz servings and mix with whole grain rice, noodles, or vegetables
7. choosing fatty meats	7. select lean cuts of meat
8. fry, saute in fats	8. bake, steam, broil, boil, or grill
9. serve French fries with hamburgers	9. prepare baked potato with chives or cut potatoes into strips and bake on ungreased cookie sheet until brown and crispy

People who wish to monitor fat intake more closely or people who count calories might want to count their weekly intake of grams of fat. This method requires that a person know the approximate daily calorie intake. The daily allotment of fat (30% of total calories) is determined by multiplying 0.30 times a person's daily calorie intake and dividing by 9 (fat contains 9 calories/gram). For example, a daily intake of 2,000 calories times 0.30 = 600, divided by 9 calories/1 gram of fat = 67 grams of fat/day. The number of grams of fat in various foods can be found in a variety of books available at most bookstores (Table 45).

Table 45.
DETERMINING CALORIES FROM PROTEIN, CARBOHYDRATE, AND FAT

A serving of nonfat milk (90 calories) contains the following:

	Grams per serving		Calories per gram	Calories	Percentage of total Calories
Protein	9.3	X	4 calories/gram =	37.2	37.2 divided by 90 = 41%
Carbohydrate	12.5	X	4 calories/gram =	50	50 divided by 90 = 55%
Fat	0.4	X	9 calories/gram =	3.6	3.6 divided by 90 = 4%

THE LOW-FAT DIET AND MEATS. In many cases, selecting low-fat foods from the Meat and Legume Group is easy. Red meats (beef, pork, or lamb) should be infrequent inclusions in the diet, perhaps used no more than two to three times a week. Select lean cuts of meat (especially those labeled 15% or less fat) and avoid fatty selections such as "Prime" or "Choice" grades and other heavily-marbled cuts, corned beef, pastrami, short ribs, spare ribs, porterhouse steaks, T-bone steaks, club steaks, rib eye roast or steak, frankfurters, sausage, bacon, and other luncheon meats. Many of these processed meats contain more than 70% fat calories. The percentage of fat listed on the label is deceiving as it refers to the amount of fat by weight, not by calories. For the remaining breakfasts, lunches, snacks, and dinners use fish, the white meat of chicken and turkey, cooked dried beans and peas, or pasta dishes such as spaghetti or macaroni.

Adults need no more than 4 to 6 ounces of lean meat, chicken, and fish each day. A 3 ounce serving is equivalent to ½ breast of chicken, a chicken leg and thigh together, 2 thin slices of lean roast beef, or ½ cup flaked fish. Rather than planning meals around the meat, serve pasta or rice and use small pieces of lean meat, chicken, or fish in the sauce. Mix small amounts of lean meat, chicken, or fish into casseroles or soups consisting primarily of grains, cooked dried beans and peas, and vegetables. For example, choose lentil soup with small pieces of chicken, Chinese pork and vegetables over rice with a small amount of pork and generous portions of vegetables and rice, linguine with clam sauce, tuna casserole with extra noodles and vegetables, or vegetables and fish sauteed in defatted chicken stock and wine over rice.

In addition to visible fat in meats, hidden fat and cholesterol are contained throughout the muscle tissue. This fat marbling makes meat juicy, tender, and high in saturated fat, the type of fat associated with an increased risk for developing cardiovascular disease. If the visible fatty exterior is removed but the serving size is increased, the total fat and cholesterol content of the meat serving will remain about the same, so an individual needs to carefully monitor serving size. Lean cuts of meat contain less fat marbling, but often are less tender. They can be "tenderized" with slow cooking, unsalted meat tenderizers, or moist methods of food preparation, such as stewing, sauteing in wine or defatted chicken stock, and poaching.

THE LOW-FAT DIET AND DAIRY PRODUCTS. Dairy products are important inclusions in the diet because of their high calcium and vitamin B_2 content. Low-fat selections provide the same, if not more, nutrients, but with less saturated fat and cholesterol. Skim or non-fat milk and yogurt are the best selections and low-fat milk and yogurt are better than whole milk and yogurt. The fat as a percentage of weight, as listed on the label, is misleading as milk is mostly water. Actually, low-fat milk is closer to whole milk than non-fat milk in its fat content. For those people who dislike non-fat milk, non-fat dry milk powder can be added to the liquid beverage to give it more "body" and a higher vitamin and mineral content, without adding fat.

Cheese varies in fat content from less than 5% to more than 70% fat calories. The hard cheeses, such as cheddar, Swiss, muenster, and American, and the soft cheeses such as gruyere and havarti have a fat content of approximately 70%. The serving size for cheese is usually 1½ ounces, not 3 ounces as with meat, and several low-fat varieties are available. Dry curd or low-fat cottage cheese; low-fat natural cheese, such as jarlsberg and partially-skimmed mozzarella or Swiss; or some processed special cheeses contain less fat than do other cheese varieties. Part-skim ricotta is 50% fat calories and sapsago and mysost cheeses are very low in fat (Table 46 and Table 47).

Table 46.
Rating The Cheeses for Fat Content (1 oz serving)

Cheese	Fat (grams)	Calories
Cream	10	100
Cheddar	9	110
American processed	9	110
Colby	9	110
Parmesan, grated	9	130
Swiss	8	110
Cheddar-flavored cold pack cheese food	7	90
Pasteurized, processed American cheese spread	6	90
Mozzarella, part-skim	5	80
Cottage (4%) (½ cup)	5	120
Edam, low-fat	3	62
Cottage, low-fat (½ cup)	1	90
Mysost	0.4	70

Table 47.
Reducing Fat in the Diet: Dairy Products

Rather than . . .	Choose to . . .
1. using butter to saute	1. saute foods in defatted chicken stock, use non-stick pans or PAM
2. putting butter on toast	2. use low-Calorie jams or low-fat cottage cheese
3. using sour cream	3. use non-fat yogurt with a dash of lemon for dips. Place non-fat yogurt in cheesecloth overnight, drain, and use yogurt curd as substitute for sour cream

Table 47. (*continued*)
REDUCING FAT IN THE DIET: DAIRY PRODUCTS

RATHER THAN . . .	CHOOSE TO . . .
4. using fruited yogurt	4. select plain, non-fat yogurt. Mix with fresh fruit
5. using cream or whole	5. use non-fat milk with non-fat milk dry milk solids or evaporated non-fat milk. Partially frozen evaporated non-fat milk can be whipped into a foam for desserts or as a replacement for whipping cream
6. using full amount of cheese	6. reduce portion of cheese in sauces to ¹/₃ to ¹/₂
7. preparing fat and flour for "roux"	7. prepare cream sauces with cornstarch and non-fat milk, water, or juice

THE LOW-FAT DIET AND WHOLE GRAIN BREADS AND CEREALS. The most misunderstood foods in the American diet are grains and other starches. These items have been falsely accused as being high-calorie reasons for excessive weight gain, poor sources of nutrients, and the primary foods to avoid. Nothing could be farther from the truth.

Whole grains are low-calorie, low-fat, low-cholesterol, low-sugar, low-salt, nutrient-dense, high-fiber additions to the diet. It is the sauces, butter or margarine, sour cream, and other fats added to grains and starches that increase the calorie toll and reduce the relative nutrient content. Whole grain breads and cereals and other starchy foods should be increased to replace calories lost when fat is removed and to add fiber and essential vitamins and trace minerals to the diet.

Low-fat breads and rolls include whole wheat, rye, or raisin breads, English muffins, buns, bagels, rolls, pita bread, and tortillas. Low-fat crackers and snacks include animal, graham, Wassa, Akmak, rye, saltine, oyster, and matzo crackers; bread sticks; melba toast; flatbread; pretzels; and air-popped popcorn.

All whole grain hot cereals, such as oatmeal, multi-grain cereal, or cracked wheat cereal, are low-fat, nutrient-dense selections. Most cold cereals, except granola, which contains as much as 35% fat often from highly saturated coconut oil, are low in fat. Low-sugar, whole-grain varieties include Grape Nuts, Shredded Wheat, and NutriGrain. Whole grain varieties of pasta, including macaroni, spaghetti, linguine, ravioli, lasagna, and ribbon noodles, are excellent selections. Egg noodles will contain varying amounts of cholesterol.

The variety of whole grain cereals is endless. Americans are accustomed to oatmeal, white rice, and wheat flour, and sometimes use rye, cornmeal, and wild rice, but often ignore many other important whole grains. For example, millet, whole wheat berries, wheatgerm, buckwheat, triticale, potato flour, oat flour, kasha, barley, cracked wheat or bulgar, and brown rice can add a variety of tastes and textures, as well as essential vitamins, minerals, and fiber to the diet. Serve whole wheat berries instead of noodles, add barley to soups, use brown instead of white rice in casseroles, or add cooked cracked wheat or wheatgerm to pancake mixes.

Some grain products contain hidden fats. Biscuits, muffins (beware of commercial bran muffins, which can contain 35% or more fat calories and large amounts of sugar), banana and other fruit breads, pancakes, French toast and waffles, croissants, pie crusts, and cornbread contain moderate to high amounts of fat. Homemade products can be adjusted to contain one-half the fat recommended in the original recipe. Substitute safflower oil, whenever possible, for more saturated fats, such as margarine, shortening, and butter. Finally, limit or avoid the following: butter rolls, egg bagels, egg breads, commercial doughnuts and other sweetened breakfast rolls, muffins, buttered popcorn, high-fat commercial crackers, any grain product containing coconut or palm oil, or commercial bread and muffin mixes. Any bread listed as "flaky," that appears shiny or oily on the surface, or that leaves an oily feel in the mouth contains too much butter or other fats.

In general, the more processed a grain or starchy food the higher its fat or sugar content and the lower its vitamin, mineral, and fiber content. Frozen entrees that contain rice or noodles also might contain more than 60% fat calories. Canned or dried soups, entrees, and other convenience foods with grain products might contain large quantities of salt or fat, or recommend the addition of fatty dairy products or oils in preparation. Individuals should read labels and choose those varieties low in salt and fat.

THE LOW-FAT DIET AND VEGETABLES AND FRUITS. Fresh fruits and vegetables contain the most vitamins for the fewest calories of any other food group. Almost all fresh or frozen plain fruits and vegetables are low-fat, nutrient-dense selections. Avocados and olives are high in fat. Olives are also high in salt, as are pickles. Vegetables canned or frozen in sauces usually contain fat or salt. Read labels and select vegetables that contain no more than 2 to 3 grams of fat for every 100 calories.

THE LOW-FAT DIET AND DESSERTS. Desserts can be an excellent source of vitamins and minerals. Fresh fruit, fruit canned without sugar, and plain gelatin with fruit are sources of vitamin A, vitamin C, iron, and fiber. Plain air-popped popcorn, pretzels, sherbet, ice milk, frozen or fruited non-fat yogurt, and angel food cake contain little or no fat and some nutrients. Gelatin desserts can be prepared with plain gelatin and unsweetened fruit juices for a low-fat, low-sugar dessert (Table 48).

Table 48.
REMOVING THE FAT FROM THE DIET

Instead of . . .	Choose . . .
BREAKFAST	
Scrambled eggs and bacon	Oatmeal with low-fat milk, raisins, and nuts
Toast with butter	Whole wheat toast with low-sugar jam
Coffee with cream	Coffee with non-fat condensed milk
Orange juice	Orange juice
LUNCH	
Hamburger on bun with sauce	Broiled chicken sandwich, no mayonnaise
French fries	Tossed green salad with low-fat dressing
Milkshake	Milk, non-fat or low-fat
Chocolate cake	Fresh fruit
DINNER	
Fried chicken	Baked or broiled chicken without the skin
Baked potato with sour cream and butter	Baked potato with Butter Buds and chives
Sauteed vegetables	Steamed vegetables
Macaroni salad	Spinach salad with low-fat dressing
Ice cream	Sherbet or plain low-fat yogurt with fruit

THE NEW FOODS: CONVENIENCE, FAST, AND SNACK

Several factors influence modern food choices. One trend affecting food choices is the need for convenience. Food and food preparation methods sometimes need to be fast because people often do not have the time for elaborate and lengthy meal planning. Another trend is eating in restaurants. There is nothing wrong with the concept of convenience, fast, or snack foods; these foods can be nutritious, low-fat, high-fiber additions to the menu. However, many of the commercial selections are high in fat and sugar and low in fiber, vitamins, and minerals.

Convenience Foods

Since the 1940s thousands of new "convenience" foods have entered the marketplace. These new foods either attempt to replicate traditional homemade items, such as macaroni and cheese, or replace them, such as fruit drinks. Convenience foods are prepared at home from foods that already have been cooked or processed at the "factory." These foods include:

- Cold breakfast cereals
- Powdered or condensed beverages
- Frozen entrees, breakfasts, vegetables, and other foods
- Pre-prepared meals and desserts that require the addition of water, milk, or another ingredient before serving
- Canned foods that require opening, possibly heating, and serving

In general, the more a food is processed the higher its fat, salt, or sugar content and/or the lower its vitamin, mineral, and fiber content. For example, whole wheat bread made from 100% whole wheat flour is an excellent source of B vitamins, trace minerals, and fiber, while bread made from enriched white flour contains significantly less fiber, trace minerals (except iron), and many of the B vitamins.

Frozen entrees can be either high or low in fat. To meet the National Cancer Institute's and the American Heart Association's guidelines for fat consumption (no more than 30% of total calories should come from fat), a food item should not contain more than 3 grams of fat for every 100 calories (3 grams × 9 calories/gram = 27% of total calories). Pasta dishes can be deceiving as the sauce often adds considerable fat and calories to the otherwise low-calorie noodles. Many frozen foods are also moderate to high in salt (sodium). New frozen lines, such as Healthy Choices and Right Course, have developed an array of low-fat, low-sodium entrees.

Other new "fad" foods might be marketed as "healthy," but could be high in fat or low in vitamins, minerals, or fiber. For example, croissants can be mistaken for a nutritious grain selection, when as much as 60% of their calories come from fat. In contrast, whole grain breads contain only 1% to 10% fat calories. Commercial quiche is another example. The pie crust of quiche is the same as any other used for creamed pies or meat fillings; it contains approximately 55% to 60% fat calories, most of which comes from lard or other highly saturated fats. The "lighter" the crust, the higher the fat content. The cheese and egg filling increases the fat and cholesterol content of most quiches and brings the total fat content of one moderate serving to approximately 21 to 27 grams of fat, a fat content equivalent to 4 to 6 pats of butter. Many homemade recipes for quiche contain equivalent or greater amounts of fat and cholesterol, but these can be modified by reducing the amount of butter, cream (use canned non-fat milk instead), whole eggs (use two egg whites for every whole egg and discard yolk), and cheese (substitute low-fat varieties and reduce the amount).

VITAMINS, MINERALS, AND HEALTH FOOD

All foods should be health foods. People have a right to accessible, pure food that is not adulterated, contaminated with insecticides and other poisons or cancer-causing substances, or altered in any way as to compromise the nutritional or sanitary quality of the food. People also should be able to choose from lean meats that are not exposed to steroid hormones, antibiotics, or other growth-promoting substances. Industrial waste products and toxic chemicals should not be allowed to contaminate the water supply and soil, thus entering the food chain. Food should not need to be labeled "health food" to be of this quality. In addition, many claims of "health food" are more promise than substance.

There is no evidence that "natural" or "organic" foods are more healthful than other foods. In fact, in many states there is no regulation or legal definition for these words; industry can use them on any item, regardless of its contents. It is assumed that "organic" foods are grown on soil fertilized with organic fertilizers and without chemical fertilizers or pesticides. However, pesticides from neighboring farms, added directly to the food, or remaining in the soil from past use are found in "organic produce."

There is no evidence that foods grown on soil fertilized with compost, manure, or other natural fertilizers are more nutritious than foods grown on chemically fertilized soil. In fact, the soil fertilized with organic fertilizers is more likely to be deficient in trace minerals. The nutrient content of foods depends on the variety of food, the climate, the nutrients available for growth, and the stage of maturation when the food is harvested. For example, the vitamin C content of oranges varies widely in different areas of the United States and at different times of the year.

There are no guarantees that foods labeled "natural" or "organic" are free from additives, preservatives, or other "unnatural" substances. Many foods called "natural" are highly processed and often contain additives, colorings, synthetic flavorings, or preservatives.

The greatest sales in health foods have been for snack items and convenience foods. Many of these foods are considered unhealthful when sold in a supermarket, but are touted as healthful when packaged and sold in a health food store, regardless of their high-fat, high-sugar (often listed as "natural sweeteners"), high-salt (often listed as "sea salt"), high-cholesterol, or low-vitamin/mineral content. "Natural" butter, granola bars, protein bars, coconut and coconut oil, cream cheese, "fertilized" eggs, granola, cheese, honey, miso, tamari or soy sauce, and many candies or snack items fit this description. In addition, a product advertised as containing no preservatives might be high in fat, salt, or some other unhealthful ingredient.

Another disadvantage to "health foods" is that they usually cost more than the same food purchased in a supermarket. Even the foods placed in special "health food" sections of the supermarket cost more than similar foods found on other shelves.

Some health food companies are sincere in their attempts to provide quality foods and some items in health food stores are an inexpensive alternative to more conventional items. Items sold in bulk bins, such as oatmeal, flour, nuts, beans, and dried fruits, are often less expensive than the same items prepackaged or sold in supermarket sales. Some distributors and growers provide legal statements that their foods are grown or handled according to "organic" principles. The consumer should request to see those statements prior to purchasing an item promoted as "organic" or "natural."

Reading labels and finding a reputable health food store manager can assist the consumer in sorting fact from the fiction. For example, a store that promotes "natural" vitamin supplements over other supplements should be viewed with a suspicious eye as there is no evidence that "natural" is better, only more expensive. Beware of the credibility of salespersons who promote items that are not usually found in the diet, such as bee pollen, algae, protein powders, enzymes (superoxide dismutase or digestive enzymes), and hormonal extracts, or who falsely promote a substance as a vitamin or essential nutrient, such as pangamic acid as vitamin B_{15} or bioflavonoids as vitamin P. (See Chapters 3 and 4 for a list and description of the essential vitamins.) These people are often self-taught and are not credible or reliable sources of sound nutrition information.

The same principles for selecting foods and meal planning apply to health food purchases and conventional food purchases.

- Read labels and avoid products that contain excessive amounts of fats, sugars, salt, additives, or refined ingredients.

- Select foods that have been minimally processed.
- Choose foods from the modified Four Food Groups: whole grain breads and cereals, fresh fruits and vegetables, cooked legumes or lean meats, and low-fat or non-fat dairy products.
- Avoid promotional claims that increase the price, but do not improve the nutritional quality of a food, such as "organic," "natural," or "therapeutic."
- Comparison shop and choose the nutritionally best item for the least amount of money.

SPECIAL DIETS

The principles of menu and diet planning are consistent regardless of age, gender, the presence or absence of degenerative disorders such as heart disease or diabetes, or food preferences. However, certain conditions, lifestyle patterns, or food-intake patterns require minor adjustments or considerations for an individual to maintain optimal health. The three general categories presented here are athletes, people following vegetarian diets, and people on weight-loss diets.

Athletes

No group, except dieters, is more vulnerable to nutrition mythology than athletes. Runners are sure there is a certain food combination that will improve their endurance, wrestlers are convinced there is a pill or powder that will increase their strength, weight-lifters believe extra protein will increase muscle mass, and football players think zinc will make them "tougher." The dangerous use of steroid hormones and other potentially harmful or even lethal substances in the attempt to improve athletic performance attests to the athlete's belief in the magical properties of foods, vitamins, and minerals (Table 54, pages 310–311).

In reality, athletes require the same nutrients as anyone else, although they sometimes require more calories or a little more of a few vitamins and minerals. It is seldom necessary to increase protein intake, even for athletes building muscle mass, since the American diet already contains two to four times more protein than most people need. Extra protein, as steak, raw eggs, or protein powders, does not build extra muscle—only training builds muscle.

The same dietary guidelines outlined at the beginning of this chapter should be followed by all athletes. For example, the carbohydrate needs are high for the endurance athlete, such as swimmers, runners, and bicyclists, because this form of energy is an important storage fuel source during long-distance events. The modified Four Food Group plan recommends at least two-thirds of the diet come from foods high in starch, such as whole grain breads and cereals, fresh fruits and vegetables, and cooked dried beans and peas. The daily diet for the endurance athlete will provide ample amounts of complex carbohydrate (starch) if this diet plan is followed. In the few days prior to a marathon or triathalon or any event lasting more than 2 hours, the athlete might want to further increase the intake of these carbohydrate-rich foods to three-quarters of the food intake to guarantee optimal storage of carbohydrate as glycogen in the muscle and liver tissues. There is no evidence that "carbo-loading" prior to all athletic events will improve performance in events lasting less than $1\frac{1}{2}$ hours, i.e. 10K races or swimming events.

Wrestlers concerned about "making weight" for weekend wrestling matches or football players concerned about weight gain during the off-season should continue to follow the modified Four Food Group plan, but adjust calorie intake to gain or lose weight.

Calorie intake should never fall below 2,000 calories and no more than two pounds should be lost each week unless supervised by a physician. A faster weight loss means muscle tissue, rather than fat tissue, is being lost with the extra danger of dehydration and heat exhaustion. In addition, extreme weight loss, especially in women, is associated with cessation of the menses and bone loss.

A primary concern for athletes is adequate fluid intake. Wrestlers purposely dehydrate themselves in an attempt to make weight, football players and other athletes workout in warm weather often wearing heavy uniforms, tennis players and most athletes lose fluids when perspiring, and long-distance runners exercise for extended periods of time without frequent water stops. Thirst is not an accurate indicator of fluid losses and often an athlete becomes dehydrated during several days of exercise because fluid intake only replaces a portion of the water lost in perspiration during training. The results of chronic fluid deficit and progressive dehydration include muscle fatigue, reduced athletic performance, heat exhaustion, heartbeat irregularities, and possibly heat stroke and even death.

To guarantee adequate fluid intake, drink twice as much water as it takes to quench thirst. A minimum of 8 glasses of water should be consumed each day, in addition to other beverages such as low-fat or non-fat milk, fruit juices, tea, and soft drinks. Athletes should not take sodium or salt tablets, especially prior to first replacing fluid losses. Salt tablets increase the effects of dehydration on the body and are unnecessary since the minimal amounts of electrolytes, such as sodium and potassium, lost in perspiration are easily replaced in the normal diet. Salt tablets or electrolyte replacement beverages should be considered only if more than 4 quarts of water have been lost as perspiration (1 quart of water = 2 pounds of body weight, so a person must lose more than 8 pounds during an athletic event or training session to warrant consideration of salt replacement). A gram of sodium (usually the equivalent of one salt tablet) can be consumed for every quart of water lost above the initial 4 quarts. Athletes should always replace water first and electrolytes second and should begin an athletic event or training session fully hydrated.

Mineral needs might be higher for some athletes. Strenuous exercise alters trace mineral metabolism and increases the loss of several minerals, such as chromium and zinc, in the urine and iron in sweat. Magnesium loss in the urine increases after endurance events and is associated with a brief increase in blood levels of the mineral, suggesting magnesium loss from damaged muscle tissues. Low blood levels of magnesium persist for several months following the athletic event.

Iron is a particular concern for athletes, especially females, engaged in endurance, weight-bearing sports. Blood iron levels appear to decrease in runners, although this is partially explained by the increased blood volume which dilutes the concentration of red blood cells and gives a false reading for iron. However, the repeated pounding of some sports might result in destruction of some red blood cells and a condition called "runner's anemia." The iron status of some female marathon runners is poor and increased iron intake might be necessary for these athletes.

Vitamin needs might increase above the RDAs for some athletes. Some forms of muscle damage in athletes has been attributed to free radical damage to muscle cell membranes. Increased intake of vitamin E might help prevent this damage and soreness. Laboratory studies on animals support this finding and conclude exercise increases the need for vitamin E. Female bicyclists show an increased dietary need for vitamin B_2 to maintain normal tissue and blood levels of the vitamin. Poor intake of other vitamins, such as vitamin B_1, vitamin B_6, and vitamin C, also impair athletic performance.

The diets of athletes are not always optimal. In addition, there are no adequate measurements of nutritional status in athletes. The RDAs, designed for a "reference person," are a poor guideline for assessing adequate nutrient intake for the competition athlete who is a 280-pound football player, a 7-foot-tall basketball player, or a marathon runner with 5% body fat. Intake of vitamin B_6, iron, magnesium, and zinc is reported to be below 70% of the RDA in many athletes and some athletes do not consume adequate amounts of calcium, iron, and vitamins A, D, E, B_2, B_{12}, C, and niacin. An athlete must carefully plan the diet to meet the requirements of the modified Four Food Groups. Whole grain breads and cereals should be chosen, rather than refined varieties. Extra calories to meet the demands of exercise should be provided by additional servings of grains, vegetables, fruits, and other nutrient-dense foods. A vitamin/mineral supplement might be useful (see pages 293–298 for guidelines in choosing a supplement). However, megadoses of vitamins and minerals do not improve athletic performance.

Vegetarian Diets

Vegetarian diets are not new. Accounts of these diets date from 2,000 B.C. Some vegetarian diets might be more healthful than the conventional American diet. Numerous studies have found meat consumption linked to an increased risk for heart disease and other degenerative disorders, whereas a vegetarian diet reduces heart disease risk. The high fiber intake characteristic of the vegetarian diet also improves glucose tolerance in diabetics and lowers blood pressure. Finally, vegetarian diets tend to be low in sugar, whereas the high sugar intake characteristic of American diets is possibly linked to an increased risk for heart disease and cancer. (Tables 28 and 29, pages 150 and 158; and page 164).

The vegetarian diet is actually a blanket term for a variety of diets. The vegan diet is the most restrictive and includes only foods of plant origin, such as nuts, seeds, vegetables, fruits, grains, and legumes. The lactovegetarian diet includes all the foods included in the vegan diet, plus dairy products, such as cheese, milk, and yogurt. The lacto-ovo vegetarian diet includes all of the above foods plus eggs. Variations on the vegetarian diet include fruitarians who eat only fruit, nuts, olive oil, and honey, and the macrobiotic diet that includes seven progressively more restrictive diets with the final diet consisting only of brown rice. These latter diets are too restrictive to guarantee optimal intake of all vitamins, minerals, protein, and calories and are not recommended. People who consume chicken or fish are not considered vegetarians.

A vegetarian diet, whether it be vegan, lactovegetarian, or lacto-ovo vegetarian, can supply all the necessary vitamins, minerals, protein, and other nutrients essential to health, if careful planning is followed. The more restrictive a diet is the more likely nutrient deficiencies will result, especially in pregnant and lactating women and small children. For example, dairy products supply as much as 50% of the daily need for calcium and vitamin B_2. Other foods, such as dark green leafy vegetables and broccoli, are good sources of these nutrients, but large quantities must be consumed each day to meet the RDA levels. Children have small stomachs and finicky appetites, which makes it difficult for them to consume the RDA for calcium obtained from 4 to 6 cups of dark green leafy vegetables necessary in the vegan diet. Calcium-fortified soymilk can meet part of the calcium needs, but other nutrient deficiencies still are possible. In addition, vitamin E needs might be higher with these diets than with conventional diets, because of the increased intake of polyunsaturated fats from nuts, seeds, and vegetable oils.

THE VEGAN DIET. It is not recommended that children less than 18-years-old follow a vegan diet, because of the high nutrient demands and either limited capacity to consume volumes of food or the sporadic eating habits of children. The nutrients most likely to be deficient in the vegan diets of adults include protein, calcium, vitamin B_2, vitamin B_{12}, iron, zinc, and calories.

The vegan diet must be planned carefully to include adequate amounts of protein. The 8 to 10 essential amino acids are found in protein-rich foods, such as lean meat, chicken, fish, eggs, milk, cheese, and yogurt. These foods are called high-quality protein foods because they provide all the essential amino acids in the proper ratio for optimal absorption and use. The vegan diet excludes these foods and individuals following this diet must combine lower quality protein foods, such as nuts, seeds, legumes, and grains, to obtain the proper amount and proportion of the essential amino acids. Each of these foods are excellent sources of amino acids, but usually are lacking in one or more of the essential amino acids.

A high-quality protein can be obtained by combining two or more of these foods. For example, legumes, such as kidney beans or split peas, are low in the amino acids methionine and cystine but are high in the amino acid lysine. Grains, such as corn or wheat, are high in lysine but low in methionine and cystine and are an excellent "complement" to the legumes. The combination of corn and beans, such as the corn tortilla and beans in a burrito, supply high-quality protein. Grains combined with nuts and seeds do not provide the complement of amino acids to constitute a high-quality protein source. Other complementary protein combinations include:

1. Legumes and Grains
   - peanut butter sandwich
   - baked beans and brown bread
   - lentil and rice soup
   - black beans and rice pilaf
2. Seeds/Nuts and Legumes
   - lentil and cashew loaf
   - tofu and sesame burgers
   - stuffed cabbage rolls, with split peas and sunflower seeds

Calcium needs are more difficult to meet on the vegan diet than on less restrictive diets that include dairy products. A glass of milk provides 36% of the adult RDA for calcium; a cup of legumes provides 12%; and nuts, seeds, and grains provide even less. However, daily calcium needs can be met with planning. Dark green leafy vegetables, such as mustard greens, beet greens, collards, kale, and broccoli, are excellent sources of calcium and contain between 50% to 100% of the calcium in a glass of milk (300 mg). Some greens, such as spinach, contain calcium but the mineral is not well absorbed because of other calcium-binding substances, called oxalates, in spinach. Calcium-fortified soymilk is the best source of calcium for vegans. Soymilk can be included in the diet as a base for soups, as an ingredient in homemade breads, as the fluid for rice and other cereals, and as a beverage. Powdered calcium carbonate can be added to flour for baking or calcium supplements can be taken. A source of vitamin D also must be identified, since fortified milk is the only reliable source of this essential vitamin.

A main source of vitamin B_2 is dairy products. The vegan must be particularly careful in diet planning to meet daily needs for this water-soluble vitamin. The foods of plant origin in the following list supply approximately the same amount of vitamin B_2 as does one cup of milk (0.395 mg), and a minimum of three servings each day should be consumed to meet the adult RDA.

- avocado, 1 medium
- fortified cereal, one ounce
- fresh mushrooms, $1^{1/4}$ cups
- cooked turnip greens, $1^{1/4}$ cups
- cooked broccoli, $1^{1/3}$ cups
- winter squash, $1^{1/2}$ cups
- cooked asparagus, $1^{3/4}$ cups
- cooked spinach, $1^{3/4}$ cups
- Brussels sprouts, 2 cups
- okra, $2^{1/4}$ cups

The only reliable dietary sources of vitamin B_{12} are foods of animal origin. A few kinds of algae and some fermented soybean products, such as tempeh and miso, are the only plant sources of this vitamin, but contain varying amounts. Vitamin B_{12}-fortified soymilk or supplements should be consumed regularly to prevent deficiencies.

Although many foods of plant origin are high in iron, the iron from these sources is not as well absorbed as the iron in meat (called "heme" iron). In addition, the high fiber content of the vegan diet might interfere with optimal absorption of some trace minerals, such as iron and zinc. To increase absorption of iron, the vegan should consume a vitamin C-rich food with meals, cook in cast iron pots, and include several servings each day of iron-rich foods.

The best sources of zinc are lean meats, oysters, herring, milk, and egg yolks. Whole grain breads and cereals are the best source of zinc in the vegan diet, but this form of zinc is poorly absorbed. Frequent daily servings of whole grain breads and cereals must be included in the vegan diet to increase zinc intake or a multi-vitamin/mineral supplement that includes zinc should be taken.

The modified Four Food Group plan must be adapted for the vegan diet. The daily food guide for people on this type of vegetarian diet is as follows:

Vegetables   4 servings
(At least 1 dark green leafy vegetable and 1 raw salad for calcium, vitamin B_2, vitamin A, and folic acid. A serving size is 1 cup.)
Fruits   3 servings
(At least 1 iron-rich selection and 1 vitamin C-rich selection. Servings include juice or whole fruit.)
Grains   5 servings
(Whole grain varieties only. A serving size is 2 slices of bread; 4–6 crackers; 1 cup cooked cereal, noodles, or rice; or 2 ounces of ready-to-eat cereal.)
Beans and Nuts, including soymilk   3 servings
(At least 1 cup calcium-fortified soymilk. Beans are preferable to nuts as a low-fat protein source. A serving size is 1 cup cooked beans, 2 cups soymilk, 6 ounces tofu, 2 ounces nuts, or 4 tablespoons peanut butter.)

THE LACTOVEGETARIAN AND THE LACTO-OVO VEGETARIAN DIETS. These vegetarian diets easily can meet the RDA for all vitamins, minerals, protein, and other nutrients. Inclusion of dairy foods guarantees adequate intake of protein, calcium, vitamin D, vitamin B_{12}, and vitamin B_2. The vegetarian should not rely too heavily on cheese as a source of calcium and protein, since it contains a high percentage of saturated fat. Zinc and iron intake might be low since meat is not included in the diet.

In addition, combining the high-quality protein in eggs or low-fat dairy products with other plant sources of protein improves the quality of protein in beans, nuts, grains, and seeds. For example, the amino acids in eggs and milk products complement the plant proteins in the following foods:

• Cereals and milk . . . . whole grain breakfast cereal and milk
• Pasta and cheese . . . . macaroni and cheese

- Bread and cheese . . . . cheese sandwich on whole wheat bread
- Beans and cheese . . . . bean and cheese burrito
- Rice and milk . . . . brown rice pudding
- Bread and egg . . . . scrambled eggs and whole wheat toast
- Peanuts and milk . . . . peanut butter sandwich and yogurt

The modified Four Food Group plan remains the same for the lactovegetarian or lacto-ovo vegetarian. The only alteration is for the meat and legume group. Rather than the four recommended servings equally divided between lean meats and legumes, now all four servings each day must come from cooked dried beans and peas, nuts and seeds, or eggs. A serving of beans or peas is one cup, a serving of nuts or seeds is 2 ounces, and a serving of eggs is one egg. (Table 37, page 251) The balanced diet for a lacto-ovo vegetarian might resemble the following:

- 2 servings low-fat or non-fat milk or milk products
- 4 servings protein-rich cooked dried beans and peas, peanut butter, seeds, or nuts
- 4+ servings of whole grain breads and cereals
- 4+ servings of fruits and vegetables, especially dark green selections

The Weight Loss Diet

Weight loss and weight maintenance are dependent on identifying and following a diet and exercise program that balances calories (energy) consumed with calories (energy) used. This regime will vary from individual to individual based on age, gender, history of dieting, genetic conditions, and hormonal or neurochemical variations. Not everyone can maintain the "thin" look promoted by today's fashion magazines and still remain healthy. But each person can find a personal and optimal weight that also maintains health.

There are no pills, powders, combination of foods or order of food intake, injections, individual foods, or machines that will produce long-term weight loss and maintenance. The only effective long-term eating pattern is a lifelong diet and exercise program. Consuming only fruit for breakfast, eating grapefruit at every meal, eliminating carbohydrate foods, eating a high-protein diet, eating "diet candy" before each meal, or any other quick weight-loss technique usually results in an initial loss of a few pounds (mostly water and muscle tissue, seldom fat tissue), but none of these techniques produce long-term weight loss or weight maintenance. In all cases, the reason any weight is lost is because of the reduced calorie intake.

Some quick weight-loss techniques can be dangerous. Some herbal diet pills might cause overactive thyroid. Tryptophan supplements have shown inconsistent results as weight loss aids and recent reports show even moderate doses could cause liver damage or a rare blood disorder. Very low calorie diets (VLCD) that contain less than 800 calories must be monitored by a physician because of potential adverse changes in potassium. People who consume a diet that contains less than 1,200 calories also might be deficient in vitamin B_1, vitamin B_6, vitamin B_{12}, iron, magnesium, and zinc. Even high-protein weight loss diets that contain less than 1,000 calories per day do not provide adequate amounts of protein, since the low calorie intake results in dietary protein being used as energy. In contrast, many high-protein diets contain excessive amounts of fat and cholesterol, increase blood fat levels, or increase a person's risk for developing cardiovascular disease or cancer. Finally, weight loss that exceeds 2 pounds a week results in loss of water and lean body tissue (muscle and internal organs) rather than fat tissue.

The best "diet" for weight loss is based on the Four Food Groups plan plus a minimum of 3 aerobic exercise sessions each week (at least 30 minutes in length). The minimum number of servings (four whole grains, four fruits and vegetables, two milk, and two meat or legume) provides approximately 1,600 calories. The high fiber intake from these foods or from fiber products such as guar gum reduces hunger, possibly by reducing drastic fluctuations in blood sugar levels. In addition, secondary benefits from this low-fat, high-fiber diet are enhancement of the immune system and reduced risk for developing diabetes, cardiovascular disease, hypertension, and cancer. If weight is not lost on this diet, then exercise levels must be increased to either more or longer sessions each week. Further reductions in calorie intake should only be considered with the advice and supervision of a physician. Repeated weight loss and weight gain cycles—called "yo-yo dieting"—results in increasing body fat, making it more and more difficult to lose weight and maintain the weight loss. In other words, repeated unsuccessful attempts to lose weight make a person "fatter."

The use of artificial sweeteners is questionable. Saccharin and cyclamates produce cancer in laboratory animals. The safety of aspartame in NutraSweet™ has been challenged since studies show aspartame and beverages containing the non-nutritive sweetener might stimulate appetite, promote weight gain, or cause seizures in some individuals. Until more information is gathered, aspartame should be consumed in moderate amounts.

Weight-loss diets must be followed at home and away from home. Suggestions for those watching their weight when eating in restaurants include the following:

1. Eat something to take the edge off the appetite before leaving home.
2. Locate restaurants where the management will tailor their menu items to meet your needs and prepare each meal to order.
3. Order half-orders or split an order with a friend.
4. Order à la carte.
5. Focus on salad bars, but avoid marinated vegetables, pasta salads, and other ingredients mixed with mayonnaise or other fats.
6. Be assertive. Ask for foods steamed, baked, or broiled dry. Send orders back if they are not prepared to order.
7. Decide ahead of time what to order.
8. Order without looking at the menu.
9. Order mineral water, herb tea, or tomato juice to sip while waiting for the meal.
10. Ask for salad dressing on the side.
11. Avoid the following words: refried, sauteed, au gratin, gravied, fried, à la mode, prime, pot pie, au fromage, hollandaise, crispy, creamed, or cheese sauce.
12. Choose fresh fruit, steamed or raw vegetables, baked potatoes with chives, baked or boiled lean meats and fish, whole grain breads, consommé, barley or vegetable soups, seafood cocktails, pasta with marinara sauce, and fruit ices.
13. Call the local American Heart Association for a local guide to restaurants that serve low-calorie foods.
14. Pay more attention to the conversation than to the food or hors d'oeuvres.

Summary

Many variations on the conventional American diet still can provide adequate amounts of all the essential vitamins and minerals if planned carefully. All diets should contain a variety of foods and all foods should be consumed in moderation. Regardless of whether a vegetarian diet, a diet for athletes, a weight-loss diet, or a more conventional diet is desired, the foundation for food choices is a moderate calorie, nutrient-dense diet that is low in fat, low in cholesterol, low in sugar, low in salt, and high in fiber, vitamins, and minerals. A well-balanced supplement might be needed to guarantee optimal intake of all vitamins and minerals if the daily energy intake is less than 2,000 calories. (See pages 293–298 for guidelines in choosing a supplement.)

CHAPTER 8

Understanding Supplements

No other topic in nutrition has created such heated debates as vitamin-mineral supplements and the appropriateness of their inclusion in the diet. Everyone agrees the best place to obtain the daily needs for essential vitamins and minerals is from a well-balanced diet. However, not everyone is able or wants to consistently consume a diet based on these recommendations, and vitamin-mineral status might suffer unless an alternative source of these nutrients is found.

UNDERSTANDING THE TERMINOLOGY

Vitamin-mineral supplements are a multi-billion dollar industry. The great variety of formulas, single-nutrients, or combination preparations in numerous dosages line an entire wall or aisle in many stores. This diversity and variation in products is more confusing than helpful to most shoppers. The hundreds of bottles, jars, individually-wrapped "packs," cans, and envelopes can be overwhelming to someone looking for a vitamin-mineral preparation to meet his or her needs. Words, such as "organic," "therapeutic," "natural," "buffered," or "time-released," further complicate the choice. Choosing a vitamin-mineral supplement to best meet individual needs is simple once the words are defined and a few guidelines for selecting a supplement are provided.

Dietary Supplements Versus Nonprescription Drugs

Most vitamin-mineral preparations are called *dietary supplements*. These products are designed for use as supplements to a normal diet and to increase the total daily intake of one or more vitamins or minerals. The Food and Drug Administration (FDA) classifies a product as a nonprescription drug if it is promoted on the label or in accompanying literature to cure or treat health conditions or if the ingredients produce dangerous side effects. For example, experts at the FDA determined from the scientific literature that vitamin K could be dangerous for people on anticoagulant (blood thinning) medications. Consequently, supplementation with this fat-soluble vitamin is recommended only with the supervision of a physician. Therefore, vitamin K supplements are classified as a drug rather than a dietary supplement. Laetril, a substance promoted to treat cancer and sold as vitamin B_{17}, was banned by the FDA because of the therapeutic claims used to sell the substance and because laetril contains potentially dangerous quantities of cyanide.

Megavitamin Supplements

Megavitamin therapy is the use of one or more vitamins in amounts exceeding the RDA by 10-fold or more. Megavitamin dosages became popular because of the misconception that if a small amount of a nutrient is good for health, more must be better.

Megavitamin therapy is usually unnecessary and can be expensive and potentially harmful. For example, many of the water-soluble vitamins perform specific functions, usually in conjunction with an enzyme made in the body. These vitamins have no metabolic function by themselves. The amount of a vitamin-dependent enzyme that a cell can make in a day is limited. To consume more of the vitamin than can be used in the manufacture or use of the related enzyme will not stimulate a greater production of the enzyme; instead it will increase urinary excretion of the unused water-soluble vitamin.

Fat-soluble vitamins (A, D, E, and K) potentially can accumulate to toxic levels in the tissues because they are not readily excreted in the urine. Vitamins A and D have shown toxicity symptoms in healthy individuals and vitamin K might be toxic to people on anticoagulant medications when consumed in large amounts over long periods of time. Although megadoses of vitamin E have not been proven toxic, no benefits of large doses of this fat-soluble vitamin have been proven.

Large doses of certain minerals (several times the RDA) can be toxic if they accumulate in tissues or cause secondary deficiencies of other minerals and only should be taken with the supervision of a physician and dietitian. For example, large doses of iron can cause constipation and other stomach or intestinal upsets and, in some people, can cause hemosiderosis, a disorder characterized by abnormal iron accumulation in the liver, pancreas, and other organs. Large doses of selenium or copper also produce toxic symptoms including nervous system disorders and liver or kidney malfunction. Long-term megadoses of zinc can produce a copper deficiency because the two trace minerals compete in the small intestine for absorption.

In general, dietary intakes of no more than three times the RDA are probably safe. Doses of 10 to 1,000 times the RDA for long periods of time of even the water-soluble vitamins might have detrimental effects on health. For example, megadoses of:

- vitamin A (retinol) might cause liver damage
- vitamin D might contribute to atherosclerosis, liver damage, and kidney disease
- niacin (nicotinic acid) might cause liver damage
- vitamin B_6 might cause irreversible nerve damage
- pantothenic acid might cause diarrhea
- folic acid can mask an underlying vitamin B_{12} deficiency and result in irreversible nerve damage
- vitamin C might encourage the formation of kidney stones and suppress the immune response
- iron can interfere with zinc absorption
- zinc can suppress the immune response

Size, genetic individuality, age, gender, and numerous other factors contribute to tolerance to megadoses of a nutrient. What is safe for one person could be toxic for another.

Buffered Vitamins

Some vitamins, especially vitamin C, are acidic and, although not strong acids like the hydrochloric acid in the stomach or sulfuric acid, they can irritate the digestive tract when consumed in megadoses. A compound that buffers or "neutralizes" the acidity of vitamin C can be added to a supplement to counteract the irritating effects. Ascorbate is a form of buffered vitamin C. Sodium ascorbate should be avoided by people who must restrict their salt (sodium) intake, such as people with high blood pressure.

Chelated Minerals

A chelated mineral is one attached to another substance, such as an amino acid, called a *chelator*. The chelator can be a natural or synthetic substance. Gluconate, as in zinc gluconate, is a common chelator. Chelated minerals are promoted as better absorbed and more available than other minerals. Supposedly the attached substance, such as the amino acid, enhances the absorption of the mineral from the intestines into the bloodstream. This argument in favor of chelation is based on incomplete information and might be incorrect.

Chelation forms a weak bond between the mineral and the other compound or chelator. This bond is easily broken in the highly acidic environment of the stomach. Once detached from its chelator, the mineral floats freely and independently in the intestine and is absorbed no better (but no worse) than any other supplemental or dietary form of the mineral. The only benefit of chelated minerals, such as iron fumarate or zinc gluconate, is that they are less irritating to the stomach and intestine and less likely to cause stomach upsets or constipation than are other minerals, such as zinc sulfate or iron sulfate, when taken in large amounts. One exception to this general rule is chromium picolinate, which is a chelated form of chromium that is very well absorbed.

Chelation is less important to absorption and utilization of a mineral than are the circumstances associated with taking the supplement. Minerals, in general, are better absorbed if taken with a meal. The presence of other dietary ingredients, such as protein and carbohydrate, stimulate the release of digestive enzymes and juices that facilitate the breakdown and absorption of all nutrients, including minerals. An exception to this rule is iron, which is better absorbed on an empty stomach.

Chewable Vitamins

The most common vitamin available in chewable form is vitamin C. No harm will come from infrequent small doses of this form of the water-soluble vitamin. However, frequent exposure of the tooth enamel to an acidic substance, such as vitamin C, can wear away the enamel and increase the likelihood of dental cavities.

Parents should closely monitor children's consumption of chewable multivitamins. These supplements are sweetened, taste like candy to a child, and if consumed in quantities could approach toxic levels. Children are more susceptible than adults to vitamin toxicities and should not consume more than the RDAs from the combination of wholesome foods, fortified cereals and convenience foods, vitamin-mineral supplements, or other potential sources of nutrients.

Natural, Organic, or Synthetic Vitamins?

Despite the implied wholesomeness of the words "natural" and "organic," in most cases the quality or usefulness of a vitamin is not dependent on its source. The definitions and distinction between these words are either nonexistent or vague.

Vitamins and minerals do not exist alone. They are either manufactured by a plant or microorganism or are synthesized in a laboratory. In many cases both processes occur at one time. For example, vitamins or minerals often are "synthesized" by using bacteria or yeast to manufacture the substance or incorporate a nutrient from their environment into a more biologically available form. Selenomethionine, the "natural" form of selenium, and GTF chromium, the "natural" form of chromium, are synthesized by yeast in the laboratory. Does that make them synthetic or natural?

Other "natural" vitamins are extracted from foods, such as wheatgerm, by exposure to numerous chemical solvents during both the removal from the original food source and the concentration of the vitamin into a tablet, capsule, or pill. For example, vitamin E is obtained from natural sources, such as the vegetable oils from soy beans, corn, or wheatgerm. Several chemical solvents are required to separate the vitamin from the oil and concentrate it in a capsule small enough to swallow. In addition, preservatives are included in many preparations to prevent decay of the capsule. What began as natural ends up a highly refined and processed product. Does that make them natural or synthetic?

In other cases, the word "natural" is used on a vitamin-mineral supplement but the product is manufactured in the laboratory with only a small addition of the natural source. For example, small amounts of bioflavonoids and rose hips are added to large amounts of synthetic vitamin C and the product is called "natural." In reality, natural rose hips contain approximately 2% vitamin C and a vitamin C supplement that relied entirely on this source of the vitamin would be too big to swallow.

In contrast, some nutrients are often synthetic vitamins added to a yeast or other natural base. Selenomethionine, a "natural" form of selenium, is only formed if selenium is added to the yeast culture and is absorbed and converted to the natural form within the yeast. However, selenium mixed with yeast is often sold as a "natural" form of the mineral. Natural B vitamins often are sold this way.

Theoretically, supplements should be manufactured only from

"organic" food sources. The lack of regulation, however, allows such a loose interpretation of the word that it becomes useless, especially in the case of supplements. Some credibility does exist for organically produced sources of supplemental selenium and chromium. Both "organic" and "natural" are used to describe the process where these minerals are added to a yeast base where they are absorbed and incorporated into the structure of the yeast. These sources of selenium and chromium might be better absorbed and used by the human body. Otherwise, "organic" promises no more than increased cost. In addition, no scientific evidence exists showing that the body uses organic vitamins and minerals better than it does synthetic forms. Except for selenium, chromium, and possibly vitamin E, the nutrients are identical and no reliable tests exist to discern a natural from a synthetic vitamin or mineral.

Water-Solublized Fat-Soluble Vitamins

The fat-soluble vitamins A, D, E, and K require small amounts of dietary fat, special fat-digesting enzymes from the pancreas, and bile from the liver and gallbladder to be digested and absorbed. The fat-soluble vitamins are easily absorbed by most people, but deficiencies can develop in people with intestinal diseases, such as celiac disease, tropical sprue, cystic fibrosis, or ulcerative colitis. In these disorders, a physician might recommend a water-solublized form of vitamins A, D, E, or K. The vitamin is attached to a water-soluble compound that is easily absorbed in the intestine without the need for the fat-digesting enzymes and bile. Once in the bloodstream, the vitamin portion splits from the attached compound and is used like any other form of the vitamin.

Some fat-soluble vitamins, especially vitamin A, are available in an emulsified form. The emulsifier separates the fat-soluble vitamin into tiny beadlets that remain suspended in a watery base, much like the lecithin added to commercial salad dressings that keeps the oil and vinegar from separating. Emulsified vitamin A dissolves more readily in the watery medium of the intestine and is easier for people with the above mentioned intestinal disorders to digest and absorb. Emulsified vitamin A might be toxic at lower doses than other forms of the vitamin and no more than the RDA should be consumed unless monitored by a physician.

Time-Released Supplements

The theory supporting time-released vitamins makes sense. In reality, however, time-released vitamins might be no better, and even might be less effective, than regular supplements.

The time-release theory is based on two important considerations about vitamin and mineral absorption:

1. Vitamin-mineral supplements taken in large doses cause blood levels of the nutrients to rise abruptly. A substantial amount of the nutrient is lost in the urine because the kidneys increase urinary excretion to remove the abnormally high blood concentrations.
2. Anything that slows the absorption of vitamins and minerals would eliminate the rapid rise in blood levels and more of the nutrient would be available for longer periods of time for use in body processes.

Time-released supplements were developed in an attempt to solve this problem. They were to dissolve slowly in the intestine, increase the amount of absorption of a vitamin or mineral, and hopefully reduce the dramatic fluctuations in blood levels. Vitamins and minerals are absorbed at very specific spots along the intestinal tract, however, and unless they dissolve and are available at that point of absorption, they continue to travel down the digestive tract and are excreted. It is chance that a time-release tablet requiring 4 to 8 hours to dissolve will release each nutrient at the appropriate spot for absorption.

In reality, nutrients from time-release preparations are often poorly absorbed. In one study, when niacin as either a time-released or regular supplement was given to patients with high blood cholesterol levels, the regular niacin supplement was more effective in lowering blood cholesterol and other fats than was the time-released tablets.

CHOOSING A VITAMIN AND MINERAL SUPPLEMENT

Vitamin and mineral needs vary widely from one individual to another and even within the same person from week to week. Nutrient needs fluctuate depending on individual variation in the absorption and use of specific nutrients, the adequacy of the diet, age, sex, and confounding factors such as disease, medications, tobacco use, alcohol consumption, and stress (Worksheet 1).

Worksheet 1.
RATE THE DIET

	Usually	Sometimes	Seldom
1. I eat a variety of foods such as fresh fruits and vegetables, whole grain breads and cereals, lean meats, cooked dried beans and peas, low-fat dairy products, and nuts and seeds, and consume at least 2,000 calories worth of these foods every day.	4	1	0
2. I limit the amount of fat in the diet, including meats, oil, butter, cream, desserts, fried foods, salad dressings, mayonnaise, and other fatty foods.	2	1	0
3. I avoid sugar and sugary foods, including soft drinks, candy, desserts, hidden sugars in processed foods, and ready-to-eat cereals.	2	1	0
4. I include at least one dark green leafy vegetable, one citrus fruit, and two to three calcium-rich foods in the diet each day.	2	1	0
5. I am not on long-term prescription or non-prescription medications.	2	1	0
6. I avoid quick-weight loss diets.	2	1	0
7. I avoid alcohol and tobacco or use them in moderation.	2	1	0

Add the circled numbers.

- A score of 11 to 16 is excellent. It is unlikely you need to take a supplement.
- A score of 7 to 10 is good, but some changes need to be made in eating habits and a multiple vitamin-mineral supplement might improve the daily nutrient intake.
- A score of 4 to 6 indicates a health risk. Dietary changes and the inclusion of a multiple vitamin-mineral supplement in the daily nutrient intake should begin immediately.
- A score less than 4 indicates a high risk to health and nutritional status. Major dietary changes are required that include supplementation and possible dietary advice from a registered dietitian or physician.

In general, a low-dose, broad spectrum, multiple vitamin and mineral preparation would meet the needs of most people and would avoid the problems of supplement abuse and nutrient toxicities. The following guidelines are designed to guarantee safety and economy when choosing an all-purpose vitamin-mineral supplement.

1. Choose a multiple vitamin-mineral preparation and avoid numerous individual supplements that contain a few nutrients, unless individual nutrients are prescribed by a physician or dietitian. A multiple vitamin-mineral supplement should include the following:

   - the fat-soluble vitamins: A, D, and E
   - the water-soluble vitamins: B_1, B_2, B_6, B_{12}, niacin, pantothenic acid, biotin, folic acid, and vitamin C
   - the minerals: chromium, copper, iron, manganese, molybdenum, selenium, and zinc

   Multiple vitamin-mineral supplements usually do not provide adequate amounts of calcium and magnesium and a separate supplement might be needed if these two minerals are a concern in the diet.
2. Choose a supplement that provides approximately 100% (no more than 300%) of the USRDA for all the vitamins and minerals listed. The delicate balance of nutrients necessary for optimal health is upset by both deficiencies and excesses. Although not always toxic, these excesses can negatively influence other nutrients. For example, a multiple preparation that supplies 50 times the USRDA for pantothenic acid can increase niacin loss. Large intakes of either iron, copper, or zinc affects the absorption and use of the other two minerals. These nutrient-nutrient interactions can be avoided if a supplement is chosen that supplies approximately the same percentage of the USRDA of each vitamin and mineral.
3. Avoid supplements that contain unrecognized substances, such as "vitamin B_{15}" or pangamic acid, bee pollen, cytochrome C, herbs, octacosanol, hormones, enzymes, or spirulina. Avoid supplements that provide nutrients in minute amounts (less than 15% of the USRDA). If a substance is listed, such as bioflavonoids, but no amounts are given, assume little or none of the substance is contained in the product.
4. Carefully read labels on supplement products and purchase only those products that contain the vitamins and minerals needed. Avoid "extras," the vitamins or minerals not needed in a supplement, such as sodium, phosphorus, or chloride. Avoid potentially

unsafe inclusions, such as glandular products, hormones, and dessicated organs, that increase the cost, but not the health benefits, of a product. In general, avoid promotional words such as "natural," "organic," "therapeutic," "balanced," "sustained or time-released," "super potency," or "stress formula."

Table 49 is an example of a vitamin-mineral preparation that meets the above recommendations.

Table 49.
SAMPLE MULTIPLE VITAMIN-MINERAL SUPPLEMENT

2 tablets daily provide the following nutrients:

	Amount		% of the USRDA
Vitamin A (retinol)	2,500	IU	50
Beta Carotene	2,500	IU	50
Vitamin D	400	IU	100
Vitamin E (d-alpha tocopherol)	30	IU	100
Vitamin B₁ (Thiamin)	1.5	mg	100
Vitamin B₂ (Riboflavin)	1.7	mg	100
Niacin (Niacinamide)	20	mg	100
Vitamin B₆ (Pyridoxine)	2	mg	100
Vitamin B₁₂ (Cobalamin)	6	mcg	100
Folic Acid (Folacin)	400	mcg	100
Biotin	300	mcg	100
Pantothenic Acid (Calcium Pantothenate)	10	mg	100
Vitamin C (Ascorbate)	90	mg	150
Calcium (Calcium carbonate)	162	mg	15*
Chromium (GTF-Chromium)	200	mcg	**
Copper	3	mcg	**
Iron (Ferrous)	18	mg	100
Magnesium	60	mg	15*
Manganese	5	mg	**
Molybdenum	20–50	mcg	**
Selenium (Selenomethionine)	200	mcg	**
Zinc (Zinc gluconate)	15	mg	100

* This supplement would not supply adequate amounts of calcium and magnesium, and additional supplements of these two minerals might be necessary if calcium and magnesium intake is low in the diet.

** No USRDA has been established for these nutrients. The amounts recommended are based on the Food and Nutrition Board's Safe and Adequate daily amounts.

Supplementation: A Word of Caution

Supplementing the diet with vitamins and minerals has its limitations. Supplements cannot substitute for a nutritious and wholesome diet, especially as many substances in foods, other than vitamins and minerals, have been and continue to be identified that promote health and protection against disease. For example, compounds called "indoles" found in vegetables in the cabbage family, such as broccoli, asparagus, and cauliflower, apparently protect against certain forms of cancer. Substances in garlic might help lower blood cholesterol levels and aid in the prevention of heart disease and atherosclerosis. These non-nutrient substances are not found in supplements.

Supplements also can be harmful if taken indiscriminately or in large doses. Vitamins and minerals move from the realm of nutrition into the realm of pharmacology and drugs when taken in doses exceeding 10 times the RDAs. Until recently, the fat-soluble vitamins were the primary source of concern for toxicity. Now it is recognized that even water-soluble vitamins and many minerals have toxic effects when taken in unusually high doses. Little information is available on the long-term effects of supplement abuse, but some of the effects identified can be irreversible.

Supplements will not bestow immunity from disease or prevent premature aging in an otherwise unhealthy body. They are, however, an economical and practical way to ensure adequate nutrition when combined with a nutritious diet or during those times when a person cannot eat the perfect diet (Worksheet 2).

Worksheet 2.
PERSONALIZED SUPPLEMENTATION SHEET

Design a personalized supplementation program based on the analysis of your diet on page 294 and the Sample Multiple Vitamin-Mineral Supplement on page 296. Review the guidelines for choosing a vitamin and mineral supplement discussed on pages 295–296. After completion of the Personalized Supplementation Sheet, visit the vitamin-mineral supplement section of the local drug store, supermarket, or health food store. Identify a multiple preparation or combinations of multiple and individual supplements that provide approximately the amounts of each nutrient listed on the sheet. Use the suggested dosage on the Sample Multiple Vitamin-Mineral Supplement table if a USRDA is not listed on the supplement's label.

Nutrient	Amount (mg,mcg,IU)	USRDA	% of the USRDA
FAT-SOLUBLE VITAMINS			
Vitamin A/Beta Carotene	_____	5,000 IU	_____
Vitamin D	_____	400 IU	_____
Vitamin E	_____	30 IU	_____

Worksheet 2. (*continued*)
PERSONALIZED SUPPLEMENTATION SHEET

Nutrient	Amount (mg,mcg,IU)	USRDA	% of the USRDA
WATER-SOLUBLE VITAMINS			
Vitamin B$_1$	_____	1.5 mg	_____
Vitamin B$_2$	_____	1.7 mg	_____
Niacin	_____	20 mg	_____
Vitamin B$_6$	_____	2 mg	_____
Vitamin B$_{12}$	_____	6 mcg	_____
Folic Acid	_____	400 mcg	_____
Biotin	_____	300 mcg	_____
Pantothenic Acid	_____	10 mg	_____
Vitamin C	_____	60 mg	_____
MINERALS			
Calcium	_____	1,000 mg	_____
Chromium	_____	50–200 mcg*	_____
Copper	_____	2 mg	_____
Iron	_____	18 mg	_____
Magnesium	_____	400 mg	_____
Manganese	_____	5 mg*	_____
Molybdenum	_____	15–50 mcg*	_____
Selenium	_____	50–200 mcg*	_____
Zinc	_____	15 mg	_____

* No USRDA has been established for these nutrients. The Safe and Adequate ranges determined by the Food and Nutrition Board, National Research Council are used instead.

CHAPTER 9

Questions on Vitamins and Minerals

The following pages provide answers to the most frequently asked questions on vitamins and minerals. This information can assist an individual in determining his or her own vitamin and mineral needs and in making informed choices about how to obtain and maintain optimal nutrition and health for a lifetime.

GENERAL NUTRITION QUESTIONS

1. What are nutrient-dense foods?

Nutrient-dense foods provide a large amount of vitamins and/or minerals for a relatively small amount of calories. Examples of nutrient-dense foods include fruits and vegetables, whole grain breads and cereals, cooked dried beans and peas, low-fat or non-fat dairy products, fish, chicken without the skin, and lean meats. Foods steamed, baked, or broiled with no added butter, margarine, or other fats are nutrient-dense.

2. What is a calorie-dense food?

A calorie-dense food is one that supplies small amounts of vitamins and/or minerals and relatively large amounts of calories. Examples of calorie-dense foods include high-fat and high-sugar foods, such as butter, oils, candy, bacon, hot dogs, cookies, or fried foods.

3. What is a balanced diet?

A balanced diet is one where all vitamins, minerals, and other nutrients are supplied in optimal amounts. The typical balanced diet contains a variety of foods from the following selections: fresh fruits and vegetables, whole grain breads and cereals, cooked dried beans and peas, low-fat or non-fat dairy products, lean meat, chicken, fish, and nuts and seeds.

4. What is a nutrient?

A nutrient is an substance obtained from the diet and used in the body to promote the growth, maintenance, and repair of tissues.

5. What is an essential nutrient?

An essential nutrient is one that cannot be produced by the body in adequate amounts to meet daily needs and must be obtained from the diet. Many nutrients are essential to health, but essential nutrient refers to vitamins, minerals, fatty acids, amino acids, and other nutrients that must be supplied by food.

6. What is a calorie?

A calorie is a measurement of energy in food. A calorie (or more accurately a kcalorie) is the amount of heat energy required to raise the temperature of 1,000 grams of water 1° C. (Calor means "heat" and kilo means "1,000.") The proteins and carbohydrates in food provide 4 calories/gram, whereas fats provide 9 calories/gram and alcohol 7 calories/gram. Vitamins and minerals do not supply calories.

7. What is a secondary deficiency?

A secondary deficiency is a vitamin or mineral deficiency caused by something other than poor dietary intake of the nutrient. A secondary deficiency can be caused by a disease that reduces the absorption or utilization of a vitamin or mineral, or excessive intake of one nutrient that interferes with the absorption or use of another.

8. What is an enzyme?

An enzyme is a compound that acts as a catalyst in starting a chemical reaction. All enzymes are produced from amino acids in the body. The millions of different enzymes speed up chemical reactions without being destroyed or altered in the process. Many of the B vitamins and several minerals work closely with specific enzymes.

9. What is mineral water?

No legal definition or standardization exists for the term "mineral water." In some cases, commercial products are obtained from underground spring water and contain trace to substantial amounts of certain minerals, such as calcium and magnesium. Other bottled waters sold as mineral water are actually distilled water with added minerals. Some mineral waters contain large amounts of sodium, others contain little or no sodium. The Food and Drug Administration (FDA) loosely regulates bottled water, but accurate information on the mineral content of these products is difficult to obtain and information provided on the label is not always accurate.

10. What is the difference between gram (gm), milligram (mg), and microgram (mcg)?

The gram is a metric unit of weight, equal to 1/28th of an ounce (28 grams = 1 ounce). Protein, complex and simple carbohydrates (starch and sugars), and fat are called the *macronutrients* because they are needed by the body in the greatest quantity, which is measured in grams (gm).

Vitamins and minerals are called the *micronutrients* because they are needed in relatively small amounts, measured in milligrams (mg) and micrograms (mcg). A milligram is 1/1,000th of a gram; a microgram is 1/1,000 of a milligram or one millionth of a gram. For example, the RDA for calcium is 800 mg to 1,200 mg (0.8 gm to 1.2 gms) and the RDA for folic acid is 400 mcg (0.4 mg or 0.0004 grams). These amounts are minute when compared to the 5 grams in 1 teaspoon.

11. What is an International Unit (IU)?

International Units (IU) are arbitrary units of measurement used for the fat-soluble vitamins A, D, and E. These units standardize the biological activity (potency) of the vitamin, rather than measure the weight. However, IUs for each fat-soluble vitamin can be converted to a weight measurement, such as milligrams or micrograms. For example, 3.33 IU of vitamin A (retinol) are equivalent to 1 microgram of the vitamin; 40 IU of vitamin D are equivalent to 1 microgram; and 1.00 IU of synthetic vitamin E (dl-alpha tocopherol) or 1.49 IU of natural vitamin E (d-alpha tocopherol) are equivalent to 1 milligram.

12. What is a Retinol Equivalent (RE)?

Retinol equivalents (RE) are another way to measure the amount of vitamin A. One RE is equivalent to 1 mcg or 3.33 IU of vitamin A as retinol or 6 mcg or 10 IU of vitamin A as beta carotene. An average of one RE for every 5 IU is used for convenience as a mixture of vitamin A and beta carotene occur in the diet. For example, the adult female RDA for vitamin A is 800 RE or 4,000 IU.

13. What is an antioxidant?

An antioxidant is a compound produced in the body or a nutrient supplied in the diet that neutralizes harmful substances called *free radicals* that are associated with degenerative disease, such as cardiovascular disease and cancer, and premature aging. Vitamin E, selenium, beta carotene, and vitamin C are examples of antioxidant nutrients.

14. What is a free radical?

Free radicals are highly reactive substances found in air pollution, tobacco smoke, rancid foods, and produced in the body. They damage cell membranes and result in tissue destruction and possibly disease.

15. At what level is vitamin A toxic?

Toxic symptoms from vitamin A consumption will vary on the length of time large doses are consumed, the type of vitamin A consumed, and the size and possibly the age of the individual.

The adult RDA for vitamin A is 4,000 IU for women and 5,000 IU for men. Long-term consumption of 50,000 IU to 100,000 IU preformed vitamin A (retinol) found in fish liver oils, liver, and some supplements, can cause nausea, vomiting, joint and abdominal pain, bone abnormalities, hair loss, and liver damage in some people. For this reason, the Committee on Dietary Allowances recommends an upper limit for vitamin A (retinol) consumption at 25,000 IU. Beta carotene in fruits and vegetables appears to be safe at any dose.

Infants and children should consume no more than their RDA of 1,400 IU to 3,300 IU, depending on age and gender. Regular consumption of vitamin A in amounts exceeding 10,000 IU should be done only with the supervision of a physician.

16. Can a person manufacture enough vitamin D from the sun without a dietary source?

A dietary source of this fat-soluble vitamin might be necessary if a person is usually indoors during the daytime; wears clothing outdoors that covers most of the body; lives where there is frequent smog, fog, or air pollution; or is exposed to sunlight primarily through a screen, window, or filtered glass. Dark-skinned people are most dependent on dietary sources of vitamin D as their skin can screen out as much as 95% of the vitamin D-producing ultraviolet rays. The ability to manufacture vitamin D diminishes as a person ages and dietary sources of the vitamin become more important in later years.

17. Does vitamin E improve fertility?

Research in the 1920s identified an "antisterility" food substance that prevented infertility and degeneration of the sex organs in rats. Research on animals continued to support the association between inadequate dietary intake of vitamin E (tocopherol) and reproduction and sexual dysfunction, such as reduced production of sperm, degeneration of the sex organs, an increase in miscarriage, and infertility. However, this association has not been observed in humans and vitamin E appears to have a role in fertility or sexual dysfunction only in certain animals.

18. *What is the difference between niacin, niacinamide, and nicotinic acid?*

Niacin is a general name for a family of compounds that includes niacinamide (or nicotinamide) and nicotinic acid. These compounds are easily converted after absorption to the biologically active (potent) form of the water-soluble vitamin. Only nicotinic acid produces flushing and tingling when large doses are consumed.

19. *What are the bioflavonoids?*

The bioflavonoids are a family of related compounds that includes rutin, flavones, flavonols, and the flavonones. The bioflavonoids are not vitamins, although they were at one time called vitamin P or substance P. They are found in the inner peel of citrus fruits, the white core of green peppers, buckwheat, and leafy vegetables.

20. *What function do the bioflavonoids serve?*

Bioflavonoids, in conjunction with the vitamin C found in these foods, help strengthen blood vessel walls and help prevent the breakage or leakage from these tissues that results in hemorrhoids and varicose veins. Limited evidence shows bioflavonoids might also prevent bruising and damage to artery walls caused by free radical attack. No deficiency symptoms in humans or animals have been identified when bioflavonoids are removed from the diet and there is no evidence these compounds are essential to humans.

21. *How much calcium is enough?*

The RDAs for calcium vary throughout an individual's lifecycle between 800 mg and 1,200 mg. An average daily intake of 1,000 mg for women in the childbearing years or women after menopause who are on estrogen replacement therapy is probably sufficient to aid in the prevention of osteoporosis if combined with a well-balanced diet; regular weight bearing exercise, such as walking, jogging, or jumping rope; and a healthy lifestyle that includes avoidance of tobacco and limited use of alcohol. A daily intake of 1,000 mg to 1,500 mg of calcium either from dietary sources or supplements should be maintained to prevent excessive bone loss in post-menopausal women who are not on estrogen replacement therapy (Table 50).

Table 50.
FACTORS ASSOCIATED WITH THE PREVENTION OF OSTEOPOROSIS

- Adequate intake of calcium, magnesium, zinc, vitamin D, manganese, vitamin A, protein, phosphorus, and copper
- Weight-bearing exercise
- Avoidance or moderate use of alcohol and tobacco
- Maintain ideal body weight and avoid quick-weight loss diets
- Limit use of diet soft drinks
- Limit use of caffeine-containing foods and beverages
- Minimize stress
- Avoid excessive fiber intake

22. How do I know if my diet is adequate in calcium?

National nutrition surveys show many Americans are not consuming adequate amounts of calcium. One cup of non-fat or low-fat milk or yogurt, 1½ ounces of low-fat cheese, 2 cups of cottage cheese, or 2 cups of broccoli provide 300 mg of calcium each. At least three servings a day of these or other calcium-rich foods or a combination of food and other calcium sources should be consumed to aid in the prevention and treatment of osteoporosis.

23. Can taking too much calcium cause arthritis and calcium deposits in the joints?

Calcium deposits in the joints and arthritis (osteoarthritis) result from long-term or severe injury to the joint or a problem with a gland in the body, called the *parathyroid gland*, that regulates calcium metabolism. Dietary intake of calcium is not a cause of these disorders.

24. Are foods cooked in an iron skillet a good source of iron?

Cooking foods, especially acidic foods such as spaghetti or tomato sauce, in an iron pan increases their iron content by as much as 300-fold. The iron leaches from the pot into the food during the cooking; the longer a food is cooked, the higher its iron content. A seasoned cast iron pot supplies less iron because the process of seasoning seals the pores of the pot and reduces the amount of iron that migrates into the food.

25. Is selenium an essential nutrient or a toxic substance?

Selenium is both toxic and essential to health and the prevention of disease. Large doses of selenium over long periods of time cause slowed growth, eye damage, loss of hair, faulty bone formation, tooth decay, and increased risk for heart and liver damage. In contrast, regular small amounts of this trace mineral, daily doses between 50 mcg and 200 mcg, protect the body against free radical attack and its associated diseases, such as heart disease, some forms of cancer, and cell damage similar to that seen in rheumatoid arthritis. The upper safe limit for selenium is estimated at 500 mcg/day.

26. *Is sea salt better than regular salt?*
All salt originates from the ocean. Sea salt is no better, but it is more expensive, than regular table salt. Prior to processing, sea salt contains small amounts of other minerals, such as magnesium and calcium, but these minerals are never supplied in appreciable amounts and are lost during processing.

QUESTIONS ON SPECIAL DIETS, VITAMINS, AND MINERALS

27. *Should a vegetarian take a vitamin B_{12} supplement?*
Vitamin B_{12} is only found in foods of animal origin, such as meat, milk, eggs, chicken, and fish. When a plant supplies vitamin B_{12} it is because the plant has been contaminated with microorganisms (germs) that produce the B vitamin, such as the fermented soybean product miso. A vegetarian diet that includes eggs and/or dairy products (lacto-ovo vegetarian) provides ample amounts of vitamin B_{12}. A vegetarian diet that avoids all foods of animal origin (strict vegetarian or vegan) and relies entirely on grains, dried beans and peas, fruits, vegetables, and nuts for nourishment will not provide enough vitamin B_{12} to meet the RDA. Body stores of the vitamin last for months to years, however, and vitamin B_{12} deficiency from poor nutrient intake is uncommon. Many vegetarian products are fortified with vitamin B_{12}, including some commercial soymilk products. A supplement of vitamin B_{12} might be necessary if a strict vegetarian diet is followed for years and no fortified foods are consumed (Table 51).

Table 51.
VEGETARIAN TERMS

AGAR-AGAR. A sea gelatin used to make puddings and as a thickener in recipes.
AMSAKE. A very smooth and sweet rice wine.
JINENJO. A rare root grown in Japan.
KOKKOH. A food made from roasted rice, sweet rice, oatmeal, soybeans, and sesame seeds.
MISO. A paste made from fermented soybeans, salt, wheat, barley, and water.
TAMARI. An ancient form of soy sauce, fermented for at least 18 months and made from the same ingredients as miso.
TOFU. A curd or "cheese" made from soybeans.

28. *Do vegetarians need to supplement with zinc?*
Lean meats and shellfish are a primary source of zinc in the diet. Avoidance of these foods coupled with a high-fiber diet that inter-

feres with zinc absorption might increase a vegetarian's risk for developing zinc deficiency. Foods high in zinc in the vegetarian diet include cooked dried beans and peas, nuts, whole grain breads and cereals, and seeds. Daily consumption of these foods and a diet that supplies at least 2,000 calories will help prevent zinc deficiency in strict vegetarians (Table 52).

Table 52.
POSSIBLE NUTRIENT DEFICIENCIES FOR ADULT VEGANS

Nutrient	Common Sources	Vegan Sources
Vitamin D	Fortified milk, fish oil	Sunshine, fortified foods, supplements
Vitamin B_{12}	Meat, chicken, fish, milk eggs	Fortified soymilk, supplements
Calcium	Milk, cheese, canned salmon or sardines	Dark green leafy vegetables, supplements
Zinc	Meat, liver, eggs, seafood, chicken	Cooked dried beans and peas, wheatgerm, whole grain breads and cereals
Iron	Meat, chicken, fish, leafy greens, "enriched" breads and cereals	Leafy greens, cooked dried beans and peas, dried fruit, iron cookware, supplements
Vitamin B_2	milk and milk products, meat, chicken, "enriched" breads and cereals, eggs	Leafy greens, brewer's (nutritional) yeast, cooked dried beans, whole grain breads and cereals
Protein	Milk, milk products, meat, chicken, fish, eggs	Complementary vegetable proteins, soybean products

29. Should a person on a low-sodium diet avoid supplements that contain sodium, such as sodium ascorbate?

A person on a sodium-restricted diet should monitor the total sodium intake in the diet, regardless of the source, especially if the diet has been severely restricted in sodium (i.e., below 1,000 mg sodium) by a physician. The sodium from sodium ascorbate is the same sodium as the sodium in table salt (sodium chloride) and should be considered in the day's allotment for this mineral. The sodium contribution will depend on the amount of the vitamin taken; a 10 gram dose of sodium ascorbate will contribute one gram or 1,000 mg of sodium to the diet, whereas 150 mg of sodium ascorbate contributes only 15 mg of sodium.

30. Are there any alternatives to sodium ascorbate?

Sodium ascorbate is often used by people who develop upset stomachs from other forms of the vitamin. If this is the reason for using the supplement, try calcium ascorbate or ascorbate with magnesium or potassium as a low-sodium alternative.

31. Does a diet high in soft drinks increase a person's risk for vitamin and mineral deficiencies?

The total daily intake of sugary foods, including soft drinks, should not exceed 10% of total calories. Consumption of more than this amount of sugar is likely to cause obesity or reduce intake of more nutritious foods and produce deficiencies of one or more vitamins and minerals.

32. How do diet soft drinks affect vitamin and mineral status?

Although diet soft drinks are low in calories, they contain ample amounts of phosphoric acid, a dietary source of phosphorus. A high phosphorus intake reduces calcium absorption, increases urinary loss of calcium, and reduces the calcium content of the bones, potentially resulting in osteoporosis and other bone disorders.

33. What vitamins and minerals are low in the typical fast food diet?

Vitamins, minerals, and other important food factors low in these foods include vitamin A, vitamin D, vitamin E, vitamin C, folic acid, biotin, pantothenic acid, calcium, copper, magnesium, and fiber. Other nutrients that have not been tested, but might be low in these foods, include chromium, manganese, molybdenum, and selenium (Table 53).

Table 53.
MAKING WISE FOOD CHOICES AT FAST FOOD RESTAURANTS

Wise food choices can be made at fast food restaurants. According to The Center for Science in the Public Interest the best selections are:

McDonald's hamburger	35% fat calories
Roy Roger's Potato	0%
Potato with oleo	24%
Roast beef sandwich	29%
Wendy's Chicken Sandwich on whole wheat bun	28%
Arby's Roasted Chicken breast (no bun)	25%
Long John Silver's Baked fish	12%
Corn-on-the-cob	20%
Jack-in-the-Box Shrimp salad	8%
Salad bars (lettuce, vegetables, fruit, and beans)	0%

34. Does coffee or tea consumption harm mineral status?

Both tea and coffee interfere with the absorption of iron and possibly other minerals. Tea reduces the absorption of iron from a meal by more than 85%. Coffee consumed with food reduces iron absorption by 39% to 83%, and a second cup of coffee further reduces iron absorption. Coffee and tea apparently affect mineral absorption the most when consumed with or within 1 hour after a meal or after ingesting an iron-containing supplement.

35. What vitamins or minerals are likely to be low in a weight-loss diet?

The possibility of inadequate intake of any or all vitamins and minerals is possible when dietary intake is less than 2,000 calories. The more restrictive the food selection and the fewer meals consumed each day also add to the likelihood of poor dietary intake of one or more vitamins and minerals.

36. Which vitamins or minerals will help me lose weight?

No pill, powder, capsule, special food, or particular order of eating foods will "burn" fat or increase weight loss. A diet that includes a wide variety of nutrient-dense foods and restricts calorie intake by reducing foods high in fat or sugar, combined with a regular aerobic exercise is the only effective and safe means to weight loss and maintenance of ideal body weight.

QUESTIONS ON LIFESTYLE HABITS, VITAMINS, AND MINERALS

37. Does smoking cigarettes or inhaling other's cigarette smoke interfere with vitamin status?

Tobacco smoke might affect nutritional status in smokers and nonsmokers. Inhalation of tobacco smoke depletes the tissues of vitamin C and increases the daily need for this water-soluble vitamin. Smokers are two to three times more likely to show signs of vitamin C deficiency than are nonsmokers and a normal dietary intake might not be adequate to maintain body stores of this vitamin in smokers.

In addition, vitamin E reduces the damage to lung tissue from outside air pollution. Whether this fat-soluble vitamin reduces damage to the tissues of the lungs and mouth from indoor air pollution, such as tobacco smoke, is unclear. Other nutrients that protect against the development and progression of lung cancer include selenium, vitamin E, vitamin A, beta carotene, and vitamin C. In particular, inadequate intake of vitamin A and beta carotene (the building block for vitamin A found in dark green or orange fruits and vegetables) is associated with an increased risk for developing lung cancer, and adequate intake of this vitamin reduces cancer risk even in people who smoke or chew tobacco.

38. *What dietary guidelines should a smoker follow?*

Besides following the modified Four Food Group Plan, smokers and nonsmokers exposed to tobacco smoke should consume at least four servings a day of fresh fruits and vegetables high in vitamin A and vitamin C.

39. *Does frequent consumption of alcohol affect vitamin or mineral status?*

The risk for developing several vitamin and mineral deficiencies increases with increased use or abuse of alcohol. Poor eating habits and consequently reduced intake of vitamins and minerals often accompany excessive alcohol consumption. However, deficiencies develop even when nutrient intake approaches the RDAs. Alcohol damages the lining of the stomach and intestine and alters or reduces vitamin and mineral absorption. Alcohol damages the liver, an important organ in the storage, conversion, and metabolism of several nutrients, including the fat-soluble vitamins, folic acid, vitamin B_{12}, and iron. Alcohol consumption reduces the ability of the immune system to combat invading microorganisms, and the additional stress of infection and disease increases the body's need for nutrients at a time when inadequate amounts are consumed or available. Greater amounts than the RDA for several B vitamins are required by the liver for detoxification of alcohol.

Nutrient deficiencies associated with alcohol abuse include vitamin A, vitamin B_1, vitamin B_2, niacin, vitamin B_6, vitamin B_{12}, vitamin C, magnesium, iron, selenium, and zinc. (See pages 229–230 for more information on alcohol and nutrition.)

40. *Are copper cooking utensils a source of copper in the diet?*

Copper pots, pans, and other cooking utensils are a source of dietary copper if the food comes in direct contact with the metal. Most copper pots are lined with another metal, such as tin or stainless steel, and copper leakage into the food occurs only when the metal lining is scratched or worn away, exposing the underlying copper. The amount of copper that transfers into food will depend on the length of exposure time, the acidity of the food, and the age of the pot or utensil.

Copper is an essential trace mineral, but also is toxic if consumed in large amounts. Copper in large amounts also destroys vitamin C and gives foods an off color and flavor. For these reasons, old or damaged copper pots should be relined before using. The greenish-blue film or tarnish that develops on copper pots exposed to air is called *verdigris* and is poisonous. Food should not contact this tarnish and copper pots should be kept clean to avoid build up of verdigris.

41. Are there any cooking methods that improve the chromium content of the diet?

Cooking in stainless steel cookware increases the chromium content of food, because chromium leeches out of the pot.

42. Does all handmade pottery contain lead?

Only some types of low-fired pottery are fired with lead-containing glazes. Stoneware pottery is a high-fired cookware, exposed to temperatures exceeding 2,000° F. Lead is not used in the stoneware glazes, and even if it was it would burn off at these high temperatures.

Earthenware pottery is fired at lower temperatures, usually under 2,000° F and, if lead is present in the glaze, it might remain in the finished pot. Brief exposure of foods to this form of pottery, even if lead is present, probably is safe, but if acid drinks, such as orange juice, are stored in lead-containing earthenware pots, significant amounts of lead can leach into the food.

A general guideline for using handmade pottery is to have the pottery checked for lead prior to using if the pot is old or from a foreign country. This type of pottery is more likely to have been fired in an inefficient kiln or glazed with lead-containing glazes. Ask if the pottery is low-fired earthenware with lead glaze or high-fired stoneware when purchasing new pottery. In many cases, the pottery is marked when it is safe for cooking and serving food.

43. Do athletes need extra vitamins and minerals?

Endurance athletes might require extra amounts of certain minerals, such as iron, chromium, magnesium, and zinc. Increased calorie consumption requires increased amounts of the B vitamins, vitamin B_1, vitamin B_2, niacin, and vitamin B_6. However, these nutrients will be consumed in adequate amounts if the extra calories come from nutrient-dense foods (Table 54).

Table 54.
NUTRITION AND ATHLETICS: FACTS AND FALLACIES

FACT	Complex carbohydrates, such as breads and cereals, are the best form of fuel for endurance sports.
FALLACY	Sugar is the perfect fuel for sports.
FACT	The athlete needs little or no more protein than is provided in the typical American diet.
FALLACY	Athletes require more protein than is provided in the diet and protein powders are necessary to meet this daily need.

FACT Vitamin and mineral requirements for competition athletes are similar to or only slightly greater than the RDAs.

FALLACY Everyone who exercises needs large amounts of additional vitamins and minerals beyond the recommendations established by the RDAs.

FACT Water should be consumed every 15 to 20 minutes during exercise.

FALLACY It is best to restrict fluids during training.

FACT Salt tablets and electrolyte replacements are usually not necessary unless more than 4 quarts of body water have been lost during training or an endurance event. Water always should be replaced before salt tablets are taken.

FALLACY Salt tablets are beneficial for replacing sodium lost in sweat and commercial "activity" drinks are better fluid replacements than is water.

FACT Physically active people should follow the same low-fat, high-fiber dietary guidelines established by the Four Food Groups Plan and the American Heart Association.

FALLACY Physically active people can eat anything they want, because exercise "burns" excess cholesterol.

---

44. Do senior citizens require more vitamins and minerals than do other adults?

Seniors are one of the most nutritionally vulnerable groups. In addition, the aging process often masks or overlaps the recognized signs of vitamin and/or mineral deficiencies. Seniors who do not take supplements often are low in vitamins A, E, C, B_1, B_2, B_{12}, and folic acid, and in calcium, selenium, and chromium. These deficiencies are not as common when the diet is high in these nutrients, or supplements containing them are taken. Finally, greater amounts than the RDAs might be necessary for some nutrients if seniors are taking medication, are ill, or are under long-term stress.

45. Does stress increase the need for vitamins and minerals?

Nutrition and stress are closely related. Stressful times deplete the body of essential nutrients and poor nutrition reduces the ability to cope with stress. Stress has a negative impact on the immune system, and the nutrients important in maintaining this system, such as vitamin C, zinc, vitamin B_6, and beta carotene, might be required in increased amounts during times of stress. The body's stores of certain nutrients, including magnesium, the B vitamins, chromium, and vitamin C, are low during stressful times. (See pages 221–223 for more information on vitamins, minerals, and stress.)

QUESTIONS ON HEALTH ISSUES, VITAMINS, AND MINERALS

46. Are feelings of fatigue or irritability signs of vitamin or mineral deficiencies?

Fatigue or mood changes such as irritability or depression are common symptoms of numerous lifestyle or health disorders, including nutritional deficiencies. Almost all clinical and marginal deficiencies of the B vitamins include feelings of fatigue and mood changes. However, these symptoms also can result from lack of sleep, emotional or physical stress, problems at work or school, or other situations. Chronic fatigue might be a warning signal of a health disorder and if the fatigue persists, a physician should be consulted regarding not only possible nutrient deficiencies, but other underlying emotional or physical problems.

47. What vitamins or minerals are good for the skin?

The skin is one of the largest organs in the body and the one most susceptible to signs of vitamin or mineral deficiencies. All vitamins and minerals related to normal production and maintenance of healthy blood cells are important to the skin because these cells supply oxygen to and remove waste products from the skin. These nutrients include iron, copper, vitamin B_6, folic acid, vitamin B_{12}, vitamin E, and vitamin K. Other nutrients that affect the softness, tone, color, moisture, or strength of the skin include vitamin B_1, vitamin B_2, niacin, biotin, pantothenic acid, vitamin C, vitamin A, vitamin D, and zinc.

48. Can vitamins and minerals prevent aging?

The natural aging process cannot be halted by diet; however, a nutritious diet that supplies optimal amounts of the antioxidant nutrients, combined with regular exercise, avoidance of tobacco smoke, moderate alcohol consumption, limited exposure to sunlight and wind, frequent use of moisturizers, and effective coping of stress will help prevent premature aging of the skin.

49. Is dull or dry hair a sign of vitamin or mineral deficiencies?

Changes in hair color, texture, and luster can be a sign of vitamin deficiencies. Several nutrients are important for shiny, healthy hair including protein, vitamin A, niacin, vitamin B_{12}, vitamin C, iron, and zinc, and deficiencies of one or more of these nutrients might result in hair that is thin, dry, brittle, or lifeless. Severe deficiencies of zinc or certain B vitamins can result in hair loss or balding. Normal hair loss or balding also can be inherited and can be a natural consequence of aging. A lifetime of excellent eating habits will slow the process but cannot prevent the inevitable.

50. Does vitamin or mineral intake affect the nails?

Several nutrients are important in the maintenance of healthy nails. Nails become brittle, develop ridges, and crack easily when a person is deficient in iron. A long-term deficiency results in spoon-shaped nails. In addition, niacin maintains healthy nails. Nutrients that maintain a constant supply of nutrient-rich blood to the nails and nailbed are important for the strength and appearance of nails. The oxygen-carrying capacity of the blood is reduced and nails are more likely to grow slowly, split, peel, or break without an adequate supply of vitamin B_6, vitamin B_{12}, folic acid, vitamin C, copper and iron.

QUESTIONS ON VITAMIN-MINERAL SUPPLEMENTS

51. Is there ever a need to take individual vitamins or mineral supplements instead of a multiple?

Individual vitamin or mineral supplements are sometimes useful when tailoring nutrient intake to personal needs. For example, a pregnant woman might need extra iron or folic acid, someone on a diuretic medication for hypertension (high blood pressure) might need additional magnesium or potassium if the medication does not spare potassium, or a female athlete might need extra vitamin B_2.

Many diets and all multiple supplements do not provide all of the essential vitamins and minerals in adequate amounts to meet the RDA. Usually a number of nutrients, especially calcium and magnesium, are missing or are supplied in insignificant amounts in multiple preparations. Even a well-balanced diet might be low in one or more nutrients, especially if food intake or Calories are restricted.

52. Should I take a supplement that provides both vitamins and minerals?

Yes. The body requires more than 45 nutrients for optimal functioning and health. These nutrients function in teams. For example, strong bones depend on calcium, magnesium, vitamin A, vitamin D, and several other nutrients. For this reason, if a person feels his or her diet warrants supplementation, it is likely both vitamins and minerals are needed. It would be rare for any diet to need only a multiple vitamin preparation. A supplement must state vitamins *and* minerals are contained in the preparation. No minerals are present if the label only states the product is a multivitamin preparation.

53. Do vitamin and mineral supplements lose their potency if stored for a long time?

Minerals remain basically unchanged even if they disintegrate into a powder and vitamins retain their potency if stored in a cool, dark place in a tightly sealed container. However, vitamin supplements or combined vitamin and mineral supplements will lose some vitamin potency if they have passed their expiration date; have been stored in warm, well-lit places; or have been exposed to air for long periods of time.

54. Do vitamin or mineral supplements increase appetite?

No scientific evidence exists supporting claims that supplements increase appetite. Several nutrient deficiencies, such as vitamin A, the B vitamins, iron, magnesium, potassium and zinc result in loss of appetite that is corrected when the intake of the missing nutrient is increased. However, increased intake is only effective if the loss of appetite is caused by a pre-existing nutrient deficiency.

55. Why do some people say their appetite increases when they take supplements?

Appetite is somewhat subjective and is influenced by a variety of factors. For example, a renewed interest in nutrition and diet that might result from beginning a supplement program could enhance the appreciation for food and temporarily increase appetite.

56. Are chewable vitamins safe for children?

Some brands of children's chewable vitamins contain sugar in the form of sucrose (table sugar), glucose, or fructose. These sugars promote tooth decay. The claim stating a supplement is "naturally sweetened" only means the product contains some form of sugar. Parents should monitor the intake of children's vitamin-mineral supplements since their sweet taste encourages overconsumption and possible intake of a large dose of certain nutrients.

57. Does mineral oil have nutritional value?

Mineral oil contains no minerals nor does it contribute any nutrients to the daily intake. Mineral oil is a chemical byproduct of the manufacture of petroleum and is sold for its effectiveness as a laxative. Mineral oil is nondigestible and works by coating food particles and the intestinal lining so food particles are unable to be digested or absorbed and instead are excreted. Mineral oil reduces the absorption of several nutrients, including the fat-soluble vitamins A, D, E, and K and the essential fatty acid linoleic acid.

58. *What is a placebo?*

A placebo is defined as any treatment that has no specific action on the person's symptoms or disease. A placebo can be a tablet that resembles a vitamin tablet, but contains no active ingredients.

59. *What is the "placebo effect?"*

The "placebo effect" is producing an effect without the use of a biologically active (potent) substance. For example, if subjects report fewer colds after taking a tablet thought to contain vitamin C, the reduced incidence of infection might be a result of the subject's belief that vitamin C is effective. Researchers try to avoid the placebo effect by dividing subjects into two groups: one group receives the vitamin or mineral supplement and the other group receives a placebo.

60. *What is a "double-blind" study?*

In a double-blind study, neither the researchers nor the subjects know which group is taking the vitamin or mineral and which group is taking the placebo. Only after the final information is collected and tallied is that information released. This type of study helps remove prejudices or preconceived notions by the participants and the researchers about the effectiveness of a treatment.

61. *What is the difference between the vitamin A in fish oils, retinol, retinyl palmitate, and retinoic acid?*

Vitamin A is found in a variety of forms. Preformed vitamin A, or retinol, is found in foods of animal origin, such as fish liver oils, liver, and eggs. This form of vitamin A is readily absorbed and used as is in the body. Retinol can accumulate to toxic levels if consumed in large doses over long periods of time. Retinyl palmitate is retinol attached to palmitic acid. This form of vitamin A is stable and easy to store, as in a supplement.

Retinoic acid (also called vitamin A acid) and its related compound 13-cis-retinoic acid (isotretinoin), are synthetic forms of vitamin A, available by prescription only. Retinoic acid used internally and topically, as well as topical application of isotretinoin, have been used with physician supervision in the treatment of acne vulgaris.

62. *What is beta carotene?*

Beta carotene is the building block for vitamin A found in dark green and orange vegetable and fruits. Not all of the ingested beta carotene is converted to vitamin A, some remains intact. For this reason, beta carotene is not as toxic as retinol and larger amounts can be consumed with no harm to health.

63. *How is beta carotene different from carotenoids?*

Carotenoids are the pigments in vegetables that give them their color. Beta carotene is one of many carotenoids found in dark orange or green vegetables and fruits, but it is the only carotenoid converted to appreciable amounts of vitamin A. A dark orange carrot has more beta carotene than does a pale orange carrot.

64. What is canthaxanthin?

Canthaxanthin is a carotenoid, as is beta carotene, but it cannot be converted to vitamin A. Limited research shows canthaxanthin, like beta carotene, might be effective in lowering a person's risk for developing cancer.

65. Can beta carotene or the carotenoids be toxic?

Consumption of large doses of beta carotene and other carotenoids from the diet or supplements might produce a similar, but temporary, yellowing of the skin that is reversed when intake is lowered.

66. Are there any precautions to using retinoic acid?

Precautions when using retinoic acid include avoiding contact with eyes, mouth, angles of the nose, and all mucous membranes and avoiding exposure to sunlight. The medication also might cause peeling and dryness of the skin.

67. Can vitamin E be toxic if taken in large amounts?

No toxic effects of vitamin E intake have been reported in humans and long-term intake of dosages several times the RDA appear to be safe. Studies on animals show occasional toxic symptoms with large doses of vitamin E, such as altered absorption of vitamin A and vitamin K, slowing of growth, anemia, poor blood clotting, and slowed bone formation.

68. What is water-soluble vitamin E?

Water-soluble vitamin E is the same fat-soluble vitamin bound to a water-soluble compound. This form of the vitamin is effective for people with some liver disorders, cystic fibrosis, and fat malabsorption syndromes, such as celiac disease or tropical sprue.

69. What is the E complex?

Natural vitamin E in foods, such as wheatgerm and nuts, is a mixture of alpha, beta, gamma, and delta tocopherol. Purified concentrates of natural vitamin E are exclusively alpha tocopherol. The alpha tocopherol form of vitamin E is the most effective as an antioxidant, however, some preparations continue to provide the mixture of tocopherols to more closely resemble the naturally-occurring vitamin E. The supplement's label usually provides information on the biological activity (i.e., potency) of only the alpha tocopherol.

70. What form of vitamin E is better, natural or synthetic?

A long-standing debate exists whether there is a marked difference in potency between natural and synthetic vitamin E supplements.

Some evidence shows the natural source of vitamin E is more potent and better absorbed than the synthetic form. However, taking slightly larger doses of the synthetic vitamin E helps to compensate for its lower potency. Natural vitamin E supplements are more expensive than synthetic vitamin E and choosing the less expensive form of the vitamin is probably prudent until more information is gathered on the potency of both.

71. Will taking a B complex supplement give me energy?

Calories in food are what provide energy for the body and dietary protein, carbohydrate, and fat are the only nutrients that contain calories. The B complex vitamins, in conjunction with several minerals, such as cobalt, copper, iron, magnesium, manganese, phosphorus, potassium, and zinc, are important in the breakdown and conversion of these food-factors to energy. Without these nutrient co-workers, the energy in the form of calories would remained trapped inside the calorie-containing nutrients and the body would starve. In this way, the B vitamins are secondary providers of energy.

The body requires enough of these vitamins and minerals to adequately process the daily intake of the calorie-containing nutrients. Consuming more B vitamins than is needed for this purpose will not provide additional benefits or extra energy.

72. Why do supplements contain only 400 mcg or 800 mcg of folic acid?

Inadequate intake of folic acid or vitamin B_{12} produces similar deficiency symptoms, including anemia, fatigue, and irritability. Large doses of folic acid will effectively treat these symptoms, but mask a possible underlying vitamin B_{12} deficiency. The undetected deficiency progresses and can cause irreversible nerve damage. The Food and Drug Administration (FDA) limits the dosage of supplemental folic acid for children and adults to 400 mcg and for pregnant women to 800 mcg to prevent overconsumption of the B vitamin and possible consequences of vitamin B_{12} metabolism. Larger doses of folic acid are available by prescription.

73. Are vitamin B_{12} supplements effective as a "pick-me-up" for older adults?

There is no evidence that even large doses of vitamin B_{12} cure fatigue or improve endurance, unless the person has a long-term deficiency of the B vitamin that has resulted in anemia.

74. What is the vitamin C complex?

A supplement that contains vitamin C, various related compounds such as bioflavonoids, and rose hips is called a "vitamin C complex." No legal definition or standardization exists for the term, and the type and amount of ingredients will vary greatly from one product to another.

75. Are large doses of vitamins or minerals harmful to my health?

What is normally an essential nutrient in small doses becomes a pharmacologic agent, acting more like a drug than a nutrient, when taken in megadoses. Unless prescribed and monitored by a physician, avoid vitamin and mineral intakes greater than three times the RDA, since some nutrients produce toxic symptoms that might be irreversible or can cause secondary deficiencies of other nutrients.

76. Can supplements of water-soluble vitamins be toxic?

Little is known about the long-term effects of megadosing with nutrients. Until recently, only the fat-soluble vitamins were thought to be potentially toxic if taken in large amounts over long periods of time. Now it is recognized even water-soluble vitamins, such as vitamin B_6, can be produce irreversible nerve damage if taken in large amounts. Other B vitamins, such as niacin, pantothenic acid, and vitamin B_1, also might be toxic at large doses.

77. Can mineral supplements be toxic?

Calcium, chromium, copper, iron, selenium, and zinc have produced toxic symptoms when taken in large amounts.

78. Do I need calcium supplements?

Calcium supplements might be necessary at any stage in life if dietary intake is inadequate. Bone tissue and density develop during the early years and reach a maximum in the early to middle 30s. Calcium intake should be optimal during the first 35 years to maximize bone strength and density, so the bones will be less susceptible to frailty and fracture in later years. After age 35, calcium intake should be optimal to maintain strong, dense bones and limit the progressive bone loss associated with later symptoms of osteoporosis. Bone loss accelerates after menopause in women not taking estrogen replacement therapy. Calcium intake is important after menopause to prevent this rapid bone loss.

79. What is the best calcium supplement?

The best supplemental sources of calcium are: calcium lactate, calcium gluconate, calcium carbonate, calcium citrate and calcium citrate-malate. The absorption of calcium lactate is slightly better than the other supplements. (Lactate is similar to milk sugar lactose and both substances increase calcium absorption.) The amount of calcium in each tablet of calcium lactate, however, is small and often more than nine tablets must be taken each day to meet the RDA of 800 mg. Calcium gluconate also contains small amounts of calcium and requires several tablets to supply adequate amounts of the mineral. In contrast, calcium carbonate is a concentrated source of calcium; only two to three tablets are needed to meet the RDA. However, some people do not absorb calcium very well from this source. Calcium citrate and calcium citrate-malate are well-absorbed forms of supplemental calcium.

80. What is oyster shell calcium?
Oyster shell is a source of calcium carbonate.

81. What is calcium citrate?
The calcium in calcium carbonate is not absorbed well by people with poor secretion of stomach acid, a condition called *achlorhydria*. Calcium citrate is a concentrated source of the mineral and is better absorbed in these individuals.

82. What calcium supplements should I avoid?
Avoid chelated calcium, liquid calcium preparations, or "natural" calcium supplements, since the extra cost does not provide extra benefits (Table 55).

Table 55.
THE AMOUNT OF CALCIUM IN DIFFERENT CALCIUM SUPPLEMENTS

Calcium Supplement	Theoretical Tablet size (mg)	Percent Calcium	Calcium Content (mg)
Calcium gluconate	1,200	9%	108
Calcium lactate	1,200	13	156
Caclium phosphate	1,200	29	348
Calcium citrate	1,200	32	384
Calcium carbonate	1,200	40	480

83. Are dolomite and bone meal safe sources of calcium?
Samples of both dolomite and bone meal have been found to contain trace amounts of lead and other toxic metals, which leads researchers to question the safety of these sources of calcium.

Dolomite and bone meal are both considered "natural" sources of calcium and magnesium. Dolomite is a natural mineral combination of calcium carbonate and magnesium carbonate; bone meal is the ground powder of animal bones. The ratio of calcium to magnesium is well-balanced in dolomite. It is questionable that this ratio is important when considered in the context of the total day's dietary intake of these and other minerals. The calcium from dolomite is absorbed and used by the body the same as other less expensive sources of the mineral.

Bone meal contains a greater proportion of calcium to magnesium than does dolomite. This supplemental source of minerals is obtained from the bones of older animals who have in some cases accumulated other toxic metals in their bones over a lifetime.

84. Can a person consume too much calcium?

Little evidence exists on the possible toxicity of large doses of calcium, such as 10,000 mg a day. Excessive intake of calcium could cause a secondary deficiency of zinc. Supplementation with zinc would not alleviate this problem since excessive zinc ingestion would result in deficiencies of copper, iron, or both. There is no reason to consume daily more than 1,000 mg to 2,000 mg of calcium from dietary or supplemental sources.

85. Do calcium supplements cause kidney stones?

A high intake of calcium might encourage the development of kidney stones in those people with a history or increased susceptibility to this disorder. Optimal calcium intake from dietary sources or supplements is safe and essential to health in the absence of any kidney disorder.

86. Do I need to take potassium tablets if I perspire heavily or exercise excessively?

The body loses more water than potassium and other minerals in perspiration and is very efficient in conserving these minerals. Instead, the fluids become more concentrated with minerals after heavy losses of water in perspiration, and it is more important to replace the water than to replace the minute amounts of potassium lost. The potassium lost in perspiration is easily replaced by the inclusion of fruits and vegetables in the daily diet. There is no need to replace lost sodium by taking salt tablets or special "electrolyte" replacement drinks, since American diets are already too high in sodium (salt) and excessive consumption of this mineral is linked to hypertension.

General guidelines for fluid and mineral replacement after heavy perspiration losses are:

1. Replace water lost through perspiration. Thirst is not an accurate measure of water need, so drink approximately twice as much water as it takes to quench the thirst sensation.
2. If more than four quarts of water are needed to replace fluid losses, for every additional quart of water consumed add an extra teaspoon of salt to the daily diet.

87. What is the best form of iron supplements?

Iron is available in two forms: ferrous and ferric. The ferrous form of iron is better absorbed and less irritating to the stomach and intestine than the ferric form.

88. Are there side effects to taking iron supplements?

Ferrous sulfate in doses greater than 18 mg can cause nausea, heart-burn, and either diarrhea or constipation in some people. These side effects can be minimized by increasing the dose gradually from a few milligrams to the level of the RDA over several days, taking the sup-plement in several small doses throughout the day, or by taking less irritating, chelated forms of the supplement, such as ferrous fumarate, ferrous succinate, or ferrous gluconate.

89. Are supplements as good a source of iron as food?

Iron in supplemental form or the iron added to fortified cereals and other convenience foods is poorly absorbed in comparison to dietary iron in lean meat and other foods. However, often people cannot obtain optimal amounts of iron from dietary sources alone and must supplement this intake.

90. What is iron picolinate?

Iron picolinate is a supplemental form of iron that is very well absorbed. However, little research is available on this substance and recommended supplemental amounts have not been determined.

*91. Which is a better source of supplemental zinc, zinc sulfate or zinc
    gluconate?*

Both zinc sulfate and zinc gluconate are well absorbed, well used by the body, and are good sources of zinc. The sulfate form is more acidic and might irritate some people's stomachs. This side effect is avoided if the supplement is consumed with food or by consuming zinc gluco-nate.

92. Why is zinc added to some calcium supplements?

Limited evidence shows zinc might be important in the absorption of calcium across the intestinal lining. It is unclear whether it is the presence of zinc in the supplement or diet or the general zinc status of the body that is the determining factor in calcium absorption. The small amount of zinc in many supplements might be of little use to the body since a high ratio of calcium to zinc reduces the absorption of the latter.

*93. What are nucleic acids and why are they added to some supple-
    ments?*

Nucleic acids are the substances that constitute the genetic mate-rial in cells and are responsible for repair and growth of tissues. The two types of nucleic acids are ribonucleic acid (RNA) and deoxy-ribonucleic acid (DNA). Because they are essential to cell growth and tissue repair, nucleic acids received attention as "anti-aging" factors and were promoted for the treatment of several degenerative diseases, such as atherosclerosis, senility, and diabetes. They also were claimed to effectively treat graying hair or wrinkled skin. No evidence from well-designed studies has substantiated these claims. These substances are digested and absorbed as their component parts rather than as intact nucleic acid. In addition, the body produces RNA and DNA so it is not essential that these substances be supplied by the diet.

94. Can supplemental nucleic acids be toxic?

Large intakes of nucleic acid are not recommended to people at risk for gout and kidney disease, since the breakdown products increase blood levels of uric acid.

95. Is PABA an essential nutrient?

Para-aminobenzoic acid (PABA) is a component of folic acid. It is sometimes classified as a B vitamin, but it has no potency or nutritional significance outside of its role as a portion of folic acid. The only verified function of PABA is as a sunscreen in suntan lotions. Large doses can cause nausea and vomiting.

96. Can choline be toxic?

Chronic ingestion of large doses of choline might have toxic effects on the lymph system, liver, and spleen. Limited information is available on the toxic effects of choline and what information is available is from studies on animals. Megadoses of choline in rats destroy liver and spleen tissue and reduce the size of the thymus gland, an important tissue in the immune system.

97. What is DHEA and what does it do?

Dehydroepiandrosterone (DHEA) is a hormone produced in the adrenal gland. Recent evidence shows high levels of this hormone in the blood is related to a reduced risk of developing atherosclerosis and cardiovascular disease. Low blood levels of this hormone might be linked to increased risk for death from cardiovascular disease. The hormone inhibits the production of fats and cholesterol in the body and it is thought that low levels of it in the blood might contribute to obesity and atherosclerosis.

Over-the-counter sale of DHEA was banned by the Food and Drug Administration (FDA) after claims were made that the product would cause weight loss and prevent aging. Until these claims are substantiated and the safety of DHEA is established, DHEA will continue to be an unapproved drug.

98. Do fish oil supplements contain cholesterol?

Many of the dietary and supplemental sources of fish oils and their omega 3 fatty acids also contain cholesterol. A 3½ ounce serving of cod liver oil supplies approximately 19.2 grams of omega 3 fatty acids—eicosapentaenoic acid (EPA) and docohexaenoic acid (DHA)—

and approximately 570 mg of cholesterol. Equal weight servings of herring oil and salmon oil contain approximately 766 mg and 485 mg of cholesterol, respectively.

The first fish-oil (or omega-3 fatty acid) supplements that appeared on the market contained varying amounts of cholesterol, up to and exceeding 200 mg. Many newer products contain little or no cholesterol.

99. *Are cod liver oil supplements a good source of vitamin A and fish oils?*

Although cod liver oil is an excellent source of both the omega-3 fatty acids and the fat-soluble vitamins A and D, the concern that toxic amounts of the vitamins will be consumed warrant careful and limited use of cod liver oil.

100. *When is the best time to take a supplement?*

In general, supplemental vitamins and minerals are best absorbed with food. The exception to this rule is iron, which is best absorbed on an empty stomach. For simplicity, routinely take a supplement with breakfast or dinner. However, for maximum absorption, take smaller doses more frequently, such as with every meal and/or snack.

Appendix

BODY BASICS

Following is a brief overview of physiology and biochemistry as they relate to nutrition. This introduction is meant to provide a basic understanding of the terms, compounds, interrelationships, and processes involving vitamins and minerals discussed throughout the book.

Atoms and Molecules

The study of nutrition begins with the smallest component of life—the atom. A substance composed of only one atom is called an element. Examples of elements are oxygen, carbon, hydrogen, calcium, iron, and other minerals. The physical properties, such as smell, weight, taste, or color, of any material depend on the arrangement and composition of its atoms.

A molecule is the second smallest component of life and is formed when two or more atoms join. Examples of molecules are hormones, cholesterol, amino acids, fats, carbohydrates such as sugar and starch, all the vitamins, and any mineral joined to another compound such as calcium carbonate or sodium chloride (table salt).

Metabolism

Molecules that are also nutrients, such as vitamins, protein, and fats, are consumed in the diet and stored, broken down, and rebuilt in the body. In addition, other molecules, such as hormones, prostaglandins, neurotransmitters, and other body regulators are formed from dietary and stored nutrients. The total of all alterations in molecules that constitute growth, maintenance, and repair of body processes is called *metabolism*.

The word "metabolism" originates from the Greek word "metaballein," meaning to change or alter. In short, metabolism is all the processes that allow the body to take apart substances and put them back together in new ways as needed. Metabolic assembly lines composed of a few to thousands of chemical reactions are exact and interconnected and the accuracy of one system determines the outcome of others. The sequence of these reactions is called a *metabolic pathway*, and proceeds in a step-by-step manner, so a failure at one step affects all following steps.

For example, hemoglobin in red blood cells is a complex molecule comprised of many amino acids, iron, and other substances. The multi-stepped process of making hemoglobin includes one step where vitamin B_6 serves as a helper. If vitamin B_6 is in short supply, all reactions that follow this step are halted and the hemoglobin molecule is not made. Long-term deficiency of vitamin B_6 would result in a reduction in red blood cells and anemia. The efficiency of metabolism depends on the constant availability of all nutrients from both the diet and from body storage.

Energy

Many of the most important concepts in nutrition pertain to energy. Energy is defined as the capacity to do work. Heat, electricity, and movement are common forms of energy. There are two types of energy: active energy is used to perform work much like the active energy in a burning log or the movement of muscles, and stored energy is potential energy such as the stored energy in a wood pile or the fat tissue in the human body.

The ultimate source of energy is the sun. Chlorophyll in plants absorbs solar energy and converts it into chemical molecules, such as carbohydrates. This trapped energy is consumed by animals who further convert it to protein and fats and store these energy-containing nutrients in muscle and fat tissue. The stored energy can be converted to active energy to fuel all metabolic reactions; move muscles, digest foods, excrete waste products, or stimulate nerve cells. Humans ingest the stored energy in plants and animals and either use that energy to fuel metabolic reactions or store excess energy for later use.

Calories

The body is constantly using and producing energy. The unit in nutrition used to measure energy is the calorie (kcalorie or kcal). A calorie is equivalent to the amount of energy (heat) required to raise the temperature of one liter (1,000 grams) of water 1[degree symbol]C. All calories in the body originate from the diet and are supplied by four sources: protein (4 calories/gram), carbohydrates (4 calories/gram), fat (9 calories/gram), and alcohol (7 calories/gram). Vitamins, minerals, and other substances in foods do not supply calories and are not a source of energy.

Basal Metabolism

Most of the energy expended each day is used to maintain normal body processes, such as the beating of the heart, the inhaling of oxygen and the exhaling of carbon dioxide from the lungs, nerve transmission, the production of red blood cells and hormones, and the maintenance of body temperature. This involuntary energy expenditure is called *basal metabolism* and constitutes most of the daily energy requirement of the body. For the average woman, basal metabolism requires approximately 1,200 to 1,400 calories each day; a man's basal metabolic needs are higher. The basal metabolic rate (BMR) is influenced by many factors. The more muscle a person has and the taller he or she is, the greater will be the basal metabolic rate. Periods of rapid growth, such as pregnancy or puberty also increase BMR.

Physical activity accounts for the second greatest use of energy in the body and varies greatly between individuals. Moderate physical activity requires approximately 30% of the total day's use of calories, while the competition athlete may expend more than 60% of his or her daily energy in physical activity. This energy is used to move muscles and increase blood flow, heart rate, and breathing. The amount of energy expended during activity depends on the size of the individual and the duration and intensity of the activity. Extra calories are used or "burned" during exercise and for several hours following exercise when basal metabolism increases to repair damaged tissues, build muscle tissue, and return other body processes to pre-exercise conditions.

The third category of energy use by the body is the amount of calories used to digest food. Chewing, secretion of digestive juices, muscular movements of the gastrointestinal tract, and the activation of billions of cells that line the digestive tract account for approximately 10% of the total day's energy expenditure (Table 56).

Table 56.
THE DAY'S TOTAL ENERGY NEEDS

The day's total energy use for the average, moderately active female or male could be divided approximately as follows:

FEMALE
Basal metabolism .... 1,200 calories
Physical activity 600
Digestion of food 200
(assuming food intake of approximately 2,000 calories)
Total calories 2,000

MALE
Basal metabolism .... 1,620 calories
Physical activity 810
Digestion of food 270
(Assuming food intake of approximately 2,700 calories)
Total calories 2,700

Enzymes

Metabolism of proteins, carbohydrates (sugar and starch), and fats is regulated by molecules called *enzymes*. Enzymes are molecules made from protein that catalyze or trigger the rate of chemical reactions. Enzymes are like the equipment on an automobile production line; they speed the assembly process without becoming part of the car. An enzyme assures the two substances connect properly and quickly, so a chemical reaction that might take hours or years to occur randomly will occur several thousand times in a split second with the aid of the enzyme.

Each enzyme is designed for only one type of reaction and each of the millions of reactions that constitute metabolism requires a different, specific enzyme. For example, large food particles from the diet are broken down to their individual molecules by digestive enzymes in the mouth, stomach, and small intestine. Specific enzymes called *amylases* convert carbohydrates into sugar, other enzymes called *proteases* convert protein into amino acids. Other enzymes in the body help manufacture hormones, breakdown substances for energy, and build numerous essential substances needed for life.

Many enzymes are activated or completed by a second molecule called a *co-enzyme* or *co-factor*. Many of the B vitamins and some minerals function as co-enzymes. For example, vitamin B_1 and vitamin B_2 each work with different enzymes in the breakdown of carbohydrates and proteins for energy. Vitamin B_6 is a co-enzyme for one of the steps in the manufacture of hemoglobin, the molecule in red blood cells that carries oxygen to all the tissues. Selenium is a co-factor of an enzyme that protects the body against attack by damaging compounds called *free radicals*.

The Cell

The fundamental unit of the body is the cell. All processes of metabolism, including the breaking down and building up of every molecule and the extraction of energy from protein, carbohydrates, and fats, occur in the cell. Each cell is a minute factory, which processes nutrients for energy, growth, maintenance, and repair.

Cells reproduce and multiply by dividing. A cell grows to a specific size then divides to form two daughter cells. Six divisions later 128 cells have formed and an additional 6 divisions results in more than 8,000 cells. By this process a baby is formed, a child grows, and old or damaged tissues are repaired, while body processes monitor growth so that a person does not continue to grow uncontrollably. By the same process, abnormal and potentially cancerous cells grow and multiply into tumors.

The blueprint of cell division and therefore the growth and maintenance of all body tissues is the genetic code within the center or nucleus of each cell. Each cell contains all heredity material for the entire body, but activates only portions of the genetic code to maintain its specific processes. In this way, a kidney cell produces two kidney cells, whereas a liver cell divides to form two new liver cells. Normal functioning of the genetic code and cell replication requires the presence of several vitamins and minerals, including folic acid and vitamin B_{12}.

Cells are organized into tissues (muscle, fat, connective, or nerve tissues), which are further organized into organs, such as the liver, kidney, pancreas, or heart, that may contain hundreds of different types of specialized cells and tissues. Organs that function together are organized into body systems, such as the digestive system containing the mouth, throat, stomach, small and large intestine, and secondary organs such as the gall bladder and liver; or the immune system containing the lymph nodes and vessels, the spleen, the thymus gland, and the bone marrow. Other systems include the reproductive, respiratory, nervous, skeletal, endocrine (hormones and their glands), and excretory (kidney, ureters, bladder, and urethra) systems.

These systems are intimately related and cooperate with each other to maintain health and functioning of the total body. For example, the cells, tissues, and organs of the digestive tract break down complex foods into minute molecules that are absorbed to feed the rest of the body's cells and tissues. All of these systems comprise the human body.

The Digestive System

The digestion and absorption of food occurs along the gastro (stomach) intestinal (small and large intestine) tract or GI tract. The GI tract is similar to a tube within the body that extends about 16.5 feet in length from mouth to anus. It includes the mouth, esophagus, stomach, small intestine, pancreas, gall bladder, liver, and large intestine (colon).

The digestion of food begins in the mouth. Chewing grinds the food into smaller particles and an enzyme called *amylase* in saliva begins the chemical breakdown of carbohydrates (starch and complex sugars) to simple sugars. The sweet taste sometimes experienced when starchy foods are chewed for a long time is caused by breaking down starch to its component part, sugar. The food is swallowed, travels down the esophagus, and enters the stomach where it mixes with stomach acid and another enzyme, called *pepsin*, that begins the digestion of protein.

Most digestion and absorption occurs in the small intestine. Food slowly enters the small intestine from the stomach and is mixed with digestive enzymes from the pancreas and intestinal lining, bile from the gall bladder and liver, and other digestive juices. The digestive juices neutralize the highly acidic stomach contents and activate intestinal enzymes. Bile is essential for the emulsification or breaking apart and holding in suspension of fat particles, such as cholesterol, fats, and the fat-soluble vitamins A, D, E, and K.

The small intestine is lined with billions of cells specialized to digest and absorb the end products of digestion—amino acids from protein, sugar from carbohydrates, fatty acids from fats, cholesterol, vitamins, and minerals. Every vitamin, mineral, and other essential nutrient must be recognized and transported across these cells in order to enter the bloodstream and be available to the cells of the body.

The material entering the large intestine is comprised of water, undigested fibers, end products of digestion that were not absorbed, minerals, bile, and other waste products. The large intestine serves primarily as a site for the absorption of water and sodium. No nutrients are absorbed here except for a few vitamins, such as biotin and vitamin K that are manufactured by bacteria living in the large intestine (Table 57).

In general, if a nutrient is not recognized or absorbed in the small intestine it travels into the large intestine, is excreted, and is useless to the maintenance of a healthy body. For this reason, the GI tract is considered a separate tube within a tube (the body) and eating food does not always guarantee the nutrients will nourish the body.

Table 57.
DIGESTION OF NUTRIENTS

Digestive Tract	Digestive Action
Mouth	Food mashed by teeth and mixed with saliva. Small amount of breakdown of carbohydrates to sugars.
Esophagus	No digestive action.
Stomach	Food mixed with hydrochloric acid and enzymes. Small amount of breakdown of protein to small protein fragments called polypeptides.
Small Intestine	Starch and sugar broken down to simple sugars (glucose, fructose, and galactose). Fat broken down to fatty acids, cholesterol, and small fat fragments. Protein and polypeptides broken down to amino acids. Vitamins and minerals released from food as protein, fat, and carbohydrates are broken down to basic parts. Final end products of digestion (sugar, fatty acids, cholesterol, amino acids, vitamins, and minerals) are absorbed.
Large Intestine	Fiber and unabsorbed nutrients excreted. Water reabsorbed into bloodstream. Bacteria synthesize biotin and vitamin K.

The Circulatory System

Each of the billions of cells in the body needs a constant supply of oxygen, water, energy, and nutrients. Body fluids, such as the blood, lymph, and the fluid that bathes the individual cells (interstitial fluid) supply the cells with essential oxygen, water, and nutrients, and remove waste products such as carbon dioxide.

The blood is comprised of water, red blood cells, white blood cells, blood cell fragments called *platelets*, proteins, carriers of fat-soluble substances, minerals, vitamins, and numerous other compounds. Red blood cells are the carriers of oxygen in the blood. White blood cells are important components of the immune system, the body's natural defense system against disease. Platelets are cell fragments important for normal blood clotting and initiate the healing process after an injury such as a cut or a scraped knee.

The circulatory system, comprised of the heart and blood vessels (arteries, capillaries, and veins), is the carrier of blood and its nutrients. The heart pumps blood rich in oxygen and nutrients through the arteries into the tiny blood vessels called *capillaries* where oxygen and nutrients are released to the cells and the waste products of metabolism are absorbed into the blood. The "deoxygenated" blood is returned to the heart by way of the veins. This blood leaves the heart and is filtered through the tissues of the lungs where carbon dioxide is released and more oxygen is absorbed into the blood. The "oxygenated" blood returns to the heart and is again pumped out to the body to repeat the continuous cycle. The cycle of blood flow is as follows:

Heart → body → heart → lungs → heart → body. . . .

Some blood vessels pass by the digestive system and pick up nutrients entering from the small intestine. Water-soluble nutrients, such as the B vitamins and vitamin C, enter directly into the blood. The fat-soluble nutrients, such as vitamins A, D, E, and K, are packaged in water-soluble "bubbles" so they will remain suspended in the watery medium of the blood.

These nutrient-laden blood vessels stop at the liver, which filters the blood and releases only the proper amount of any one nutrient so a constant blood level of nutrients is maintained at all times. Excesses of nutrients are stored in the liver or are converted to other compounds for later release into the blood. This cycle of blood flow is as follows:

Heart → digestive tract → liver → heart → lungs → heart →
digestive tract. . . .

In addition to oxygen and nutrients, the blood also carries other molecules that function as messengers and regulators of body processes. Hormones, such as insulin, adrenaline, or estrogen, are chemicals produced and secreted from specialized glands in the body called *endocrine glands*, such as the pancreas, the adrenal glands, or the ovaries. Hormones are released into the blood and influence the activity of another tissue or organ. For example, insulin is released from the pancreas when blood sugar levels are too high. Insulin with the help of chromium stimulates the cells to absorb the excess blood sugar, supplies the cells with a usable form of energy, and returns blood sugar levels to normal.

Prostaglandins are compounds produced from fats, such as the fats in fish oils and vegetable oils. Prostaglandins are transported in the blood and regulate numerous body processes, including heart and muscle contraction and blood pressure.

The Excretory System

The body needs a system to dispose of waste products and nutrient excesses produced in the normal metabolism of foods and other body processes. The kidneys serve as the blood purifying and detoxifying system. Blood is constantly filtered through the sieve-like structures of the kidneys where waste products, such as urea, and excess water-soluble vitamins, potassium, and sodium, are removed and the purified blood is returned to the circulation. Waste products and excess fluids are held in the urinary bladder for periodic removal during urination.

The Nervous System

The nervous system is the body's telephone service. Messages from the brain are transported from one nerve cell to another much like voices are carried through telephone wires. Messages also travel from the body back to the brain so that a constant communication system between the body and the brain is maintained. Touching a hot stove sends signals from the nerve cells at the tip of the finger to the brain and back to the finger, and, in a fraction of a second, the hand is pulled away from danger.

Neurotransmitters are chemicals that transport messages from one nerve cell to another or from a nerve cell to another tissue, such as a muscle. Neurotransmitters are powerful chemicals in the body responsible for numerous physical and behavioral processes, including sleep, pain, mood, and many of the stress responses including increased heartbeat and perspiration. An example of a neurotransmitters is serotonin. Several nutrients are needed to create the neurotransmitters, including vitamin B_6.

Conclusion

Most of the body's work is conducted automatically with no help from the conscious mind. Sometimes, however, higher centers in the brain ignore body needs and it is important to do a routine check of the body's health by "listening" to how the body is feeling and acting. Paying attention to how the body responds to foods, the environment, other people, and internal processes, such as stress, is useful in determining the body's needs and in designing an individualized lifestyle that promotes optimal health.

References

CHAPTER 1

1. Dietary levels of households in the United States, Spring 1965. Agriculture Research Service, US Department of Agriculture, 1968, pp 12–17.
2. Ten State Nutrition Survey. US Department of Health, Education, and Welfare, Health Series and Mental Health Administration Center for Disease Control. DHEW Publication No (HSM) 72-8130-8134, Atlanta, GA.
3. First Health and Nutrition Examination Survey. Public Health Service, Health Resources Administration, US Department of Health, 1971–1972.
4. Nationwide Food Consumption Survey, Spring 1980. US Department of Agriculture, Science and Education Administration, Beltsville, MD.
5. Dietary Intake Source Data: United States 1976–1980. Data from the National Health Survey, Series 11, No. 231, DHHS Publication No (PHS) 83-1681, March 1983.
6. Pennington J, Young B, Wilson D, et al: Mineral content of foods and total diets: The selected minerals in foods survey, 1982–1984. *JAMA* 1986;86:876–891.
7. Somer E: Consumer reports vitamin story inaccurate and outdated. *Nutr Rep* 1986;4:50.
8. Morgan K, Stampley G, Zabik M, et al: Magnesium and calcium dietary intakes of the US population. *J Am Col N* 1985;4:195–206.
9. Polley D, Willis R, Folkers K: Dietary vitamin B$_6$ in college women. *Nutr Rep In* 1985;31:281–285.
10. Ricketts C, Kies C, Garcia P, et al: Manganese and magnesium utilization of humans as affected by level and kind of dietary fat. *Fed Proc* 1985;44:1850.
11. Seelig M: Magnesium requirements in human nutrition. *Cont Nutr* 1982;7:1–2.

12. Anderson R, Kozlovsky A: Chromium intake, absorption and excretion of subjects consuming self-selected diets. *Am J Clin Nutr* 1985;41:1177–1183.
13. Pennington J, Young B: Total diet study nutritional elements, 1982–1989. *J Am Diet Assoc* 1991;91:179–183.

CHAPTER 2

14. Brin M: Dilemma of marginal vitamin deficiency. Proc 9th Int. Congr Nutrition, Mexico, 1972. Karger, Basel 1975;4:102–115.
15. Brin M: Erythrocyte as a biopsy tissue in the functional evaluation of thiamine status. *J Am Med Assoc* 1964;187:762.
16. Brin M, Soe D: Drug-diet interactions. *J Fla Med Assoc* 1979;66:422.
17. Sidell N, Gamitiga E, Golub S: Immunological aspects of retinoids in humans: II. Retinoic acid enhances induction of hemolytic plaque-forming cells. *Cell Immun* 1984;88:374–381.
18. Pollitt E, Greenfield D, Leibel R: Behavioral effects of iron deficiency among preschool children in Cambridge, MA. *Fed Proc* 1976;37:487.
19. Garrison R, Somer E: *The Nutrition Desk Reference*. New Canaan, CT, Keats Publishing Co, 1985, pp 66–68.
20. Borel M, Smith S, Brigham D, et al: The impact of varying degrees of iron nutriture on several functional consequences of iron deficiency in rats. *J Nutr* 1991;121:729–736.
21. Hambidge K, Walravens P, Brown R, et al: Zinc nutrition of preschool children in the Denver Head Start Program. *Am J Clin Nutr* 1976;29:734.
22. Bistrain B, et al: Prevalence of malnutrition in general medical patients. *JAMA* 1976;235:1567–1570.
23. Axelrod A: Immune processes in vitamin deficiency status. *Am J Clin Nutr* 1971;24:265.
24. Dreizen S: Nutrition and the immune response: A review. *Int J Vita Nutr Res* 1978;49:220–228.
25. Brozek J: Physiological effects of thiamine restriction and deprivation in young men. *Am J Clin Nutr* 1973;26:150.
26. Abou-Saleh M: The biology of folate in depression: Implications for nutritional hypotheses of the psychoses. *J Psych Res* 1986;20:91–101.
27. Sterner R, Price W: Restricted riboflavin: Within subject behavioral effects in humans. *Am J Clin Nutr* 1973;26:150.
28. Siminoff M: Chromium deficiency and cardiovascular risk: A review. *Cardio Res* 1984;18:591–596.
29. Mertz W: Chromium: An Essential micronutrient. *Cont Nutr* 1982;7:1–2.
30. Potter J, Levin P, Anderson R, et al: Glucose metabolism in glucose intolerant older people during chromium supplementation. *Metabolism* 1985;34:199–204.
31. Rabinowitz M, Gonick H, Levin S, et al: Clinical trial of chromium and yeast supplements on carbohydrate and lipid metabolism in diabetic men. *Biol Tr El Res* 1983;5:449–466.

32. Roden D: Magnesium teatment of ventricular arrhythmias. *Am J Card* 1989;63:43G–46G.
33. Lindeman R: *Magnesium in Health and Disease.* Jamaica, NY, SP Medical and Science Books, 1980.
34. Altura B: Hypomagnesemia and vasocontriction: Possible relationship to etiology of sudden death ischemic heart disease and hypertensive vascular diseases. *Artery* 1981;9:212–280.
35. Willett W: Vitamin A and lung cancer. *Nutr Rev* 1990;48:201– 211.
36. Stryker W, Stampfer M, Stein E, et al: Diet, plasma levels of beta-carotene and alpha tocopherol, and risk of malignant melanoma. *Am J Epidem* 1990;131:597–611.
37. Burton G: Beta carotene: An unusual type of lipid antioxidant. *Science* 1984;224:569.
38. Stich H, Hornby A, Dunn B: Beta carotene levels in exfoliated mucosa cells of population groups at low and elevated risk for oral cancer. *Int J Canc* 1986;37:389–393.
39. Grobbee D, Waal–Manning H: The role of calcium supplementation in the treatment of hypertension. *Drugs* 1990;39:7–18.

CHAPTER 3: VITAMIN A

40. Patty I, Benedek P, Deak G, et al: Cytoprotective effect of vitamin A and its clinical importance in the treatment of patients with chronic gastric ulcer. *Int J Tiss* 1983;5:301–305.
41. Nuwayri-Salti N, Murad T: Immunologic and anti-immunosuppressive effects of vitamin A. *Pharmacol* 1985;30:181– 187.
42. Shapiro S, Bendich A: Effect of dietary carotenoids on lymphocyte responses to mitogens. *Fed Proc* 1985;44:544.
43. Stehr P, Gloninger F, Kuller L, et al: Dietary vitamin A deficiencies and stomach cancer. *Am J Epidem* 1985;121:65–70.
44. Van Eenwyk J, Davis F, Bowen P: Dietary and serum carotenoids and cervical intraepithelial neoplasia. *Int J Cancer* 1991;48:34–38.
45. Byers T, Graham S, Haughey B, et al: Diet and lung cancer risk: Findings from the Western New York Diet Study. *Am J Epidem* 1987;125:351–363.
46. Menkes M, Comstock G: Serum and dietary carotene levels and lung cancer risk. *Am J Epidem* 1986;124:502.
47. Barros J, Silveira F, Coelho R: Vitamin A in colon cancer. *Dig Dis Sci* 1986;31:172S.
48. Verreault R, Chu J, Mandelson M, et al: A case-control study of diet and invasive cervical cancer. *Int J Cancer* 1989;43:1050–1054.
49. Ziegler R: A review of epidemiologic evidence that carotenoids reduce the risk of cancer. *J Nutr* 1989;119:116–122.
50. Palan P, Mikhail M, Romney S: Decreased B-carotene tissue levels in uterine leiomyomas and cancers of reproductive and nonreproductive organs. *Am J Obst G* 1989;161:1649–1652.

51. McCormick M, van Rensburg S: Retinol and carotene in head and neck cancer. *Clin Otolar* 1984;9:310–311.

52. Mugliston T: Vitamin A and squamous cancer of the larynx. A preliminary report. *Clin Otolar* 1987;12:59–60.

53. Wald N, Boreham J, Bailey A: Serum retinol and subsequent risk of cancer. *Br J Canc* 1986;54:957–961.

54. Edes T, McDonald P: Combined cancer risk factors: Vitamin A status in cigarette smokers. *Clin Res* 1988;36:A710.

55. Sumner S, Liebman M, Wakefield L: Vitamin A status of adolescent girls. *Nutr Rep In* 1987;35:423–431.

56. Kummet T, Meyskens F: Vitamin A: A potential inhibitor of human cancer. *Sem Oncol* 1983;10:281.

57. White W, Roe D: Effect of in vivo irradiation on plasma levels of carotenoids and vitamin A. *Fed Proc* 1986;45:831.

58. Rybski J, Grogan T, Genster H: Reduction of UVB-tumor-infiltrating T-lymphocytes by dietary canthaxanthin. *Lab Inv* 1989;60:A82.

59. Micozzi M, Beecher G, Taylor P, et al: Carotenoid analysis of selected raw and cooked foods associated with a lower risk for cancer. *J Natl Ca Insti* 1990;82:282–285.

60. Corbett J, Selhorst J, Waybright E, et al: Liver lover's headache: Pseudotumor cerebri and vitamin A intoxication. *J Am Med A* 1984;252:3365.

61. Solomons N, Russel R: The interaction of vitamin A and zinc: Implications for human nutrition. *Am J Clin Nutr* 1980;33:2131– 2140.

CHAPTER 3: VITAMIN D

62. MacLaughlin J, Holick M: Aging decreases the capacity of human skin to produce vitamin D3. *J Clin Invest* 1985;76:1536–1538.

63. Vitamin D: New perspectives. *Dairy Council Digest* 1990;61(3):13–18.

64. Kummerow F, Holmes R: The relationship of adequate and excessive intake of vitamin D to health and disease. *J Am Col Nutr* 1983;2:173–199.

65. Palmieri G, Pitcock J, Brown P, et al: Effect of calcitoin and vitamin D on osteoporosis. *Clin Res* 1988;36:A884.

66. Vitamin D and insulin. *Nutr Rev* 1982;40:221.

67. Lointier P, Levin B, Wargovich M, et al: The effects of vitamin D on human colon carcinoma cells in vitro. *Gastroenty* 1986;90:1526.

68. Cunningham D, Gilchrist N, Cowan R, et al: Vitamin D as a modulator of tumor growth in low grade lymphoma. *Scot Med J* 1985;30:193.

69. Pence B, Buddingh F: Inhibition of dietary fat promotion of colon carcinogenesis by supplemental calcium and vitamin D. *P Am Assoc Ca* 1987;28:154.

70. Tsoukas C: 1–25 dehydroxycholecalciferol vitamin D3: A novel immunoregulatory hormone. *Science* 1984;224:1438.

71. Irwin J: Hearing loss and calciferol deficiency. *J Laryng Ot* 1986;100: 1245–1247.

72. Brookes G: Vitamin D deficiency: A new cause of cochlear deafness. *J Larngology Oncol* 1983;97:405–420.
73. Loomis W: Skin-pigment regulation of vitamin D biosynthesis in man. *Science* 1967;157:501.
74. Hathcock J: Nutrition: Toxicology and pharmacology. In: Nutrition Reviews' Present Knowledge In Nutrition, fourth editon, Washington DC, Nutrition Foundation, 1976, pp 504–515.
75. Santos F, Smith M, Chan J: Hypercalciuria associated with long-term administration of calcitriol (1,25-dihydroxyvitamin D3). *Am J Dis Ch* 1986;140:139–142.
76. Agwu D, Holub B: The proaggregatory effect of 25-hydroxycholecalciferol (25-(OH)D3) on human platelets. *Nutr Res* 1984;4:823–827.
77. Mahajan S, Abu-Hamdan D, Prasad A, et al: Zinc metabolism. *Kidney Int* 1990;34:473.

CHAPTER 3: VITAMIN E

78. Calabrese E: Influence of dietary vitamin E on susceptibility to ozone exposure. *Bull Environ Contam* 1985;34:417–422.
79. Howard L: The biological syndrome of vitamin E deficiency: Laboratory and electrophysiologic assessment. *Nutr Res* 1990;48:169–177.
80. Wartanoxicz M, Panczenko-Kresowska B, Ziemlanski S, et al: The effect of alpha-tocopherol and ascorbic acid on the serum lipid peroxide level in elderly people. *Ann Nutr Metab* 1984;28:186–191.
81. Meydani M, Verdon C, Blumberg J: Effect of vitamin E, selenium and age on lipid peroxidation events in rat cerebrum. *Nutr Res* 1985;5:1227–1236.
82. Knedt P: Serum vitamin E and risk of female cancers. *Int J Epidem* 1988;17:281–288.
83. Shklar G, Schwartz J, Trickler D, et al: Regression of experimental cancer by oral administration of combined alpha tocopherol and beta-carotene. *Nut Cancer* 1989;12:321–325.
84. Bierenbaum M, Noon F, Machlin L, et al: The effect of supplemental vitamin E on serum parameters in diabetic, post coronary and normal subjects. *Nutr Rep In* 1985;31:1171–1180.
85. Jandak J, Steiner M, Richardson P: Reduction of platelet adhesiveness by vitamin E supplements in humans. *Thromb Res* 1988;49:393–404.
86. Srivastava K: Vitamin E exerts antiaggregatory effects without inhibiting the enzymes of the arachidonic acid cascade in platelets. *Pros Leuk Med* 1986;21:177–185.
87. Sundaram G, Manimekalai S, London R, et al: Changes in fractionated high density lipoprotein cholesterol in response to ingestion of different doses of vitamin E. *Clinical Chemistry* 1984;30:942.
88. Haeger K: Long-time treatment of intermittent claudication with vitamin E. *Am J Clin Nutr* 1974;27:1179.

89. Bolton-Smith C, Woodward M, Casey C, et al: Dietary antioxidant vitamins and odds ratios (OR) for coronary heart disease. *FASEBJ* 1991;5:A715.
90. Ayres S: Vitamin E therapy and lupus erythematosus. *Nutr Rep* 1986;4:44–45.
91. Munthe E, Aaseth J: Treatment of rheumatic arthritis with selenium and vitamin E. *Scand J Rheum* 1984;103:S53.
92. Vitamin E deficiency. *Lancet* 1986;I:423–424.
93. Bjorneboe G, Johnsen J, Bjorneboe A, et al: Diminished serum concentration of vitamin E in alcoholics. *Ann Nutr Med* 1988;32:56–61.
94. Karmali R, Bhagavan H: Plasma levels of retinol, alpha-tocopherol, and beta carotene in women at high risk for breast cancer: Effect of fish oil. *Clin Res* 1988;36:A761.
95. Quintanilha A: Effects of physical exercise and/or vitamin E on tissue oxidative metabolism. *Biochem Soc Trans* 1984;12:403–404.
96. Lehmann J, Martin H, Lashley M, et al: Vitamin E in foods from high and low linoleic acid diets. *J Am Diet A* 1986;86:1208–1216.
97. Possible role of vitamin E in the conversion of cyanocobalamin to its coenzyme form. *Nutr Rev* 1979;37:332–333.
98. Machlin L, Gabriel E: Interactions of vitamin E with vitamin C, vitamin B12, and zinc. In: Micronutrient interactions: Vitamins, Minerals and Hazardous Elements. Levander O, Cheng L, eds. New York, Annals of the New York Academy of Sciences, 1980, vol. 355.
99. Bunk M, Dnistrian A, Schwartz M: Dietary zinc deficiency lowers plasma concentration of vitamin E. *P Soc Exp M* 1989;4:379–384.
100. Omaye S: Heavy metal-nutrient interactions. Interaction between nutrients and toxicants. *Food Tech* 1982; October.
101. Ganther H: Interactions of vitamin E and selenium with mercury and silver. In: Micronutrient Interactions: Vitamins, Minerals, and Hazardous Elements. Levander O, Cheng L, eds. New York, Annals of the New York Academy of Sciences, 1980, vol. 355.
102. Arnich L, Arthur V: Interactions of fat soluble vitamins in hypervitaminosis. In: Micronutrient Interactions: Vitamins, Minerals, and Hazardous Elements. Levander O, Cheng L, eds. New York, Annals of the New York Academy of Sciences, 1980, vol. 355.

CHAPTER 3: VITAMIN K

103. Chlebowski R, Dietrich M, Akman S, et al: Vitamin K3 inhibition of malignant murine cell growth and human tumor colony formation. *Canc Tr Rep* 1985;69:527–532.
104. Noto V, Taper H, Yihua J, et al: Effects of sodium ascorbate (vitamin C) and 2-methyl-1-4-naphthaquinone (vitamin K) treatment on human tumor cell growth in vitro. *Cancer* 1989;63:901–906.
105. Suttie J, Mummah-Schendel L, Shah D, et al: Vitamin K deficiency from dietary vitamin K restriction in humans. *Am J Clin Nutr* 1988;47:475–480.

CHAPTER 3: VITAMIN B₁

106. Lonsdale D, Shamberger R: Red cell transketolase as an indicator of nutritional deficiency. *Am J Clin Nutr* 1980;33:205–211.
107. Ruenwonasa P, Pattanavibag S: Decrease in activities of thiamine pyrophosphate dependant enzymes in rat brain after prolonged tea consumption. *Nutr Rep Int* 1983;27:713–721.
108. Unna K: Pharmacology and toxicology. In: The Vitamins, second editon. Sebrell W, Harris R, eds. London, Academic Press, 1968, vol 2, pp 150–155.
109. Miller D, Hayes K: Vitamin excess and toxicity. In: Nutritional Toxicology. Hathcock J, ed. New York, Academic Press, 1982, vol 1, pp 81–133.

CHAPTER 3: VITAMIN B₂

110. Powers H: The relative effectiveness of iron and iron with riboflavin in correcting a microcytic anaemia in men and children in rural Gambia. *Human Nutr: Clin Nutr* 1983;37:413–425.
111. Kaul L, Heshmat M, Kovi J, et al: The role of diet in prostate cancer. *Nutr Cancer* 1987;9:123–128.
112. Prasad A, et al: Effect of oral contraceptive agents on nutrients. II: Vitamins. *Am J Clin Nutr* 1975;28:385.
113. Belko A, Roe D: Exercise-riboflavin relationship. *Fed Proc* 1984;43:870.
114. Garrison R, Somer E: *The Nutrition Desk Reference.* New Canaan, CT, Keats Publishing Company, 1985, p 46.
115. Sauberlich H: Interactions of thiamin, riboflavin, and other B vitamins. In: Micronutrient Interactions: Vitamins, Minerals, and Hazardous Elements. Levander O, Cheng L, eds. New York, Annals of the New York Academy of Sciences, 1980, vol 355, pp 80–97.

CHAPTER 3: NIACIN

116. Odetti P, Cheli V, Carta G, et al: Effect of nicotinic acid associated with retinol and tocopherols on plasma lipids in hyperlipoproteinaemic patients. *Pharmathera* 1984;4:21–24.
117. Berge K, Canner P: Coronary Drug Project: Experience with niacin. *Eur J Cl Ph* 1991;40:549–551.
118. Cohen L, Morgan J: Effectiveness of individualized long-term therapy with niacin and probucol in reduction of serum cholesterol. *J Fam Pract* 1988;26:145–150.

119. Scheulen M, Schmitt-Graff A, Schmidt C: Reduction of adriamycin cardiotoxicity by niacin and isocitrate. *Proc Am Assoc Canc Res* 1983;24:251.

120. Bourgeois B, Dodson W, Ferrendelli J: Potentiation of the antiepileptic activity of phenobarbital by nicotinamide. *Epilepsia* 1983;24:238–244.

121. Blom W, van den Berg G, Huijmans J: Successful nicotinamide treatment in an autosomal dominant behavioral and psychiatric disorder. *J Inh Met D* 1985;8:107–108.

122. Miller D, Hayes K: Vitamin excess and toxicity. In: Nutritional Toxicology. Hathcock J, ed. New York, Academic Press, 1982, vol 1, pp 81–133.

123. Bean W: Some aspects of pharmacologic use and abuse of water-soluble vitamins. In: Nutrition and Drug Interrelations. Hathcock J, Coon J, eds. New York, Academic Press, 1978.

124. Einstein N, Baker A, Galper J, et al: Jaundice due to nicotinic acid therapy. *Am J Dig Dis* 1975;20:282–286.

125. The Coronary Drug Project Research Group: Clofibrate and niacin in coronary artery disease. *J Am Med Assoc* 1975;231:360–381.

CHAPTER 3: VITAMIN B₆

126. Reynolds R, Natta C: Depressed plasma pyridoxal phosphate concentrations in adult asthmatics. *Am J Clin N* 1985;41:684–688.

127. Reynolds R, Natta C: Depressed plasma and erythrocyte pyridoxal phosphate in asthmatics. *Fed Proc* 1984;43:470.

128. Groves P, Schlesinger K: *Introduction to Biological Psychology*, second edition. Dubuque, Iowa, Wm C Brown Company, 1982.

129. Bender D: B vitamins in the nervous system: A review. *Neurochem I* 1984;6:297–321.

130. Bassler K: Megavitamin therapy with pyridoxine. *Int J Vit Nutr* 1988;58:105–118.

131. Driskell J, Wesley R, Hess I: Effectiveness of pyridoxine hydrochloride treatment on carpal tunnel syndrome patients. *Nutr Rep In* 1986;34:1031–1040.

132. Amadio P: Pyridoxine and carpal tunnel syndrome. *Nutr Rep* 1988;6:65, 70,72.

133. Jackson D: Pyridoxine modification of vincristine toxicity. Proceedings of the American Association of Cancer Research. 1984;25:313.

134. Slavik M, Bland O, Smith K, et al: Prevention of 6-azauridine triacetate (6-Azurd-TA) biochemical side effects by administration of pyridoxine. *Inv New Dr* 1984;2:115.

135. Serfontein W, Ubbink J, DeVilliers L, et al: Plasma pyridoxal-5-phosphate level as risk index for coronary artery disease. *Atherosclerosis* 1985;55:357–361.

136. Kok F, Schrijver J, Hofman A, et al: Low vitamin B₆ status in patients with acute myocardial infarction. *Am J Card* 1989;63:513–516.

137. Meydani S, Ribaya-Mercado J, Russell R, et al: Vitamin B$_6$ deficiency impairs interleukin 2 production and lymphocyte proliferation in elderly adults. *Am J Clin Nutr* 1991;53:1275–1280.
138. Gridley D, Shultz T, Stickney D, et al: In vivo and in vitro stimulation of cell-mediated immunity by vitamin B$_6$. *Nutr Res* 1988;8:201–207.
139. Manore M, Vaughn L, Carroll S, et al: Plasma pyridoxal 5'-phosphate concentration and dietary vitamin B$_6$ intake in free-living, low-income elderly people. *Am J Clin Nutr* 1989;50:339–345.
140. Watts R, Veall N, Purkiss P, et al: The effect of pyridoxine on oxalate dynamics in three cases of primary hyperoxaluria (with glycollic aciduria). *Clin Sci* 1985;69:87–90.
141. Williams M, Harris R, Dean B, et al: Controlled trial of pyridoxine in the premenstrual syndrome. *J Int Med R* 1985;13:174–179.
142. Hagen I, Nesheim B, Tuntland T: No effect of vitamin B$_6$ against premenstrual tension. *Acta Obst Sc* 1985;64:667–670.
143. Chrisley B, Hendricks T, Driskell J: Vitamin B$_6$ status of a group of cancer patients. *Nutr Res* 1986;6:1023–1029.
144. Gridley D, Stickney D, Shultz: Evaluation of cancer patients leukocyte responses in presence of physiologic and pharmacologic pyridoxine and pridoxal levels. *J Cl Lab An* 1989;3:95–100.
145. Shideler C: Vitamin B$_6$: An overview. *Am J Med Te* 1983;49:17–22.
See also references 9 and 115.

CHAPTER 3: VITAMIN B$_{12}$

146. Garrison R, Somer E: *The Nutrition Desk Reference.* New Canaan, CT, Keats Publishing Company, 1985, pp 116–118.
147. Bhatt H, Linnell J, Matthews D: Can faulty B$_{12}$ (cobalamin) metabolism produce diabetic neuropathy? *Lancet* 1983;II:572.
148. Cole M, Prchal J: Low serum vitamin B$_{12}$ in Alzheimer type dementia. *Age and Aging* 1984;13:101–105.
149. Freedman M, Tighe S, Amato D, et al: Vitamin B$_{12}$ in Alzheimer's disease. *Can J Neur* 1986;13:183.
150. Wieland R: Vitamin B$_{12}$ deficiency in the nonanemic elderly. *J Am Ger So* 1986;34:690.
151. Lindenbaum J, Healton E, Savage D, et al: Neuropsychiatric disorders caused by cobalamin deficiency in the absense of anemia or macrocytosis. *N Eng J Med* 1988;318:1720–1728.
See also references 97 and 115.

CHAPTER 3: FOLIC ACID

152. Check W: Folate for oral contraceptive users may reduce cervical cancer risk. *J Am Med Assoc* 1980;244:633–634.

153. Butterworth C: Folate-induced regression of cervical intraepithelial neo-plasias in users of oral contraceptive agents. *Am J Clin Nutr* 1980;32:926.
154. Davis R, Nicol D: Folic acid. *Int J Biochem* 1988;20:133–139.
155. Tamura T, Stokstad E: Folic acid. *Nutr & MD* 1984;10:1–2.
156. Butterworth C: Folic acid and vitamin C in cervical dysplasia. *Am J Clin Nutr* 1983;37:332.
157. Garrison R, Somer E: *The Nutrition Desk Reference*. New Canaan, CT, Keats Publishing Co, 1985, pp 49–50.

CHAPTER 3: BIOTIN

158. Mock D, Johnson S, Holman R: Effects of biotin deficiency on serum fatty acid composition: Evidence for abnormalities in humans. *J Nutr* 1988;118:342–348.
    See also reference 115.

CHAPTER 3: PANTOTHENIC ACID

159. Lacroix B, Didier E, Grenier J: Role of pantothenic acid and ascorbic acid in wound healing processes: In vitro study on fibroblasts. *Int J Vit Res* 198;58:407–413.
160. Litoff D, Scherzer H, Harrison J: Effects of pantothenic acid on human exercise. *Med Sci Spt* 1985;17:287.
    See also reference 115.

CHAPTER 3: VITAMIN C

161. Fann Y, Rothberg K, Tremmi G, et al: Ascorbic acid promotes pros-tanoid release in human lung parenchyma. *Prostagland* 1986;31:361–368.
162. Frei B, England L, Ames B: Ascorbate is an outstanding antioxidant in human blood plasma. *Proc Natl Acad Sci* 1989;86:6377–6381.
163. Garrison R, Somer E: *The Nutrition Desk Reference*. New Canaan, CT, Keats Publishing Co, 1985, p 140.
164. Bright-See E: Vitamin C and cancer prevention. *Sem Oncol* 1983;10:294–297.
165. Vinson J, Possanza C, Drack A: The effect of ascorbic acid on galactose-induced cataracts. *Nutr Rep In* 1986;33:665–668.
166. Chandra D, Varma R, Ahmad S, et al: Vitamin C in the human aqueous humor and cataracts. *Int J Vit Nutr Res* 1986;56:165–168.

167. Stankova L: Plasma ascorbate concentrations and blood cell dehydroascorbate transport in patients with diabetes mellitus. *Metabolism* 1984;33:347–353.
168. Sinclair A, Girling A, Gray L, et al: Disturbed handling of ascorbic acid in diabetic patients with and without microangiopathy during high dose ascorbate supplementation. *Diabetol* 1991;34:171–175.
169. Chen L, Thacker R: Effects of dietary vitamin E and high supplementation of vitamin C on plasma glucose and cholesterol levels. *Nutr Res* 1985;5:527–534.
170. Garrison R, Somer E: *The Nutrition Desk Reference.* New Canaan, CT, Keats Publishing Co, 1985, pp 173–174.
171. Norden C, Heine H, Stepanauskas M, et al: The interaction between blood to vessel wall in patients with arteriosclerosis obliterans during vitamin C treatment. *Int J Micro* 1984;3:425.
172. Kennes B, Dumont I, Brohee D, et al: Effect of vitamin C supplements on cell-mediated immunity in old people. *Gerontology* 1983;29:305–310.
173. Anderson T: Large scale trials of vitamin C. *Ann NY Acad Sci* 1975;258:498.
174. Johnson A, Rathbone B, Jones C, et al: Gastric juice secretion of ascorbic acid. *Clin Sci* 1986;70:38.
175. Oldroyd K, Dawes P: Clinically significant vitamin C deficiency in rheumatoid arthritis. *Br J Rheum* 1985;24:362–363.
176. Johnson M, Murphy C: Adverse effects of high dietary iron and ascorbic acid on copper status in copper-deficient and copper-adequate rats. *Am J Clin Nutr* 1988;47:96–101.
177. Robinson M, Huemmer P: Effect of a megadose of ascorbic acid, a meal and orange juice on the absorption of selenium as sodium selenite. *NZ Med J* 1985;98:627–629.
178. Pru C, Eaton J, Kjellstrand C: Vitamin C intoxication and hyperoxalemia in chronic hemodialysis patients. *Nephron* 1985;39:112–116.
179. Zweig M, Jackson A: Ascorbic acid interference in reagent-strip reactions for assay of urinary glucose and hemoglobin. *Clin Chem* 1986;32:674–677.
180. Toxic effects of water-soluble vitamins. *Nutr Rev* 1984;42:33–40.
181. Fox M: Effects of vitamin C and iron on cadmium metabolism. In: Micronutrient Interactions: Vitamins, Minerals, and Hazardous Elements. Levander O, Cheng L, eds. New York, Annals of the New York Academy of Sciences, 1980, vol 355, pp 249–261.
182. Hill C: Interactions of vitamin C with lead and mercury. In: Micronutrient Interactions: Vitamins, Minerals, and Hazardous Elements. Levander O, Cheng L, eds. New York, Annals of the New York Academy of Sciences, 1980, vol. 355, pp 262–266.
183. Pennington E, Kies C, Fox H: Thiamin and ascorbic acid status of humans as affected by use of calcium carbonate, calcium phosphate and manganese gluconate supplements. *Fed Proc* 1986;45:820.
184. Papaioannou R, Sohler A, Pfeiffer C: Effect of ascorbic acid and other adjuvants on manganese absorption. *Fed Proc* 1986;45:484.
See also references 80, 115, and 159.

CHAPTER 3: VITAMIN-LIKE FACTORS

185. Vinson J, Bose P: Comparative bioavailablity to humans of ascorbic acid alone or in a citrus extract. *Am J Clin Nutr* 1988;48:601.
186. Yuting C, Rongliang Z, Zhongjian J, et al: Flavonoids as superoxide scavengers and antioxidants. *Fr Rad Bio Med* 1990;9:19–21.
187. Tazaki Y, Sakai F, Otomo E, et al: Treatment of acute cerebral infarction with a choline precursor in a multicenter double-blind placebo-controlled study. *Stroke* 1988;19:211–216.
188. Zeisel S, DaCosta K, Franklin P, et al: Choline: An essential nutrient for humans. 1991;5:2093–2098.
189. Clements R, DeJesus P, Winegrad A: Raised plasma myoinositol level in uraemic and experimental neuropathy. *Lancet* 1973;I:1137.

CHAPTER 4: CALCIUM

190. McCarron D, Morris C, Bukoski R: The calcium paradox of essential hypertension. *Am J Med* 1987;82:27–33.
191. Stemmerman G, Nomura A, Chyou P: The influence of dairy and non-dairy calcium on subsite large-bowel cancer risk. *Dis Colon Rectum* 1990;33:190–194.
192. Williamson R, Appelton G: The role of calcium in the prevention of colorectal cancer. *Nutr Res* 1988;6:57,64.
193. Bloom S, Ahmed A: Ca channel blockage, inhibition of (Na,K)-ATPase, and myocardial necrosis associated with dietary magnesium deficiency. 1988;2:A824.
194. Rottka H, Pierper R, von Herrath D, et al: The influence of the calcium/phosphorus ratio in the diet on human bone disease, the role of nutritive secondary hyperparathyroidism. *Int J Vit Nutr Res* 1981;51:373–379.
195. Recker R: Osteoporosis. *Cont Nutr* 1983;8:1–2.
196. Spencer H, Kramer L: NIH Concensus Conference: Osteoporosis. *J Nutr* 1986;116:316–319.
197. Somer E: Calcium supplementation: A two-edged sword? *Nutr Rep* 1986;5:34.
198. Whittaker P, Cook J: The effect of calcium supplementation on iron absorption in healthy subjects. *Am J Clin Nutr* 1988;47:773.
199. Johnson C: Myocardial tissue concentrations of magnesium and potassium in men dying suddenly from ischemic heart disease. *Am J Clin Nutr* 1979;32:967–970.
200. Resnick L, DiFabio B, Marion R, et al: Increased oral calcium intake prevents the pressor effects of dietary salt in essential hypertension. *Kidney Int* 1987;31:308.
Also see references 8 and 39.

CHAPTER 4: MAGNESIUM

201. Neglen P, Qvarfordt P, Eklof B: Peroral magnesium hydroxide therapy and intermittent claudication. *VASA* 1985;14:285–288.
202. Sherwood R, Rocks B, Stewart A, et al: Magnesium and the premenstrual syndrome. *Ann Clin Bi* 1986;23:667–670.
203. Abraham G, Lubran M: Serum and red cell magnesium levels in patients with premenstrual tension. *Am J Clin Nutr* 1981;34:2364–2366.
204. Morgan K, Stampley G, Zabik M, et al: Magnesium and calcium dietary intakes of the US population. *J Am Col N* 1985;4:195-206.
   See also references 8, 10, 11, 32, 33, and 34.

CHAPTER 4: SODIUM, POTASSIUM, AND CHLORIDE

205. Norbiato G, Bevilacqua M, Meroni R, et al: Effects of potassium supplementation on insulin binding and insulin action in human obestiy: Protein-modified fast and refeeding. *Eur J Cl In* 1984;14:414–419.
206. Khaw K: Dietary potassium and blood pressure. *Nutr Rep* 1985;3:68–69.
207. Garrison R, Somer E: *The Nutrition Desk Reference.* New Canaan, CT, Keats Publishing Company, 1985, pp 156–158.
208. Senate Select Committee on Nutrition and Human Needs: Dietary Goals for the United States. No. 052-070-04376-8. United States Senate. US Government Printing Office, December, 1977.
209. Saito N, Kuchiba A: The changes of magnesium under high salt diets and by administration of antihypertensive diuretics. *Mag Bul* 1987;9:53.

CHAPTER 4: CHROMIUM

210. Anderson R: The role of chromium in the control of high and low blood sugar. *Nutr Rep* 1988;6:41,48.
211. Press R, Geller J, Evans G: The effect of Cr picolinate on serum cholesterol and apolipoprotein factions in human subjects. *West J Med* 1990;152:41–45.
212. Gordon J: An easy and inexpensive way to lower cholesterol? *West J Med* 1991;154:3.
213. Schroeder H: The role of chromium in mammalian nutrition. *Am J Clin Nutr* 1968;21:230–244.
214. Anderson R, Kozlovsky A, Moser P: Effects of diets high in simple sugars on urinary chromium excretion of humans. *Fed Proc* 1985;44:751.
215. Somer E: Athletes at risk for chromium deficiency. *Nutr Rep* 1989;7:34.
   See also references 12 and 28–31.

348   *References*

CHAPTER 4: COPPER

216. Beach R, Gershwin M, Hurley L: Zinc, copper and manganese in immune function and experimental oncogenesis. *Nutr and Cancer* 1982;3:172–191.
217. Lampi K, Mathias M, Allen K: The role of dietary copper in prostaglandin synthesis. *Fed Proc* 1986;45:237.
218. Oleske J: Plasma zinc and copper in primary and secondary immunodeficiency disorders. *Biol Tr El Res* 1983;5:189–194.
219. Opsahl W: Scoliosis in chickens: Responsiveness of severity and incidence to dietary copper. *Science* 1984;225:440.
220. Strause L, Andon M, Howard G, et al: Dietary calcium intake, serum copper concentration, and bone density in postmenopausal women. *FASEBJ* 1991;5:A576.
221. MacFie J, Tasman-Jones C, Knight G: Effect of salazopyrine on the faecal excretion of copper and changes in colonic mucosal copper in patients with ulcerative colitis. *Br J Sur* 1985;72:398–399.
222. Hoffman H, Phyliky R, Flemming C: Zinc-induced copper deficiency. *Am J Clin Nutr* 1988;94:508–512.
See also reference 126.

CHAPTER 4: FLUORIDE

223. Dambacher M, Ittner J, Ruegsegger P: Long-term fluoride therapy of postmenopausal osteoporosis. *Bone* 1986;7:199–205.

CHAPTER 4: IRON

224. Labbe R: Iron deficiency: New diagnostic tests for a nutritional epidemic. *Nutr Rep* 1987;5:49,56.
225. Mehta B, Panjwani D, Jhala D: Electrophysiologic abnormalities of heart in iron deficiency anemia. *Act Haemat* 1983;70:189–193.
226. Tucker D, Sandstead H, Penland J, et al: Iron status and brain function-serum ferritin levels associated with asymmetrics of cortical electrophysiology and cognitive performance. *Am J Clin N* 1984;39:105–113.
227. Hunt J, Mullen L, Lykken G, et al: Ascorbic acid: Effect on ongoing iron absorption and status in iron-depleted young women. *Am J Clin Nutr* 1990;51:649–655.
228. Craig W, Balbach L, Harris S, et al: Plasma zinc and copper levels of infants fed different milk formulas. *J Am Col Nutr* 1984;3:183–186.
See also references 9, 18, 19, and 176.

CHAPTER 4: MANGANESE

229. Saltman P, Strause L: The role of manganese in bone metabolism. *Nutr Rep* 1987;5:33,40.

CHAPTER 4: SELENIUM

230. Helzlsouer K: Selenium and cancer prevention. *Sem Oncol* 1983;10:305–321.
231. Spallholz J: Selenium: What role in immunity and immune cytotoxicity? In: Selenium in Biology and Medicine. Spallholz J, Martin J, Ganther H, eds. Westport, CT, AVI Publishing, 1981, pp 103–117.
232. Tarp U, Overvad K, Thorling E, et al: Selenium treatment in rheumatoid arthritis. *Scand J Rheumatol* 1985;14:364–368.
233. Mulhern S, Taylor G, Magreuder E, et al: Deficient levels of dietary selenium suppress the antibody response in first and second generation mice. *Nutr Res* 1985;5:201–210.
234. Salonen J, Alfhan G, Huttunen J, et al: Association between serum selenium and the risk of cancer. *Am J Epidem* 1984;120:342–349.
235. Sundstrum H: Low serum selenium concentration in patients with cervical or endometrial cancer. *Int J Gynecology Obstetrics* 1984;22:35–40.
236. Sundstrom H: Serum selenium in patients with ovarian cancer during and after therapy. *Carcinogenesis* 1984;5:731–734.
237. Burney P, Comstock G, Morris J: Serologic precursors of cancer: Serum micronutrients and the subsequent risk of pancreatic cancer. *Am J Clin Nutr* 1989;49:895–900.
238. Schrauzer G, Molenaar T, Mead S, et al: Selenium in the blood of Japanese and American women with and without breast cancer and fibrocystic disease. *Jpn J Canc* 1985;76:374–377.
239. Salonen J, Salonen R, Seppanen K, et al: Relationship of serum Se and antioxidants to plasma lipoproteins, platelet aggregability and prevalent ischemic heart disease in Eastern Finnish men. *Atheroscler* 1988;70:155–160.
240. Kok F, Hoffman A, Witteman J, et al: Decreased selenium levels in acute myocardial infarction. *J Am Med A* 1989;261:1161–1164.
241. Selenium intoxication. *Morbidity and Mortality Weekly Report.* 1984;33:157–158.
    See also reference 91.

CHAPTER 4: ZINC

242. Garrison R, Somer E: *The Nutrition Desk Reference.* New Canaan, CT, Keats Publishing Co, 1985, pp 140–141.

243. Maloney G, Salbe A, Levander O: Selenium (Se) as sodium selanate (NaSeO4) is more toxic than selenium as L-selenomethionine (SeMet) in methionine deficiency rats. *Clin Res* 1988;36:A763.

244. Wahid M, Fathi S, Aboutl-Khair M: Zinc in human health and disease. *Rec Cl Lab* 1988;18:9–16.

245. Bryce-Smith D, Simpson R: Case of anorexia nervosa responding to zinc sulphate. *Lancet* 1984;II:350.

246. Safai-Kutti S, Kutti J: Zinc supplementation in anorexia nervosa (letter). *Am J Clin Nutr* 1986;44:581–582.

247. Lipman T, Diamond A, Mellow M, et al: Esophageal zinc content in human squamous esophageal cancer. *J Am Col N* 1987;6:41–46.

248. Hess J, Prasad A, Kaplan J: Zinc nutrition and cellular immunity in the elderly. *J Am Ger So* 1987;35:91.

249. Kemahli A, Babacan E, Caudar A: Cell mediated immune response in children with iron deficiency and combined iron and zinc deficiency. *Nutr Res* 1988;8:129–136.

250. Eby G: Reduction in duration of common colds by zinc gluconate lozenges in a double blind study. *Antimicrobial Agents and Chemotherapy* 1984;25:20–24.

251. Wallwork J: Zinc, brain development and function. *Nutr Rep* 1988;6:49,52,56.

252. Prasad A: Zinc metabolism in patients with the syndrome of iron deficiency anemia, hypatosplenomegaly, dwarfism and hypogonadism. *J Lab Clin Med* 1963;61:537.

253. Chandra R: Excessive intake of zinc impairs immune-responses. *Am J Clin Nutr* 1984;252:1443–1446.

254. Black M, Medeiros P, Brunett E, et al: Zinc supplementation and serum lipids in young adult white males. *Am J Clin Nutr* 1988;47:970–975.

255. Siewicki T, Sydlowski J, Van Dolah F, et al: Influence of dietary zinc and cadmium on iron bioavailability in mice and rats: Oyster versus salt sources. *J Nutr* 1986;116:281–289.

256. Teller E, Kimmel P, Watkins D, et al: Zinc (Z) nutritional status modulates the 1,25(OH)2D (1,25) response to low calcium (LC) diet (D). *Kidney Int* 1987;31:358.

See also reference 99 and 222

CHAPTER 4: ADDITIONAL TRACE MINERALS

257. Garrison R, Somer E: *The Nutrition Desk Reference*. New Canaan, CT, Keats Publishing Co, 1985, pp 78–83.

258. Allen V, Robinson K, Hembry F: Effects of ingested aluminum sulfate on serum magnesium and the possible relationship to hypomagnesemic tetany. *Nutr Rep Int* 1984;29:107.

259. Lione A: The prophylactic reduction of aluminum intake. *Food Chem Toxicology* 1983;21:103–109.

260. Lione A, Allen P, Smith J: Aluminum coffee percolators as a source of dietary aluminum. *Food Chem T* 1984;22:265–268.
261. Nielsen F: New essential trace elements for the life sciences. *Biol Tr El Res* 1990;26–27:599–611.
262. Eggleston D: Effect of dental amalgam and nickle alloys on T-lymphocytes: Preliminary report. *J Prosthetic Dentistry* 1984;51:617.
263. Abraham J: The effect of dental amalgam restorations on blood mercury levels. *J Dental Research* 1984;63:71–73
264. Carlisle E: Biochemical and morphological changes associated with long bone abnormalities in silicon deficiency. *J Nutr* 1980;110:1046–1055.
265. Carlisle E: A silicon requirement for normal skull formation. *J Nutr* 1980;110:352–359.
266. Thompson H, Chasteen D, Meeker D: Dietary vanadyl (IV) sulfate inhibits chemically-induced mammary carcinogenesis. *Carcinogenesis* 1984;5:849–851.

CHAPTER 5: INTRODUCTION

267. Cochrane C: Mechanisms of oxidant injury of cells. *Molec Aspects Med* 1991;12:137–147.
268. Dormandy T: An approach to free radicals. *Lancet* 1983;II:1010–1013.
269. Di Masco P, Murphy M, Sies H: Antioxidant defense systems: The rate of carotenoid, tocopherals, and thiols. *Am J Clin Nutr* 1991;53:1945–2005.
270. Shlafer M, Kane P, Wiggins V, et al: Possible role for cytotoxic oxygen metabolites in the pathogenesis of cardiac ischemic injury. *Circulation* 1982;66(supple I):I:85–92.
271. Nockles C: Protective effects of supplemental vitamin E against infection. *Fed Proc* 1979;38:2134–2138.
272. Banic S: Immunostimulation by vitamin C. *Int J Vit Nutr Res* 1982;23:49–52.
273. Prohaska J, Lukaswqyez D: Copper deficiency suppresses the immune response of mice. *Science* 1981;213:559–561.
274. Chandra R: Iron status, immunocompetence, and susceptibility to infection. In: Iron Metabolism. Ciba Foundation Symposium No. 51. Amsterdam, Elsevier, 1977, pp 249–268.
275. Hambridge K: The role of zinc and other trace minerals in pediatric nutrition and health. *Pediat Clin N Am* 1977;24:95.
276. Spallholz J: Importance of minerals in immunology. *Nutr Rep* 1989;8:1,8.
277. Brevard P: Beta-carotene affects white blood cells in human peripheral blood. *Nutr Rep Int* 1989;40:139–150.
278. Mickle D, Li R, Weisel R, et al: Myocardial salvage with Trolox and ascorbic acid for an acute evolving infarction. *Ann Thorac* 1989;47:553–557.

279. Bendich A: Vitamin E and immunity. *Nutr Rep* 1987;5:17,24.
280. Huwyler T, Hirt A, Morell A: Effect of ascorbic acid on human natural killer cells. *Am J Clin Nutr* 1985;10:173–176.
    See also references 17, 24, 41, 42, 58, 80, 137, 144, 162, 237, 248, 250, and 253.

CHAPTER 5: ACNE

281. Rebello T, Atherton D, Holden C: The effect of oral zinc administration on sebum free fatty acids in acne vulgaris. *Act Der Ven* 1986;55:305–310.

CHAPTER 5: AIDS

282. Jain V, Chandra R: Does nutritional deficiency predispose to acquired immune deficiency syndrome? *Nutr Res* 1984;4:537–543.
283. Dworkin B, Rosenthal W, Wormser G, et al: Selenium deficiency in the Acquired Immunodeficiency Syndrome. *J Parent En* 1986;10:405–407.
284. Kotler D, Wang J, Pierson R: Body composition studies in patients with the acquired immunodeficiency syndrome. *Am J Clin Nutr* 1985;42:1255–1265.
285. Dworkin B, Rosenthal W, Wormser G, et al: Abnormalities of blood selenium and glutathione peroxidase activity in patients with acquired immunodeficiency syndrome and AIDS-related complex. *Biol Tr El Res* 1988;15:167–177.
286. Begin M, Das U: A deficiency in dietary gamma-linolenic and/or eicosapenaenoic acids may determine individual susceptibility to AIDS. *Med Hypothesis* 1986;20:1–8.

CHAPTER 5: ALLERGIES

287. Heiner D, Singer A: Food allergy. In: Allergy and Clinical Immunology. Beall G, ed. New York, John Wiley and Sons, 1983, pp 187–200.
288. Darlington L, Ramsey N, Mansfield J: Placebo-controlled blind study of dietary manipulation therapy in the management of rheumatoid arthritis. *Br J Rheum* 1986;25:115.
289. Hughes E, Gott P, Weinstein R, et al: Migraine: A diagnostic test for etiology of food sensitivity by a nutritionally supported fast and confirmed by long term report. *Ann Allergy* 1985;55:28–32.
290. Taylor S: Food allergy and sensitivities. *J Am Diet Assoc* 1986;86:601–608.

291. Anderson J, Lessof M: Diagnosis and treatment of food allergies. *P Nutr Soc* 1983;42:257–262.
292. Zaloga G, Hierlwimmer U, Engler R: Anaphylaxis following psyllium ingestion. *J Allergy Clin Immunol* 1984;74:79–80.
See also references 161 and 168.

CHAPTER 5: ALZHEIMER'S DISEASE

293. Garrison R: From the desk of the editor. *Nutr Rep* 1984;9:58.
294. Somer E: Exploring the link between nutrition and Alzheimer's disease. *Nutr Rep* 1986;3:66,72.
295. Rosenberg G, Davis K: The use of cholinergic precursors in neuropsychiatric diseases. *Am J Clin Nutr* 1982;36:709–720.
296. Thomas D, Chung-A-On K, Dickerson J, et al: Tryptophan and nutritional status of patients with senile dementia. *Psychol Med* 1986;16:297–305.
297. Burns A, Holland T: Vitamin E deficiency. *Lancet* 1986;I:805–806.
See also references 148–150, 260, and 317.

CHAPTER 5: ANEMIA

298. Morris J: Selenium deficiency in cattle associated with heinz bodies and anemia. *Science* 1984;223:491.
299. Ono K: Effects of large dose vitamin E supplementation on anemia in hemodialysis patients. *Nephron* 1985;40:440–445.
300. Bezwoda W, Torrance J, Bothwell T, et al: Iron absorption from red and white wines. *Sc J Haemat* 1985;34:121–127.
301. Somer E: Is the iron deficiency epidemic preventable? *Nutr Rep* 1987;5:50.

CHAPTER 5: ARTHRITIS

302. Bigaoutte J, Timchalk M, Kremer J: Nutritional adequacy of diet and supplements in patients with rheumatoid arthritis who take medications. *J Am Diet Assoc* 1987;87:1687–1688.
303. Maddison P, Bacon P: Vitamin D deficiency spontaneous fractures and osteopenia in rheumatoid arthritis. *Br Med J* 1974;4:433–435.
304. Makela A, Hyora H, Vuorinen K, et al: Trace elements (Fe, Zn, Cu, and Se) in serum of rheumatic children living in western Finland. *Scand J Rheum* 1984;S53:94.

305. Simkin P: Oral zinc sulfate in rheumatoid arthritis. *Lancet* 1976;II:539.

306. UK, General Practiioner Research Group: Calcium pantothenate in arthritis conditions. *Practitioner* 1980;224:208–211.

307. Tarp U, Overvad K, Hansen J, et al: Low selenium level in severe rheumatoid arthritis. *Sc J Rheum* 1985;14:97–101.

308. Kremer J: Omega-3 fatty acids and rheumatoid arthritis: Current status. *Nutr Rep* 1988;6:33,36,40.

309. Darlington L, Ramsey N, Mansfield J: Placebo controlled, blind study of dietary manipulation therapy in rheumatoid arthritis. *Lancet* 1986;I: 236–238.

310. O'Farrelly C, Price R, Fernandes L: Immune sensitization to dietary antigens associated with IgA RF in rheumatoid arthritis. *Br J Rheum* 1986;25:89.

311. Blake D, Bacon P: Iron and rheumatoid disease (letter). *Lancet* 1982;I:623.
See also references 91, 175, 232, 288, and 317.

CHAPTER 5: ASTHMA

312. Gomaa H, Hussein H, Madkour E, et al: Plasma cortisol and vitamin C in asthmatic patients. *Ann Allergy* 1985;55:236.

313. Stone J, Hinks L, Beasley R, et al: Reduced selenium status of patients with asthma. *Clin Sci* 1989;77:495–500.

314. Lindahl O, Lindwall L, Spangberg A, et al: Vegan regimen with reduced medication in the treatment of bronchial asthma. *J Asthma* 1985;22: 45–55.
See also references 126 and 127.

CHAPTER 5: BURNS

315. Kohen I: Hypogeusia, anorexia and altered zinc metabolism following thermal burn. *JAMA* 1973;223:914.

316. Sandstead H: Zinc and wound healing. *Am J Clin Nutr* 1970;23:514.

317. Somer E: Nutrition and dementia: You've come nowhere baby. *Nutr Rep* 1990;8:34.

318. Vreugdenhil G, Wognum A, van Eijk H, et al: Anemia in rheumatoid arthritis: The role of iron, vitamin B_{12}, and folic acid deficiency, and erythropoietin responsiveness. *Ann Rheum D* 1990;49:93–98.

CHAPTER 5: CANCER

319. Doll R, Peto R: The causes of cancer: Quantitative estimates of avoidable risk of cancer in the United States today. *J Natl Cancer Inst* 1981;66:1192.

320. Lai D: Naturally occurring carcinogens in our diets. *Nutr Rep* 1989;7:1,8.
321. Willett W, MacMahon B: Diet and cancer: An overview. *N Eng J Med* 1984;310:697–703.
322. Snowdon D, Phillips R, Warren C: Diet, obesity, and risk of fatal prostate cancer. *Am J Epidem* 1984;120:244–250.
323. Newman S, Miller A, Howe G: A study of the effect of weight and dietary fat on breast cancer survival time. *Am J Epidem* 1986;1234:767–774.
324. Reddy B: Dietary fat and its relationship to large bowel cancer. *Canc Res* 1981;41:3700–3705.
325. Weinzweig J, Levenson S, Rettura G, et al: Supplemental vitamin A prevents the tumor-induced defect in wound healing. *Ann Surg* 1990;211:269–276.
326. Basu T: Vitamin A and cancer of epithelial origin. *J Human Nutr* 1979;33:24–31.
327. Shekelle R, Liu S, Raynor W, et al: Dietary vitamin A and risk of cancer in the Western Electric Study. *Lancet* 1981;II:1185–1189.
328. Band P, Deschamps M, Falardeau M, et al: Treatment of benign breast disease with vitamin A. *Prev Med* 1984;13:549–554.
329. Rettura G, Gruber K, Gruber C, et al: Supplemental vitamin A prevents radiation-induced defect in wound healing. *Surg Forum* 1983;34:116.
330. Levenson S, Gruber B, Rettura G, et al: Supplemental vitamin A prevents the acute radiation-induced defect in wound healing. *Ann Surg* 1984;200:494–512.
331. Goodman G: Phase II trial of retinol in patients with advanced cancer. *Canc Tr Rep* 1986;70:1023–1024.
332. Yunis J, Soreng A: Constitutive fragile sites in cancer. *Science* 1984;226:119–1204.
333. Prior F: Theoretical involvement of vitamin B_6 in tumor initiation. *Medical Hypothesis* 1985;16:421–428.
334. Birt D: Effects of the intake of selected vitamins and minerals on cancer prevention. *Magnesium* 1989;8:17–30.
335. Garland C, Shekelle R, Barrett-Connor E, et al: Dietary vitamin D and calcium and risk of colorectal cancer: A 19 year prospective study in men. *Lancet* 1985;I:307–309.
336. Wald N: Plasma retinol, beta carotene, and vitamin E levels in relation to the future risk of breast cancer. *Br J Cancer* 1984;49:321–324.
337. McKeowne-Eyssen G, Holloway C, Jazmaji V, et al: A randomized trial of vitamin C and vitamin E supplementation in the prevention of recurrence of colorectal polyps. *Prev Med* 1987;16:275.
338. Menkes M, Comstock G: Vitamins A and E and lung cancer. *Am J Epidem* 1984;120:491.
339. Trickler D, Shklar G: Prevention of experimental oral carcinogenesis by vitamin E. *J Dent Res* 1986;65:221.
340. London R, Murphy L, Kitlowski K: Hypothesis: Breast cancer prevention by supplemental vitamin E. *J Am Col Nutr* 1985;4:559–564.
341. Ip C: Dietary vitamin E intake and mammary carcionogenesis in rats. *Carcinogenesis* 1982;3:1453–1456.
342. Menkes M, Comstock G, Vuilleumier J, et al: Serum beta-carotene, vita-

mins A and E, selenium, and the risk of lung cancer. *N Eng J Med* 1986;315:1250–1254.

343. Fariss M: Oxygen toxicity: Unique cytoprotective properties of vitamin E succinate in hepatocytes. *Fr Rad B* 1990;9:333–343.

344. Prasad D, Edwards-Prasad J: Effects of tocopherol (vitamin E) acid succinate or morphological alterations and growth inhibition in melanoma cells in culture. *Canc Res* 1983;42:550–555.

345. Stevens R, Jones Y, Micozzi M, et al: Body iron stores and the risk for cancer. *Am J Clin Nutr* 1988;319:1047–1052.

346. Akiba S, Neriishi K, Blot W, et al: Serum ferritin and stomach cancer risk among a Japanese population. *Cancer* 1991;67:1707–1712.

347. Salonen J, Salonen R, Lappetelainen R, et al: Risk of cancer in relation to serum concentrations of selenium and vitamins A and E: Matched case-control and analysis of prospectiver data. *Br Med J* 1985;290:417–420.

348. Allen J, Bell E, Oken M, et al: Zinc deficiency, hyperzincuria and immune dysfunction in lung cancer patients. *Am J Clin Nutr* 1983;37:720.

349. Allinger V, Johnasson G, Gustafsson J, et al: Shift from a mixed to a lactovegetarian diet: Influence on acidic lipid in fecal water—a potential risk factor for colon cancer. *Am J Clin Nutr* 1989;50:992–996.

350. Messina M, Barnes S: The role of soy products in reducing risk of cancer. *J Natl Canc Instit* 1991;83:541–546.

351. Booyens J, Englebrecht P, le Roux S, et al: Some effects of the essential fatty acids, linoleic acid and alpha linolenic acid and their metabolites gamma linolenic acid, arachidonic acid, eicosapentaenoic acid, docosahexaenoic acid, and of prostaglandins A1 and E1 on the proliferation of human osteogeneic sarcoma cells in culture. *Pros Leuk M* 1984;15:15–33.

352. Bristol J, Emmett P, Heaton K, et al: Sugar, fat, and the risk of colorectal cancer. *Br Med J* 1985;291:1467–1470.

353. Seitz H, Czygan P, Simanowski U, et al: Stimulation of chemically induced rectal carcinogenesis by chronic ethanol ingestion. *Alc Alcoholism* 1985;20:427–433.

354. Dichter C: Risk estimates of liver cancer due to aflatoxin exposure from peanuts and peanut products. *Food and Chemical Toxicology* 1984;22:431–437.
See also references 38, 43–57, 67–69, 83, 103, 104, 143, 144, 153, 192, 230, 234–238, 243, 247, 266, and 280.

CHAPTER 5: CARDIOVASCULAR DISEASE

355. Lipid Research Clinics Program: The Lipid Research Clinics Coronary Primary Prevention Trial results: The relationship of reduction in incidence of coronary heart disease to cholesterol lowering. *JAMA* 1984;25:365.

356. Dawber R: *The Framingham Study*. Cambridge, MA, Harvard University Press, 1980.

357. Keys A: Coronary heart disease in seven countries. *Circulation* 1970;41(supple):1.

358. Superko H: Blood cholesterol and heart disease: A new call to arms. *Nutr Rep* 1987;5:4–5,8.
359. Hulley S: The US National Cholesterol Education Program: Adult treatment guidelines. *Drugs* 1988;36 (Supple 3):100–104.
360. Somer E: Choleserol and heart disease: Diet increases mortality risk. *Nutr Rep* 1988;6:34.
361. Garrison R, Somer E: *The Nutrition Desk Reference*. New Canaan, CT, Keats Publishing Co, 1985, pp 149–171.
362. Turner P, Tuomilehto J, Happonen P, et al: Metabolic studies on the hyperlipidemic effect of guar gum. *Atheroscl* 1990;81:1345–1350.
363. Colette C, Pares-Herbute N, Monnier L, et al: Platelet function in type I diabetes: Effects of supplementation with large doses of vitamin E. *Am J Clin Nutr* 1988;47:256–261.
364. Hennig B, Boissonneault G, Wangy: Protective effects of vitamin E in age-related endothelial cell injury. *Int J Vit Nutr Res* 1989;59:273–279.
365. McCully K, Wilson R: Homocysteine theory of atherosclerosis. *Atherosclerosis* 1975;22:215–227.
366. Brattstrom L, Israelsson B, Norrving B, et al: Impaired homocysteine metabolism in early onset cerebral and peripheral occlusive arterial disease. *Atheroscl* 1990;81:51–60.
367. Brattstrom L, Hultberg B, Hardebo J: Folic acid responsive postmenopausal homocysteinemia. *Metabolism* 1985;34:1073–1077.
368. Evans G: A review of studies with chromium picolinate in humans: Part I. *Nutr Rep* 1989;7:74,78,80.
369. Copper deficiency and developmental emphysema. *Nutr Rev* 1983;38:214–222.
370. Klevay L: Hypercholesterolemia in rats produced by an increase in the ratio of zinc to copper ingested. *Am J Clin N* 1973;26:1060.
371. Sjogren A, Edvinsson L, Fallgren B: Magnesium deficiency in coronary artery disease and cardiac arrhythmias. *J Int Med* 1989;226:213–222.
372. Kok F: Selenium and cardiovascular disease. *Nutr Rep* 1990;8:33,38,40.
373. Sammon S, Roberts D: The effect of zinc supplementation on lipoprotein and copper status. *Atheroscler* 1988;70:247–252.
374. Report of AHA Nutrition Committee: Rationale of the diet-heart statement of the American Heart Association. *Arteriosclerosis* 1982;2:177–191.
375. Masarei J, Rouse I, Lynch W, et al: Vegetarian diets, lipids, and cardiovascular risk. *Aust NZ J M* 1984;14:400–404.
376. Sparks J, Sparks C, Kritchevsky D: Hypercholesterolemia and aortic glycosaminoglycans of rabbits fed semi-purified diets containing sucrose and lactose. *Atherosclerosis* 1986;60:183–196.
377. Snowdon D: Meat consumption and chronic disease. *Nutr Rep* 1986;8:60–61.
378. Snowdon D, Phillips R, Fraser G: Meat consumption and fatal ischemic heart disease. *Prev Med* 1984;13:490–500.
379. Somer E: Do you have to give an arm and a leg to save your heart? *Nutr Rep* 1990;8:18.
380. Ferrence R: Alcohol and the prevention of coronary heart disease. *Nutr Rep* 1987;5:57,64.

See also references 33, 76, 85–88, 116–118, 136, 170, 171, 193, 199–201, 225, 239, 240, and 278.

CHAPTER 5: CARPAL TUNNEL SYNDROME

See reference 132.

CHAPTER 5: THE COMMON COLD

381. Carr A, Einstein R, Lai L, et al: Vitamin C and the common cold: A second MZ Cotwin control study. *Acta Genet Med Gemellol* (Italy) 1981;30:249–255.
382. Carr A, Einstein R, Lai L, et al: Vitamin C and the common cold: Using identical twins as controls. *Med J Aust* 1981;2:411–412.
383. Banic S: Immunostimulation by vitamin C. *Int J Vitamin Nutr Res* 1982;23:49–53.
384. Kent S: Rejuvenating the immune system. *Geriatrics* 1981;36:13–22.
See also references 172, 173, 249, 250, 253, and 276.

CHAPTER 5: CYSTIC FIBROSIS

385. Solomons N: Some biochemical indices of nutrition in treated cystic fibrosis patients. *Am J Clin Nutr* 1981;34:462–474.
386. Jacob R: Zinc status and vitamin A transport in cystic fibrosis. *Am J Clin Nutr* 1978;31:638–644.
387. Palin D: The effect of oral zinc supplements on plasma levels of vitamin A and retinol-binding protein in cystic fibrosis. *Am J Clin Nutr* 1979;32:1253–1259.
388. Chase H, Long M, Lavin M: Cystic fibrosis and malnutrition. *J Pediatr* 1979;95:337–347.
389. Stead R: Selenium deficiency, cystic fibrosis, and pancreatic cancer. *Lancet* 1985;II:862–863.
390. Goodhart R, Shils M: Modern Nutrition in Health and Disease, 5th ed. Philadelphia, Lea & Fehigue, 1978, pp 124, 155, 178, 184.
391. Dworkin B, Newman L, Berezin S, et al: Low blood selenium levels in patients with cystic fibrosis compared to controls and healthy adults. *J Parent En* 1987;11:38–41.
392. Shepard R, Cooksley W, Cooke W: Improved growth and clinical, nutritional, and respiratory changes in response to nutritional therapy in cystic fibrosis. *J Pediatr* 1980;97:351–357.
393. Shepherd R, Thomas B, Bennett D, et al: Changes in body compositon and muscle protein degradation during nutritional supplementation in

nutritionally growth-retarded children with cystic fibrosis. *J Ped Gastr* 1983;2:439–444.

CHAPTER 5: DERMATITIS

394. Schaffer H: Essential fatty acids and eicosanoids in cutaneous inflammation. *Int J Derm* 1989;28:281–290.

CHAPTER 5: DIABETES MELLITUS

395. Behrens W, Scott F, Madere R, et al: Increased plasma and tissue levels of vitamin E in the spontaneously diabetic BB rat. *Life Sciences* 1984;35:199–206.
396. Simonoff M: Chromium deficiency and cardiovascular risk: A review. *Cardio Res* 1984;18:591–596.
397. Vinson J, Bose P: The effect of a high chromium yeast on the blood glucose control and blood lipids of normal and diabetic human subjects. *Nutr Rep Int* 1984;30:911–918.
398. Evans G: A review of studies with chromium picolinate in humans: Part II. *Nutr Rep* 1989;7:81,86,88.
    See also references 74, 76, 84, 167–169, 179, and 210.

CHAPTER 5: ECZEMA

399. Neild V, Marsden R, Bailes J, et al: Egg and milk exclusion diets in atopic eczema. *Br J Derm* 1986;114:117–123.

CHAPTER 5: EMOTIONAL DISORDERS

400. Martineua J, Barthelemy C, Lelord G: Long term effects of combined vitamin B_6-magnesium administration in an autistic child. *Biol Psychi* 1986;21:511–518.
401. Podell R: Nutritional supplementation with megadoses of vitamin B_6. *Postgr Med* 1985;77:113–116.
402. Vitamin B_6 toxicity: A new megavitamin toxicity. *Nutr Rev* 1984;42:44–46.
403. Weiland R: Vitamin B_{12} deficiency in nonanemic elderly. *J Am Ger So* 1986;34:690.
404. Matchar D, Feussner J, Watson D, et al: Significance of low serum vitamin B_{12} levels in the elderly. *J Am Ger So* 1986;34:680–681.

405. Bell I, Edman J, Marby D, et al: Vitamin B$_{12}$ and folate status in acute geropsychiatric inpatients: Affective and cognative characteristics of a vitamin non-deficient population. *Biol Psych* 1990;27:125–137.

406. Murphy J, Thome L, Michals K, et al: Folic acid responsive rages, seizures, and homocystinuria. *J Inh Met D* 1985;8:109–110.

407. Conlay L, Zeisel S: Neurotransmitter precursors and brain function. *Neurosurgery* 1982;10:524–529.

408. Gelenberg A, Gibson C, Wojcik J: Neurotransmitter precursors for the treatment of depression. *Psychopharm Bull* 1982;18:7–18.

409. Rapoport J, Kruesi M: Behavior and nutrition: A mini review. *Cont Nutr* 1983;8(10):1–2.

410. Havlak D: Diet, neurotransmitters and pain. *Am Diet Assoc: Dietetics in Developmental and Psychiatric Disorders Newsletter* 1982;2:June.

411. Hartmann E: Questions and Answers: Tryptophan in psychopharmacology. *JAMA* 1980;243:1089.
    See also references 18, 19, 92, 120–122, 128, 129, 151, 226, 251, 294, and 295.

CHAPTER 5: EYE DISORDERS

412. Gerster H: Antioxidant vitamins in cataract prevention. *Z Ern Ahrungswiss* 1989;28:56–75.

413. Bhat K: Nutritional status of thiamine, riboflavin, and pyridoxine in cataract patients. *Nutr Rep In* 1987;36:685–692.

414. Chandra D, Varma R, Ahmad S, et al: Vitamin C in the human aqueous humor and cataracts. *Int J Vita Nutr Res* 1986;56:165–168.

415. Neuringer M, Connor W: N-3 fatty acids in the brain and retina: Evidence for their essentiality. *Nutr Rev* 1986;44:285–294.
    See also reference 165.

CHAPTER 5: GUM AND TOOTH DISORDERS

416. Albanese A, Lorenze E, Edelson A, et al: Calcium nutrition and skeletal and alveolar bone health. *Nutr Rep Int* 1985;31:741–755.

417. Albanese A, Edelson A, Lorenze E, et al: Problems of bone health in the elderly: A ten year study. *NYSJ Med* 1975;75:326.
    See also reference 101.

CHAPTER 5: HAIR PROBLEMS

418. Gummer C: Diet and hair loss. *Sem Derm* 1985;4:35–39.

CHAPTER 5: HEADACHES

419. de Belleroche J, Cook G, Das I, et al: Erythrocyte choline concentrations and cluster headaches. *Br Med J* 1984;288:268–270.
420. Harrison D: Copper as a factor in the dietary precipitation of migraine. *Headache* 1986;26:248–250.
421. McCarron T, Hitzemann R, Smith R, et al: Amelioration of severe migraine by fish oil (omega 3) fatty acids. *Am J Clin Nutr* 1986;43:710.
422. Diamond S: Diet and headache. *Nutr Rep* 1987;5:12–13.
423. Cornwell N, Clarke L, VanNunen S: Intolerance to dietary chemicals in recurrent idiopathic headache. *Clin Pharm* 1987;41:201.
424. Lipton R, Newman L, Cohen J, et al: Aspartame as a dietary trigger of headache. *Headache* 1989;29:90–92.
    See also references 60 and 289.

CHAPTER 5: HEARING DISORDERS

425. Davis M. Kane R, Valentine J: Impaired hearing in X-linked hypophosphataemic (vitamin D-resistant) osteomalacia. *Ann Int Med* 1984;100: 230–232.
426. Wang Y, Yang S: Improvement in hearing among otherwise normal school children in iodine-deficient areas of China. *Lancet* 1985;II:518–520.
427. Milman N, Scheibel N, Jessen O: Lysine prophylaxis in recurrent herpes simplex labialis. *Acta Derm Venereol* 1980;60:85–87.
    See also references 21 and 71.

CHAPTER 5: HERPES SIMPLEX

428. Thein D, Hurt W: Lysine as a prophylactic agent in the treatment of recurrent herpes simplex labialis. *Oral Surg* 1984;58:659–666.
429. Armstrong E, Elenbaas J: Lysine for herpes simplex virus. *Drug Intel Clin Pha* 1983;39:186.

CHAPTER 5: HYPERTENSION

430. Henry H, McCarron D: Diet and hypertension: An update on recent research. *Cont Nutr* 1982;7:1–2.
431. Berchtold P: Obesity and hypertension: Conclusions and recommendations. *Int J Obesity* 1981;5(suppl 1):183.

432. Garrison R, Somer E: *The Nutrition Desk Reference*. New Canaan, CT, Keats Publishing Co, 1985, pp 155–158.

433. Basta L: Regression of atherosclerotic stenosing lesions of the renal arteries and spontaneous cure of systemic hypertension through control of hyperlipidemia. *Am J Med* 1976;61:420–421.

434. Bompiani G, Cerasota G, Morici M, et al: Effects of moderate low sodium/high potassium diet on essential hypertension: Results of a comprehensive study. *Int J Cl Ph* 1988;26:129–132.

435. Kurtz T, Albander H, Morris R: Dietary chloride as a possible determinant of NaCl-sensitive essential-hypertension in man. *Kidney Int* 1986;29:250.

436. Resnick L, Nicholson J, Laragh J: Outpatient therapy of essential hypertension with dietary calcium supplementation. *J Am Col Cardiology* 1984;3:616.

437. Kok F, VandenBroucke J, van der Heide-Wessel C, et al: Dietary sodium, calcium, and potasssium, and blood pressure. *Am J Epidem* 1986;123:1043–1048.

438. Morris C, Karanja N, McCarron D: Dietary vs supplemental calcium to reduced blood pressure. *Clin Res* 1988;36:139A.

439. Resnick L: Divalent cations in essential hypertension—Relations between serum ionized calcium, magnesium, and plasma renin activity. *New Engl J Med* 1983;309:888–891.

440. Altura B: Magnesium ions and contraction of vascular smooth muscles: Relationship to some vascular diseases. *Fed Proc* 1981;40:2672.

441. Dyckner Y, Wester P: Effect of magnesium on blood pressure. *Br Med J* 1983;286;1847–1849.

442. Sheenan J: Magnesium deficiency and diuretics. *Br Med J* 1983;286:390.

443. Altura B, Altura B, Carella A, et al: Hypomagnesiumemia and vasocontriction: Possible relationship to etiology of sudden death ischemic heart disease and hypertensive vascular disease. *Artery* 1981;9:212–231.

444. Singer P, Wirth M, Voigt S, et al: Blood pressure and lipid-lowering effect of mackerel and herring diet in patients with mild essential hypertension. *Atheroscler* 1985;56:223–235.

See also references 190, 199, 200, 206, and 209.

CHAPTER 5: INFECTION

See references 24 and 271–277.

CHAPTER 5: INSOMNIA

See references 128 and 413.

CHAPTER 5: JET LAG

See reference 413.

CHAPTER 5: KIDNEY DISORDERS

445. Ono K: Reduced osmotic hemolysis and improvement of anemia by large dose vitamin E supplementation in regular hemodialysis patients. *Kidney Int* 1984;26:583.
446. Vathsala R, Sindhu S, Sachidev K, et al: Pyridoxine in the long-term follow up of crystalluric patients. *Urol Res* 1988;16:249.
    See also references 77, 140, 177, and 178.

CHAPTER 5: LIVER DISORDERS

447. Senoo H, Wake K: Suppression of experimental hepatic fibrosis by administration of vitamin A. *Lab Inv* 1985;52:182–194.

CHAPTER 5: LUNG DISORDERS

448. Shariff R, Hoshino E, Allard J, et al: Vitamin E supplementation in smokers. *Clin Res* 1988;36:A770.
449. Bai T, Martin J: Effects of indomethacin and ascorbic acid on histamine induced bronchoconstriction. *NZ Med J* 1986;99:163.
450. Copper deficiency and developmental emphysema. *Nutr Rev* 1983;41:318–420.
451. Gerhardsson L, Brune D, Nordberg I, et al: Protective effect of selenium on lung cancer in smelter workers. *Br J Ind Me* 1985;42:617–626.

CHAPTER 5: LUPUS ERYTHEMATOSUS

452. Tappel A: Vitamin E as the biological lipid antioxidant. Symposium on vitamin E and metabolism, Zurich, Switzerland. *Vitam Hor* 1962;20:493.
453. Silver S, Feigenbaum H: Chronic discoid lupus erythematosus successfully treated with vitamin E. *Arch Derm* 1950;61:163.

454. Ayres S, Mihan R: Lupus erthyematosus and vitamin E: An effective and non-toxic therapy. *Cutis* 1972;23:49–53.
455. Vien C, Gonzalez-Cabello R, Bodo I, et al: Effect of vitamin A treatment on the immune reactivity of patients with systemic lupus erythematosus. *J Clin Lab* 1988;26:33–35.
See also reference 90.

CHAPTER 5: OSTEOMALACIA

456. Rudolf M, Arulanantham K, Greenstein R: Unsuspected nutritional rickets. *Pediatrics* 1980;66:72.
457. Omdahl J, Garry P, Hunsaker L, et al: Nutritional status in a healthy elderly population: Vitamin D. *Am J Clin Nutr* 1982;36:1225–1233.

CHAPTER 5: OSTEOPOROSIS

458. Recker R: Osteoporosis. *Cont Nutr* 1983;8:1–2.
459. Albanese A: Diet and bone fractures. *Nutr Rep* 1986;4:84–85
460. Fanelli M: Promoting women's health. *Dietetic Currents* 1985;12–4: 19–24.
461. Osteoporosis-consensus Conference: *JAMA* 1984;252:799–802.
462. Riis B, Thomsen K, Christiansen C: Does 24R,25(OH)2-Vitamin D_3 prevent postmenopuasal bone loss? *Calcif Tis Int* 1986;39:128–132.
463. Orwoll E, McCling M, Oviatt S: Therapy of severe postmenopausal osteoporosis with 25-OH vitamin D: A two year placebo-controlled double-blinded study. *Clin Res* 1986;34:63A.
464. MacLaughlin J, Holick M: Aging decreases the capacity of human skin to produce vitamin D_3. *J Clin Inv* 1985;76:1536–1538.
465. Dodds R, Catterall A, Bitensky L, et al: Osteolytic retardation of early stages of fracture healing by vitamin B_6 deficiency. *Clin Sci* 1985;68:21P.
466. Jackson T, Ullrich I: Understanding osteoporosis. *Postgraduate Medicine* 1984;75:119–125.
467. Ettinger B, Cann C, Genant H: Menopausal bone loss: Effects of conjugated estrogen and/or high calcium diet. *Maturitas* 1984;6:108–109.
468. Wasserman S, Barzel U: Osteoporosis: The state of the art in 1987: A reveiw. *Sem Nuc Med* 1987;17:283–292.
469. Strause L, Hegenauer J, Saltman P, et al: Effects of long-term dietary manganese and copper deficiency on rat skeleton. *J Nutr* 1986;116:135–141.
470. Fluoride and osteoporosis. *Nutr and MD* 1979;5:5.
471. Brautbar N, Gruber H: Magnesium and bone disease. *Nephron* 1986;44:1–7.
See also references 65, 223, and 229.

CHAPTER 5: PREMENSTRUAL SYNDROME (PMS)

472. Abraham G: Premenstrual tension. *Curr Prob in Obstet Gynecol* 1980;3: 5–8
473. Kerr G: The managment of premenstrual syndrome. *Current Medical Research and Opinion* 1977;4(supple 4):29.
474. Block E: The use of vitamin A in premenstrual tension. *Acta Obstet el Gyne Scand* 1960;39:586.
475. Michaelsson G, Juhlin L, Vahlquist A: Effects of oral zinc and vitamin A in acne. *Arch Dermatol* 1977;113:31–36.
476. London R: Nutritional intervention and the premenstrual syndrome. *Nutr Rep* 1986;4:92–95.
477. Bradley L, Reynolds M, London R: Efficacy of a multivitamin/mineral supplement in the treatment of premenstrual syndrome. *J Am Col N* 1988;7:416.
    See also references 141, 142, 202, and 203.

CHAPTER 5: PSORIASIS

478. Newborg B: Disappearance of psoriatic lesions on the rice diet. *NC Med J* 1986;47:253–254.
479. Burton C: Disappearance of psoriatic lesions in 73 year old man treated by rice diet for 8 weeks. *NC Med J* 1986;47:255.
480. Morimoto S, Yoshikawa K, Kozuka T, et al: An open study of vitamin D_3 treatment in psoriasis vulgaris. *Br J Derm* 1986;115:421–429.
481. Kato T, Rokugo M, Terui T, et al: Successful treatment of psoriasis with topical application of active vitamin D_3 analogue, 1 alpha 24-dihydroxycholecalciferol. *Br J Derm* 1986;115:431–433.
482. Takamoto S, Onishi T, Morimoto S, et al: Effect of 1-alpha hydroxy-cholecalciferol on psoriasis vulgaris: A pilot study. *Calcif Tis* 1986;39:360–364.
483. Vahlquist C, Berne B, Boberg M, et al: The fatty acid spectrum in plasma and adipose tissue in patients with psoriasis. *Arch Dermatol Res* 1985;278:114–119.
484. Allen B, Maurice P, Goodfield M, et al: The effects on psoriasis of dietary supplementation with eicosapentaenoic acid. *Br J Derm* 1985;113:777.
485. Ziboh V, Miller C, Kragballe K, et al: Effects of an 8 week dietary supplementation of eicosapentaenoic acid in serum PMNs and epidermal fatty acids of psoriatic subjects. *J Inves Der* 1985;84:300.

CHAPTER 5: SICKLE CELL ANEMIA

486. Heyman M, Katz R, Hurst D, et al: Growth retardation in sickle cell disease treated by nutritional support. *Lancet* 1985;1:903–906.
487. Jain S, Williams D: Reduced levels of plasma ascorbic acid (vitamin C) in sickle cell disease patients: Its possible role in oxidant damage to sickle cells in vivo. *Clin Chem A* 1985;149:257–261.
See also references 110 and 228.

CHAPTER 5: STRESS

488. Nakano K, Mizutani R: Decreased responsiveness of pituitary-adrenal axis to stress in vitamin A-depleted rats. *J of Nutr Sci* 1983;29:353–363.
489. Suzuki S, Nakano K: Decrease in urinary excretion of ascorbic acid and histamine in rats after repeated immobilization stress. *J Nutr* 1984;114:441–446.
490. Christiansen L, Krietsch K, White B, et al: Impact of a dietary change on emotional distress. *J Abn Psych* 1985;94:565–579.
491. Hornig D: Metabolism of ascorbic acid. *World Rev Nutr Diet* 1975;23:225–228.
492. Kallner A: Influence of vitamin C status on the urinary excretion of catecholamines in stress. *Human Nutr: Clin Nutr* 1983;37:405–411.
493. Boosalis M, Konstantinides L, Salem F, et al: Vitamin balance in trauma/surgery: Are current multivitamin preparations adequate? *Fed Proc* 1987;46:1010.
494. Seelig M: Magnesium requirments in human nutrition. *Cont Nutr* 1982;7:1–2.
495. Classen H: Stress and magnesium. *Artery* 1981;9:182–189.
496. Chutkow J, Grabow J: Clinical and chemical correlations in magnesium-deprivation encephalopathy of young rats. *Am J Phys* 1972;223:1407–1414.
497. Dickerson R, Brown R: Hypomagnesiumemia in hospitalized patient receiving nutritional support. *Heart Lung* 1985;14:561–569.
498. Fawaz F: Zinc deficiency in surgical patients: A clinical study. *JPEN* 1985;9:364–369.
499. Anderson R, Polansky M, Bryden N: Strenuous running: Acute effects of chromium, copper, zinc and selected clinical variables in urine and serum of male runners. *Biol Trace El Res* 1984;6:327–336.

CHAPTER 5: THYROID DISORDERS

500. Dolev E, Deuster P, Solomen B, et al: Alterations in magnesium and zinc metabolism in thyroid disease. *Metab* 1988;37:61–67.

CHAPTER 6: OVERVIEW

501. Hall R: Psychiatric and physiological reactions produced by over the counter drugs. *J Psychedelic Drugs* 1978;10:423–426.
502. The big picture: Volume up, Rx activity is unchanged. *Drug Topics* 1987;16 March:36.
503. Garrison R, Somer E: *The Nutrition Desk Reference.* New Canaan, CT, Keats Publishing Co, 1985, pp 209–210.
504. Roe D: *Drug-induced Nutritional Deficiencies.* Westport, CT, The AVI Publishing Co, 1983, p 39.
505. Statistical Abstracts of the United States. US Dept of Commerce. Bureau of the Census, 1980.
506. Chien C, Townsend E, Townsend A: Substance use and abuse among the community elderly: The medical aspect. *Addict Dis* 1978;3:357–372.
507. Guttman P: Patterns of legal drug use by older Americans. *Addict Dis* 1978;3:337–356.

CHAPTER 6: ALCOHOL

508. Grummer M, Erdman J: Effect of chronic alcohol consumption and moderate fat diet on vitamin A status in rats fed either vitamin A or beta carotene. *J Nutr* 1983;113:350–364.
509. Dworkin B, Rosenthal W, Jankowski R, et al: Low blood selenium levels in alcoholics with and without advanced liver disease: Correlations with clinical and nutritional status. *Dig Dis Sci* 1985;30:838–844.
510. Johansson U, Johnsson F, Joelsson B, et al: Selenium status in patients with liver cirrhosis and alcoholism. *Br J Nutr* 1986;55:227–233.
511. Dworkin B, Rosenthal W, Gordon G, et al: Diminished blood selenium levels in alcoholics. *Alc Clin Ex* 1984;8:535–538.
512. Collipp P, Kris V, Castro-Magana M, et al: The effects of dietary zinc deficiency on voluntary alcohol drinking in rats. *Alc Clin Ex* 1984;8:556–559.
513. Milne D, Canfield W, Gallagher S, et al: Metabolism of ethanol in post-menopausal women fed a diet marginal in zinc. *Clin Res* 1986;34:A801. *See also reference 93.*

CHAPTER 6: ANTACIDS

514. Spencer H, Norris C, Coffey F, et al: Effect of small amounts of antacids on calcium, phosphorus and fluoride metabolism in man. *Gastroent* 1975;68:990.

515. Blood W, Flinchum D: Osteomalacia with pseudofractures caused by the ingestion of aluminum hydroxide. *JAMA* 1960;174:1327.
516. Goulding A, McIntosh J, Campbell D: Effect of sodium bicarbonate and 1,25 dihyroxycholecalciferol on calcium and phosphorus balances in the rat. *J Nutr* 1984;114:653–659.
517. Benn A, Swan C, Cooke W, et al: Effect of intraluminal pH on the absorption of pterylmonoglutamic acid. *Br Med J* 1971;1:148.
518. McGuigan J: A consideration of the adverse effect of cimetidine. *Gastroent* 1980;80:181.
See also reference 198.

CHAPTER 6: ANTIBIOTICS

519. Garrison R, Somer E: *The Nutrition Desk Reference.* New Canaan, CT, Keats Publishing Co, 1985, pp 209–218.

CHAPTER 6: ANTICONVULSANTS

520. Gough H, Bissesar A, Goggin T, et al: Factors associated with the biochemical changes in vitamin D and calcium metabolism in institutionalized patients with epilepsy. *Irish J Med* 1986;155:181–189.
521. Roe D: Drug-food and drug-nutrient interactions. *J Env P Tox* 1985;5:115–135.
522. Fincham R, Berg M, Ebert B, et al: The effect of various doses of phenytoin on folic acid serum concentrations in normal volunteers. *Epilepsia* 1986;27:592–593.
523. Baum C, Selhub J, Rosenberg I: Antifolate actions of sulfasalazine on intact lymphocytes. *J Lab Clin Med* 1981;97:779.
524. Werther C, Cloud H, Ohtake M, et al: Effect of long term administration of anticonvulsants on copper, zinc, and ceruloplasmin levels. *Drug Nutr* 1986;4:269–274.
525. Coppen A, Chaudhry S, Swade C: Folic acid enhances lithium prophylaxis. *J Affect D* 1986;10:9–13.
526. Stewart J: Phenelzine-induced pyridoxine deficiency. *J Clinical Psychopharmacology* 1984;4:225–226.

CHAPTER 6: ARTHRITIS MEDICATIONS

527. *Facts and Comparisons: Drug Information.* St Louis, JB Lippincott Co, 1985, p 715.

CHAPTER 6: ASPIRIN

528. Rettura G, Stratford F, Padawer J, et al: Vitamin A protects against aspirin toxicity. *J Am Col N* 1984;3:291–292.
529. Franklin J, Roseberg I: Impaired folic acid absorption in inflammatory bowel disease: Effects of salicylazosulfapyridine (Azulfidine). *Gastroenterology* 1973;64:517–525.
530. Schreurs W, Egger R, Wedel M, et al: The influence of radiotherapy and chemotherapy on the vitamin status of cancer patients. *Int J Vit Nutr Res* 1985;55:425–432.
531. Dudrick S, O'Donnell J, Claque M: Nutritional rehabilitation of the cancer patient. 13th International Cancer Congress, Part K—Research and Treatment, 1983, pp 161–170.
532. Van Eys J: Effect of nutrition on response to therapy. *Cancer Res* 1982;42:7475.
533. Klein S, Simes J, Blackburn G: Total parenteral nutrition and cancer clinical trials. *Cancer* 1986;58:1378–1386.

CHAPTER 6: MEDICATIONS FOR CARDIOVASCULAR DISEASE

534. East C, Grundy S, Bilheimer D: Preliminary report: Treatment of type 3 hyperlipoproteinemia with mevinolin. *Metabolism* 1986;35:97–98.
535. Facts and Comparisons: Drug Information. St. Louis, JB Lippincott, 1987, p 171.
536. Brown B, Albers J, Brunzell J: Normalization of elevated apoliprotein-B with niacin plus colestipol in subjects with familial-combined hyperlipidemia. *Atherosclerosis* 1983;3:A477.
See also reference 519.

CHAPTER 6: ORAL CONTRACEPTIVES

537. Adams P: Effect of pyridoxine hydrochloride (vitamin B_6) upon depression associated with oral contraception. *Lancet* 1973;I:897–904.
538. Baumblatt M, Winston F: Pyridoxine and the pill. *Lancet* 1970;I:832–833. *See also reference 519.*

CHAPTER 6: MEDICATIONS FOR HYPERACTIVITY

539. Safer D, Allan R, Barr E: Depression of growth in hyperactive children on stimulant drugs. *New Eng J Med* 1972;287:217–220.

CHAPTER 6: HYPERTENSIVE MEDICATIONS

540. Demartini F, Briscoe A, Ragan C: Effect of ethacrynic acid on calcium and magnesum excretion. *Proc Soc Exp Biol Med* 1967;124:320–324.
541. Lim P, Jacob E: Magnesium deficiency in patients on long-term diuretic therapy for heart failure. *Br Med J* 1972;3:620–622.
542. Wester P: Zinc during diuretic treatment. *Lancet* 1975;I:578.
543. McLean C, Williams R, Aviv A, et al: Effect of captopril on the metabolism of some trace elements in the rat. *Trace Elem Med* 1985;2:175–178. *See also references 439–443 and 519.*

CHAPTER 6: TOBACCO

544. Brook M, Grimshaw J: Vitamin C concentration of plasma and leukocytes as related to smoking habit, age, and sex of humans. *Am J Clin Nutr* 1968;21:1254–1258.
545. Smith J: The impact of smoking on serum vitamin C levels. *Fed Proc* 1984;43:861.
546. Davis C, Brittain E, Hunninghake D, et al: Relation between cigarette smoking and serum vitamin A and carotene in candidates for the Lipid Research Clinics Coronary Prevention Trial. *Am J Epidem* 1983;118:445.
547. Stich H, Hornby A, Dunn B: Beta carotene levels in exfoliated mucosa cells of population groups at low and elevated risk for oral cancer. *Int J Canc* 1986;37:389–393.
548. Kuhnert B, Kuhnert P, Lazebrik N, et al: The effect of maternal smoking on the relationship between maternal and fetal zinc status and infant birth weight. *J Am Col N* 1988;7:309–316.
549. Second-hand smoke. Take a look at the facts. American Lung Association. 1982.

CHAPTER 6: WEIGHT CONTROL "DIET" MEDICATIONS

550. Frewin D: Phenylpropanolamine: How safe is it? *Med J Austral* 1983;July 23:54–55.

CHAPTER 7

551. The confusing world of health foods. FDA Consumer 1979; July, HHS Publication No.(FDA) 84–2108.

552. Wilmore J, Freund B: Nutritional enhancement of athletic performance. *Nutr Abst Rev Clin Nutr* 1984;54:2–12.
553. Loucks A, Horvath S: Athletic amenorrhea: A review. *Med Sci Spt* 1985;17:56–72.
554. Bone loss and amenorrheic athletes. *Nutr Rev* 1986;44:361– 363.
555. Vallerand A: Influence of exercise training on tissue chromium concentrations in the rat. *Am J Clin Nutr* 1984;39:402–409.
556. van Rij A, Hall M, Dohm G, et al: Changes in zinc metabolism following exercise in human subjects. *Biol Tr El* 1986;10:99–105.
557. Lamanca J, Haymes E, daly J, et al: Sweat iron loss of male and female runners during exercise. *Int J Sports Med* 1988;9:52–55.
558. Stendig-Lindberg G, Shapiro Y, Epstein Y, et al: Changes in serum magnesium concentration after strenuous exercise. *J Am Col N* 1987;6:35–40.
559. Watson N: Hemoglobin levels and nutritional iron requirements in college runners. *Ohio State Med J* 1979;January:13–14.
560. Eichner E: Runner's macrocytosis: A clue to footstrike hemolysis. *Am J Med* 1985;78:321–325.
561. Lampe J, Slavin J, Apple F: Poor iron status of women runners training for a marathon. *Int J Sp M* 1986;7:111–114.
562. Jackson M: Muscle damage during exercise: Possible role of free radicals and protective effects of vitamin E. *P Nutr Soc* 1987;46:77–80.
563. Aikawa K: Exercise endurance-training alters vitamin E tissue levels and red blood cell hemolysis in rodents. *Bioscience Rep* 1984;4:253–257.
564. van der Beek B, van Dokkum W, Schrijver J, et al: Impact of marginal vitamin intake on physical performance in healthy young men. *P Nutr Soc* 1985;44:A27.
565. Gohil K, Packer L, deLumen B, et al: Vitamin E deficiency and vitamin C supplements: Exercise and mitochondrial oxidation. *J App Physl* 1986;60:1286–1991.
566. Hickson J, Schrader J, Trischler L: Dietary intakes of female basketball and gymnastics athletes. *J Am Diet Assoc* 1986;86:251–252.
567. Green D, Gibbons C, O'Toole M, et al: Trends in the nutritional intakes of triathletes. *Fed Proc* 1987;46:1165.
568. Barnett D, Conlee R: The effects of a commerical dietary supplement on human performance. *Am J Clin Nutr* 1984;40:586–590.
569. van Erp-Baart A, Saris W, Binkhorst R, et al: Nationwide survey on nutritional habits in elite athletes. II: Mineral and vitamin intake. *Int J Sports Med* 1989;10:S11–S16.
570. Vorster H, Lotter A, Odendaal I: Effects of an oats fiber tablet and wheat bran in healthy volunteers. *S Afr Med J* 1986;69:435–438.
571. Anderson J: High-fiber, hypocaloric vs very-low calorie diet effects on blood pressure of obese men. *Clin Res* 1986;34:A794.
572. Heaton K: Intestinal carcinogenesis: The role of diet. *Br J Canc* 1986;54:138.
573. Doyle R: *The Vegetarian Handbook: A Guide To Vegetarian Nutrition*. New York, Crown Publishers, 1979, pp 25–36.

574. Braunstein G, Koblin R, Sugawara M, et al: Unintentional thyrotoxicosis factitia due to a diet pill. *West J Med* 1986;145:388–391.
575. Somer E: Tryptophan supplements: Unfairly accused. *Nutr Rep* 1991;January:2.
576. Clauw D, Nashel D, Umhau A, et al: Tryptophan-associated eosinophilic connective tissue disease: A new clinical entity. *J Am Med A* 1990;263;1502–1506.
577. Fischer M, LaChance P: Nutrition evaluation of published weight reducing diets. *J Am Diet Assoc* 1985;85:45–454.
578. Blackburn G: Protein requirements with very low calorie diets. *Postg Med J* 1984;60:59–65.
579. Tognarelli M, Miccoli R, Giampietro O, et al: Guar pasta: A new diet for obese subjects? *Act Diabet* 1986;23:77–80.
580. McLaren M: *Weight Loss and Nutrition.* San Diego, Health Media of America, 1986.
581. Blundell J, Hill A: Paradoxical effects of an intense sweetener (aspartame) on appetite. *Lancet* 1986;I:1092–1093.
See also references 95, 113, 215, 349, 375–378, 439–442, and 499.

CHAPTER 8

582. Anon: Vitamin B$_6$ toxicity: A new megavitamin syndrome. *Nutr Rev* 1984;42:44–46.
583. Alhadeff L, Gualtieri T, Lipton M: Toxic effects of water-soluble vitamins. *Nutr Rev* 1984;42:33–40.
584. Garrison R, Somer E: *The Nutrition Desk Reference.* New Canaan CT, Keats Publishing Co, 1985, pp 36–83.
585. Baker H, Bhagavan H, Machlin L: Biological activities of d and dl forms of vitamin E: Comparison of plasma tocopherol levels following oral administration in humans. *Fed Proc* 1985;44:935.
586. Chan A, Luttinger-Basch C: Vitamin E inhibits platelet phospholipase A2 in vivo and in vitro: Demonstration of potency difference between RRR tocopherol and all-rac tocopherol. *Fed Appl Biol Sci Abst* 1983;302:8.
587. Horwitt M, Elliott W, Kanjanangulpan P, et al: Serum concentrations of alpha-tocopherol after ingestion of various vitamin E preparations. *Am J Clin Nutr* 1984;40:240.
588. Knopp R, Ginsaber J, Albers J, et al: Contrasting effects of unmodified and time-release forms of niacin on lipoproteins in hyperlipidemic subjects: Clues to mechanism of action of niacin. *Metabolism* 1985;34:642–650.
589. Clarke J, Kies C: Niacin nutritional status of adolescent humans fed high-dosage of pantothenic acid supplements. *Nutr Rep In* 1985;31:1271–1279.

590. American Cancer Society Special Report: Nutrition and Cancer: Cause and Prevention. New York, American Cancer Society Inc, February 10, 1984.

591. Qureshi A, Din Z, Abvirmeileh N, et al: Suppression of avian hepatic lipid metabolism by solvent extracts of garlic: Impact on serum lipid. *J Nutr* 1983;113:1746–1755.
See also references 123, 124, and 130.

CHAPTER 9

592. Borisov I: Vitamin P in the nutrition of athletes. *Vopr Pitan* 1980:1:35–38.

593. Kellis J Jr, Vickery C: Inhibition of human estrogen synthetase (aromatase) by flavones. *Science* 1984;225:1032.

594. Buell D: Potential hazards of selenium as a chemopreventive agent. *Sem Oncol* 1983;10:311–321.

595. Consumer Reports. 1979, September, p 508.

596. Shannan B, Parks S: Fast foods: A perspective on their nutritional impact. *J Am Diet Assoc* 1980;76:242.

597. Disler P: The effect of tea on iron absorption. *Gut* 1975;16:193–200.

598. Morck D: Inhibition of food iron absorption by coffee. *Am J Clin Nutr* 1983;37:416–420.

599. Stich H, Rosin M, Vallejera M: Reduction with vitamin A and beta carotene administration of proportion of micronucleated buccal mucosal cells in asian betal nut and tobacco chewers. *Lancet* 1984;II:1204–1206.

600. Dworkin B, Rosenthal W, Gordon G, et al: Diminished blood selenium levels in alcoholics. *Alc Clin Ex* 1984;8:535–538.

601. Lieber C: Alcohol-nutrition interaction. *Cont Nutr* 1983;8:1–2.

602. Swarth J: *Skin, Hair, and Nails and Nutrition*. San Diego, Health Media of America, Inc, 1986, pp 1–44.

603. Sheehan J, White A: Diuretic associated hypomagnesemia. *Br Med J* 1982;285:1157–1159.

604. Peck G, Olson T, Yoder F, et al: Prolonged remissions of cystic and conglobate acne with 13-cis-retinoic acid. *N Eng J Med* 1979;300:329.

605. Haydey R, Reed M, Denbow L, et al: Treatment of keratoacanthomas with oral 13-cis-retinoic acid. *N Eng J Med* 1980;303:560.

606. Bieri J, Corash L, Hubbard V: Medical uses of vitamin E. *N Eng J Med* 1983;308:1063–1071.

607. Traber M, Kayden H, Green J, et al: Bioavailability of vitamin E, administered orally as tocopheryl polyethylyene glycol 1000 succinate (TPGS) to a vitamin E-deficient patient with cholestasis. *Am J Clin N* 1986;43:82.

608. Dillard C: Relative antioxidant effectiveness of alpha-tocopherol and gamma-tocopherol in iron-loaded rats. *J Nutr* 1983;113:226–227.

609. Baker H, Bhagavan H, Machlin L: Biological activities of d and dl forms

of vitamin E: Comparison of plasma tocopherol levels following oral administration in humans. *Fed Proc* 1985;44:935.

610. Horwitt M, Elliott W, Kanjananggulpan P, et al: Serum concentrations of a-tocopherol after ingestion of various vitamin E preparations. *Am J Clin Nutr* 1984;40:240.

611. Herbert V: Drugs effective in megaloblastic anemias. Vitamin B_{12} and folic acid. In: Pharmacological Basis of Therapeutics, fifth editon. Goodman L, Gilman A, eds. New York, Macmillan Publishing Co, 1975, pp 1324–1338.

612. Ellis F, Nasser S: A pilot study of vitamin B_{12} in the treatment of tiredness. *Br J Nutr* 1973;30:277–283.

613. Bonemeal. FDA Consumer Update, July 5, 1982.

614. Consumer Reports, New York, Consumers Union, September, 1982.

615. Crosby W: Lead contaminated health food. *J Am Med Assoc* 1977; 237:2627–2629.

616. Hallberg L, Norrby A. Solvell L: Oral iron with succinic acid in the treatment of iron deficiency anemia. *Scand J Haematol* 1971;8:104.

617. Song M, Adham N, Ament M: A possible role of zinc on the intestinal calcium absorption mechanisms. *Nutr Rep Int* 1985;31:43–51.

618. Calcium: How much is enough? *Nutr Rev* 1985;43:345–346.

619. Kent S: Can nucleic acid therapy reverse the degenerative process of aging? *Geriatrics* 1977;32:130–136.

620. Much-Petersen S: RNA treatment of dementia. *Acta Neurologica Scand* 1974;50:553–572.

621. Zarafonetis C: Darkening of gray hair during para-aminobenzoic acid therapy. *J Invest Dermatol* 1950;15:399–410.

622. Sunscreens. *Medical Letter on Drugs and Therapeutics* 1979;2:46–48.

623. Barrett-Connor E: A prospective study of dehydroepiandrosterone sulfate, mortality, and CVD. *N Eng J Med* 1986;315:1519–1524.

624. Weiner M: Cholesterol in foods rich in omega-3 fatty acids. *N Eng J Med* 1986;315:833.

Glossary

Acetylcholine: A neurotransmitter associated with the regulation of numerous body processes including memory.

Acid: A chemical substance that contains hydrogen atoms and usually tastes sour. Hydrochloric acid in the stomach, vinegar, and acetic acid are examples of acids. An acid has a pH of less than 7.0.

Acid-Base Balance: The equilibrium between acids and bases (alkaline) in the body.

Acidosis: A disorder caused by low alkalinity of the blood and the body where the normal pH falls below 7.0.

Acromegaly: A disease of the pituitary gland that results in excessive growth of the bones.

Acute: Sharp and severe onset of disease.

Additive: A chemical substance added to food, either intentionally or unintentionally.

Adrenal Gland: A ductless gland located near the kidneys, which produces/secretes hormones, including adrenalin and the corticosteroid hormone cortisone.

Adrenalin: A hormone secreted by the adrenal glands that aids in the release of stored sugar in the liver, contraction of muscles, and increased blood supply to the muscles all in response to stress.

Aerobic: In the presence of oxygen. Aerobic exercise is any slow, steady exercise, such as walking, jogging, swimming, or bicycling, that requires constant long-term use of large muscle groups.

Aflatoxin: A carcinogenic mold found in stale nuts and other foods.

Alkaline: A chemical substance called a base that will neutralize an acid to form a salt. Baking soda is an example of an alkaline substance. Alkaline compounds have a pH of more than 7.0.

Alkalosis: A disturbance of the body's natural acid-base balance that results in sweating, vomiting, and diarrhea.

Alveolar: The jaw bone where the sockets of the teeth are situated.

Alveoli: Tiny air-filled sacs in the lungs.

Amino Acid: A building block or precursor of protein. More than 20 amino acids are used by the body to manufacture different proteins in hair, skin, blood, and other tissues.

Amphetamine: A synthetic drug used to stimulate the nervous system, reduce appetite, and increase blood pressure.

Amylase: An enzyme in saliva that aids in the digestion of carbohydrates.

Anabolic Steroids: Hormones, such as testosterone, that encourage the development of muscle.

Anabolism: The portion of metabolism where simple molecules are combined to form complex structures. For example, the joining of numerous amino acids to form a protein is an anabolic process.

Analgesic: A medication that relieves pain.

Anaphylactic Shock: An immediate and severe allergic reaction, which results in collapse of an individual and sometimes death.

Anemia: A reduction in the size, number, or color of red blood cells that results in reduced oxygen-carrying capacity of the blood.

Angina Pectoris: Chest pain after mild to vigorous exercise or excitement, caused by reduced blood supply to the heart from obstruction of the arteries.

Anorexia: The lack or loss of appetite for food, associated with weight loss and muscle wastage.

Anthropometric: Measurements of the body, such as height, weight, and skin fold.

Antibiotic: A substance that inhibits the growth of or destroys microorganisms. Medications used to treat infectious diseases in plants, animals, and humans.

Antibody: A substance in body fluids that is a component of the immune system and protects the body against disease and infection.

Anticoagulant: A substance that slows or prevents blood clotting.

Anticonvulsant: An agent that prevents or relieves convulsions.

Antineuritic: A substance that prevents or treats nervous system disorders.

Antioxidant: A compound that protects other compounds or tissues from oxygen fragments by reacting with the oxygen.

Apathy: Showing little feeling or emotion. Indifferent.

Appetite: The desire to eat that normally accompanies hunger.

Arrhythmia: Irregular heart beat.

Arteriosclerosis: A general term for hardening and thickening of the arteries.

Artery: A blood vessel that supplies blood, oxygen, and nutrients to the tissues.

Ascorbic Acid: Vitamin C.

Atherosclerosis: A form of arteriosclerosis, characterized by the accumulation of fat in the artery wall. It is the underlying cause of cardiovascular disease.

Atom: The smallest particle of nature that can exist and still retain the chemical characteristics of an element.

Autism: A condition where the individual is socially withdrawn.

Autoimmunity: A condition where the immune system attacks organs or tissues of the body as if they were foreign invaders.

Avidin: A protein in raw egg white that binds biotin in the small intestine and reduces its absorption.

Bacteria: Microscopic one-celled organism found in food, the body, and all living matter.

Balanced Diet: A diet that supplies optimal amounts in appropriate ratios to each other of all the known essential nutrients.

Basal Metabolism: Energy used for internal or cellular work, including the heart beat and the repair and maintenance of tissues. Also called basal metabolic rate.

Base: An alkaline substance.

Beriberi: A disease caused by a deficiency of vitamin B_1 (thiamin) and characterized by nerve disorders, weakness, mental disturbances, dermatitis, and heart failure.

Beta Carotene: The form of vitamin A found in dark green and orange vegetables and fruits.

Beta Cells: Specific cells in the pancreas that produce insulin.

Bile: An emulsifying fluid produced from cholesterol in the liver and stored in the gall bladder to be secreted into the intestine as a digestive aid when fatty food is present.

Biological Activity or Bioavailability: The potency of a vitamin or mineral within the body.

Blood Brain Barrier: A semi-permeable series of barriers that acts as a gatekeeper to monitor and separate the body and its supply of substances and nutrients from the brain.

Bronchial Tubes: The two main branches of the trachea leading to the lungs.

Bronchitis: Inflammation of the mucous membranes in the lungs.

Bulimia: An eating disorder characterized by excessive food intake followed by vomiting, laxative use, or fasting.

Calcify: The deposition of calcium into a tissue.

Calorie: A measurement of heat. In nutrition, calorie actually refers to kilocalorie (kcalorie) and signifies the amount of energy contained in food.

Candidiasis: An infection by a fungus called candida. The infection can occur in the lungs, heart, vagina, gastrointestinal tract, skin, nails, or other tissues.

Capillary: A tiny blood vessel that joins arteries and veins. Capillaries are the site in the blood vessel system where oxygen and nutrients are released from the blood into the tissues.

Carbohydrate: The starches and sugars in the diet.

Carbon Dioxide: One of the waste products of cellular metabolism that is carried from the cells by the blood through the veins back to the heart to be exhaled through the lungs.

Carcinogen: A substances that causes cancer.

Cardiomyopathy: Damage to the heart.

Cardiovascular Disease: A disease of the heart and blood vessels often caused by the accumulation of cholesterol in the lining of the blood vessels.

Catabolism: The breakdown of complex substances to simple molecules and atoms and the release of energy. For example, glucose is catabolized to water, carbon dioxide, and energy.

Carotene: The building block for vitamin A, called a provitamin, found in dark green and orange vegetables. See beta carotene.

Cataracts: A milky film that forms over the eye and is one of the most common forms of visual loss.

Celiac Disease: An intestinal disorder brought on by a sensitivity to a protein called gliadin, and characterized by diarrhea, weight loss, anemia, and bone pain. Celiac disease requires lifelong diet therapy.

Cell-Mediated Immunity: The aspect of the immune response that occurs in the tissues and includes T lymphocytes and interferon.

Cell Membrane: The outer covering of each cell composed of fats and proteins.

Cellulose: A plant-derived carbohydrate composed of glucose, which is indigestible to humans.

Cervix: The neck or opening to the uterus.

Chelate: To combine a metal with another compound.

Chemotherapy: The treatment of a disorder with medication; usually refers to cancer therapy.

Chlorophyll: The green color in plants where photosynthesis takes place. Chlorophyll is essential to the formation of carbohydrates in plants.

Cholesterol: A type of fat found in foods from animal origin and produced in the liver. High levels of cholesterol in the blood are associated with an increased risk for cardiovascular disease. Cholesterol, unlike other fats, does not supply calories.

Chronic: Long-term. Cardiovascular disease and diabetes are chronic diseases.

Cilia: Hair-like projections that protrude from cell membranes of the lungs and intestine and which move in a rhythmic fashion to propel substances either out of the lungs or along the intestinal tract.

Circadian Rhythm: Cycles that occur approximately every 24 hours in the body.

Cirrhosis: Inflammation or fatty infiltration of the liver, usually as a result of alcohol or drug abuse.

Clinical: Pertaining to the observable signs of a disease.

Cobalamin: Vitamin B_{12}.

Cochlea: A fundamental organ of hearing located within the ear and shaped like a snail shell.

Co-enzyme: A compound required in order for an enzyme to function. Many of the B vitamins are co-enzymes.

Collagen: A protein in connective tissues and the organ substance in teeth and bones.

Colostrum: A thin fluid secreted from the mother's breast for the first few days after birth prior to full lactation.

Complex Carbohydrate: Starches and carbohydrate-like fibers.

Complimentary Protein: Two or more proteins whose amino acid composition complement each other so that the essential amino acids missing from one are supplied by the other. Examples include whole wheat bread and cooked dried beans.

Congestive Heart Failure: A condition where the efficiency of the circulatory system declines as a result of heart failure.

Conjunctivitis: Inflammation of the mucous membrane covering the outer surface of the eye.

Connective Tissue: A web-like tissue located in every organ that binds and supports the various tissues within the organ.

Cornea: The exposed and transparent portion of the eyeball.

Corticosteroid: Any steroid which has certain chemical or biological properties characteristic of the hormones secreted by the adrenal glands.

Cretinism: Severe mental retardation of an infant caused by iodine deficiency during pregnancy.

Cystitis: Inflammation of the urinary bladder.

Dehydration: Loss of water from food or the body.

Delaney Clause: A clause in the Food Additive Amendment to the Food, Drug, and Cosmetic Act that states no substance can be added to foods that is known to cause cancer at any dose.

Dementia: Insanity or memory loss.

Dental Pulp: The soft tissue under the calcified enamel and dentin.

Dentin: The calcified tissue below the enamel of teeth that forms the greatest portion of the tooth structure.

Detoxify: To transform a toxic substance in the body into a form more easily excreted.

Diabetes: An hereditary metabolic disease characterized by inadequate supply of the hormone insulin or insensitivity of the cell's to insulin's action. The result is inability to regulate blood sugar levels.

Diastolic Blood Pressure: The blood pressure in the heart and arteries when the heart relaxes between contractions.

Diuretic: An agent that increases the flow of urine and reduces the amount of water in the body.

Dopamine: A neurotransmitter and intermediate compound in the manufacture of adrenalin.

Dowager's Hump: The hunched appearance common in people with osteoporosis. The posture is further altered by collapse of the chest and protrusion of the abdomen.

Down's Syndrome: A syndrome of congenital defects that includes mental retardation and characteristic physical deformities.

Eclampsia: A disorder that sometimes develops in the later portion of pregnancy and is characterized by high blood pressure, protein in the urine, edema, salt retention, convulsions, and sometimes coma. Also called toxemia.

Edema: The abnormal accumulation of water in the tissues.

Electrocardiogram (EKG): A graphic depiction on an electrocardiograph of the electrical impulses corresponding to the heartbeat.

Electrolyte: A substance or salt that dissolves into positive or negative charged particles and conducts an electrical charge. Sodium, potassium, and chloride are examples of electrolytes.

Electrolyte Balance: The distribution of electrolytes (salts) among the body fluids.

Emulsification: To disperse one liquid into a second liquid, such as oil into water.

Emulsifier: A compound that holds an oily substance in suspension in a watery fluid, such as lecithin used in commercial oil and vinegar salad dressings. Bile is an emulsifier.

Enamel: The hard, calcified outer layer of the teeth.

Endocrine Glands: Ductless glands that secrete hormones, which in turn have profound effects on the regulation of body processes.

Energy: The ability to do work.

Energy Nutrient: A nutrient that provides energy the body can use. Carbohydrate, protein, and fat.

Epithelial Tissue: The cells of most of the body surfaces, including the skin, eyes, and linings of the lungs, intestinal tract, and urinogenital tract. Examples of endocrine glands include, ovaries, testes, thyroid, and pancreas.

Extrinsic Factor: The name given to vitamin B_{12}.

Endorphins: A group of neurotransmitter-like substances that produce a calming effect on the brain much like morphine.

Energy: The capacity to do work.

Enkephalins: A group of neurotransmitter-like substances that have a calming effect on the brain.

Enriched: The addition to processed foods of a few nutrients to bring the level back to the original vitamin or mineral content. Not all nutrients usually are added back in the enrichment process.

Enzyme: Protein-like substances in the body that initiate and accelerate chemical reactions.

Epinephrine: Adrenalin. A hormone secreted by the adrenal glands that aids in the release of stored sugar in the liver, contraction of muscles, and increased blood supply to the muscles all in response to stress.

Epithelial: The internal and external surfaces of the body, including the skin, lining of the blood vessels, and outer surface of the eye.

Esophagus: The passageway or tube from the throat to the stomach.

Essential Fatty Acid: A fat that cannot be manufactured by the body, i.e., linoleic acid found in safflower oil.

Essential Nutrient: A substance required by the body in minute amounts for growth, maintenance, and repair and that must be supplied in the diet.

Extracellular: Outside the cells. Extracellular fluid includes the blood, lymph, and fluid between the cells (interstitial fluid).

Extrinsic: From outside the body.

Fatty Acid: A fat-soluble molecule that consists of a long chain of carbon atoms with hydrogens attached. Three fatty acids combined to a glycerol molecule comprise a triglyceride. Eicosapentaenoic acid (EPA) and linoleic acid are fatty acids.

Ferrous: Iron.

Fiber: The indigestible residue of food, composed of the carbohydrates cellulose, pectin, and hemicellulose, and the noncarbohydrate lignin.

Flatulence: Distension of the stomach or intestine with air or gas.

Folacin: Folic acid.

Follicle: A small cavity that secretes a substance.

Food and Drug Administration (FDA): An agency of the United States government responsible for monitoring the safety and effectiveness of food, drugs, and cosmetics sold in the United States.

Food Intolerance: Inability to digest a food as a result of individual chemical idiosyncrasies, food contamination, psychological factors, or digestive enzyme deficiencies. Lactose intolerance is a food intolerance resulting from inadequate amounts of the digestive enzyme lactase.

Fortified: The addition of vitamins or minerals to a processed food to levels higher than naturally found. Milk is fortified with vitamin D.

Free Radical: A highly reactive compound derived from air pollution, radiation, cigarette smoke, or the incomplete breakdown of proteins and fats. Free radicals react with fats in cell membranes to change their shape and function and cause irreversible damage.

Fructose: A simple sugar or carbohydrate sometimes known as fruit sugar.

Galactose: A simple sugar or carbohydrate. Part of the sugar lactose.

Gangrene: Inadequate blood supply to a tissue that results in the death of that tissue.

Gastritis: Inflammation of the stomach.

Gastrointestinal Tract: The stomach and intestinal tract.

Genetics: The branch of biology that studies heredity and biological variation.

Glaucoma: An eye disease characterized by increasing pressure within the eye and degeneration of the optic nerve.

Glucose: Sugar; blood sugar; the building block of starch.

Glucose Tolerance Factor (GTF): A compound containing chromium that aids the hormone insulin in regulating blood sugar levels.

Glutathione Peroxidase: An antioxidant enzyme.

Glycogen: The storage form of glucose in the body. Glycogen is formed and stored in the liver and muscles and is converted to glucose when energy is needed.

Goiter: Enlargement of the thyroid gland caused by iodine deficiency.

Goitrogen: A substance in food and in some medications that promotes goiter.

Gram: A unit of weight. Twenty-eight grams equal one ounce.

Growth Hormone: A hormone produced in the brain that promotes growth and aids in the regulation of carbohydrates, fat, and protein.

Hard Water: Water with a high calcium and magnesium concentration.

Hematocrit: The volume percent of red blood cells in blood.

Heme Iron: Iron associated with hemoglobin in red blood cells. This form of iron found in meat, chicken, and fish and is well absorbed.

Hemochromatosis: A condition where excessive absorption of iron results in altered skin coloring and abnormal iron deposition in liver and other tissues.

Hemosiderosis: A disorder of iron metabolism where excessive iron is deposited into the liver and other tissues resulting in altered functioning of these tissues.

Hemoglobin: The oxygen-carrying protein in red blood cells. Each molecule of hemoglobin contains four atoms of iron.

Hemolytic: Separation of hemoglobin from the red blood cell as in hemolytic anemia caused by a vitamin E deficiency.

Hemorrhage: Seepage of blood from the blood vessels into the surrounding tissues.

Hepatitis: Inflammation of the liver.

HDL-Cholesterol: Cholesterol packaged in high-density lipoproteins. HDL is comprised of fats and protein and serves as a transport for fats in the blood.

A high level of HDL is associated with a reduced risk for developing cardio-vascular disease.

Homeostasis: The maintenance of a balanced state in the body regulated by automatic adjustment of physiological processes and feedback mechanisms.

Homocysteine: A by-product of the amino acid methionine.

Homocysteinuria: An inherited disorder characterized by excessive amounts of homocysteine in the urine, mental retardation, and blood clot formation.

Hormone: A substance produced by an organ called an endocrine gland that is released into the blood and transported to another organ or tissue, where it performs a specific action. Examples of hormones include adrenalin and estrogen.

Humoral: Immunity and resistance to infection and disease maintained by antibodies produced by B lymphocytes and other cells in the bloodstream.

Huntington's Disease: An inherited disorder of the nervous system characterized by mental retardation and emotional disturbances in adulthood.

Hyperglycemia: High blood sugar levels.

Hyperoxaluria: Excessive accumulation of oxalates in the urine, associated with kidney stone formation.

Hypertension: High blood pressure.

Hypoglycemia: Low blood sugar levels.

Immune System: A complex system of substances and organs that protect the body against disease and infection.

Immunity: The body's resistance to disease provided by a complex system of specialized cells, tissues, organs, and chemicals, such as antibodies and interferon.

Inborn Errors of Metabolism: Inherited or congenital disorders in how the body metabolizes a substance. For example, phenylketonuria (PKU) is a disorder where the body does not metabolize the amino acid phenylalanine and its toxic metabolites accumulate in the body.

Indoles: A group of compounds in cruciferous vegetables (vegetables in the cabbage family) associated with a reduced risk for developing cancer.

Insomnia: Inability to sleep, to stay asleep, or to fall asleep.

Insulin: A hormone produced by the pancreas that regulates blood sugar levels.

Interferon: A substance in the body formed in response to a virus, or other invading agent, that prevents the virus from multiplying. A component of the cell-mediated immune response.

Intermittent Claudication: Cramps and weakness in the legs induced by walking, relieved by rest, and associated with atherosclerosis.

International Unit (IU): An arbitrary unit of measurement that signifies biological activity used for the fat-soluble vitamins A, D, and E.

Interstitial Fluid: The fluid in the spaces between the cells.

Intracellular: Inside the cell.

Intrinsic: Inside the body.

Intrinsic Factor: A factor manufactured in the stomach that attaches to vitamin B_{12} and facilitates its absorption in the intestine.

Jaundice: The appearance of bile in the blood, indicating liver disease.

Keratin: A tough form of protein found in skin, hair, nails, and feathers.

Keratinization: The formation of a toughened tissue from overproduction of keratin. A symptom of vitamin A deficiency.

Ketoacidosis: A condition where the body becomes too acidic with accompanying increases in ketones in the blood. Also called ketosis.

Ketogenic Diet: A diet where a large portion of the calories comes from fat, which are converted to ketones in the body. Sometimes used in the treatment of epilepsy.

Ketones: Intermediate products of fat metabolism, acetone, or acetoacetic acid.

Kilocalorie: The amount of heat required to raise 1,000mg of water 1 degree Centigrade. Kilocalorie (kcalorie) and calorie are used interchangably in nutrition.

Lactation: Breastfeeding.

Lactose: The sugar found in milk.

Lacto-Ovo Vegetarian Diet: A diet that omits meat, chicken, and fish and is derived from fruit, vegetables, whole grain breads and cereals, nuts, seeds, eggs, and dairy products.

Larynx: The organ of the voice located in the throat.

L-Dopa: A neurotransmitter and intermediate metabolite of adrenalin.

Lecithin: A fatty substance that also contains a water-soluble component containing phosphorus. Lecithin is a constituent of cell membranes, is manufactured in the liver, and is found in food.

Legume: A plant of the bean or pea family having roots that can "fix" nitrogen, thus making these plants a good source of protein. Examples of legumes include dried beans and peas.

Lethargy: Tired, sluggish, lack of energy.

Leukotriene: A group of hormone-like substances involved in inflammation and produced from polyunsaturated fatty acids.

Linoleic Acid: An essential polyunsaturated fatty acid.

Lipid: Fat, including triglycerides, phospholipids, and cholesterol.

Lipoprotein: A compound comprised of fat and protein that carries fats, such as triglycerides and cholesterol, in the blood.

LDL-cholesterol: Low density lipoprotein. A molecule comprised of fats and protein that transports cholesterol in the blood. A high level of LDL is associated with an increased risk for developing cardiovascular disease.

Lymph: The fluid in the lymphatic vessels and lymph sacs. A colorless fluid derived from the blood that is filtered through special vessels and nodes to remove debris and cellular waste products. The filtered lymph is returned to the blood.

Lymphocyte: A specialized white blood cell that is a component of the immune system and aids in the protection of the body against disease and infection. There are B lymphocytes and T lymphocytes.

Lymphoma: Cancer of the lymph tissue.

Macrocytic: Large cell.

Macrophages: A large blood cell involved in the immune response and the body's resistance to infection and disease.

Megadose: Large intake of a nutrient; more than ten times the RDA for a vitamin or mineral.

Megaloblastic Anemia: Anemia characterized by large, misshapen red blood cells that results from a deficiency of folic acid or vitamin B_{12}.

Major Mineral: An essential mineral found in the body in amounts greater than 0.0005% of body weight.

Menstrual: Pertaining to menstruation or the monthly discharge of blood and tissue from the uterus occurring between puberty and menopause.

Menstruation: The monthly discharge of blood and tissue from the uterus.

Metabolism: The total of all body processes, whereby the body converts foods into tissues and breaks down and repairs tissues and converts complex substances into simple ones for energy.

Metabolite: Any product of metabolism.

Metastasis: The migration of a disease from the original site to a distant tissue by way of the bloodstream or lymph system.

Microgram (mcg): A metric unit of weight equivalent to 1/1000th of a milligram or one millionth of a gram.

Microorganism: Minute plants or animals, such as bacteria or viruses, that are visible only through a microscope.

Milligram (mg): A metric unit of weight equivalent to 1/1000th of a gram.

Mineral: An inorganic, fundamental substance found naturally in the soil with specific chemical and structural properties. Many minerals are essential nutrients for growth, maintenance, and repair of tissues.

Minimum Daily Requirements: An outdated system of nutrient requirements based on the minimum amount of nutrient necessary to prevent clinical signs of deficiency.

Molecule: Two or more atoms. The number and type of atoms varies with the compound. Examples of molecules include amino acids, calcium carbonate, the vitamins, carbohydrate, glucose, and fatty acids.

Monocytes: A specialized white blood cell important in the immune response.

Monounsaturated Fat: A type of fat that has one spot on the fatty acid for the addition of a hydrogen atom. An example of a monounsaturated fat is oleic acid in olive oil.

Mucus: A substance secreted by epithelial cells composed of carbohydrates called mucopolysaccharides.

Myelin: A sheath surrounding nerve cells that speeds the transmission of nerve impulses.

Myoglobin: An oxygen-storing compound within some cells, especially muscle cells.

Nasal: Pertaining to the nose.

Neuritis: Inflammation or infection of the nerves.

Neuromuscular: The junction where a nerve cell meets a muscle cell.

Neuropathy: Any non-inflammatory disease of the peripheral (hands and feet) nerves.

Neurotransmitter: A chemical that serves as a communication link between nerve cells or between a nerve cell and a muscle or organ. Serotonin and dopamine are examples of neurotransmitters.

Niacin Equivalent: The unit of measure of the niacin activity in food, computed by adding the amount of niacin preformed in the food plus the amount the body produces from ingested tryptophan.

Night Blindness: A symptom of vitamin A deficiency.

Nitrosamine: A carcinogenic substance found in foods and cigarette smoke and formed in the stomach from nitrites in foods.

Norepinephrine: A neurotransmitter that aids in the regulation of blood pressure and numerous body processes.

Nucleic Acid: A component of deoxyribonucleic acid (DNA) and ribonucleic acid (RNA), the genetic code found in every cell.

Nucleus: The center of each cell that contains the genetic code.

Nutrient: A substance in food that provides the body with energy, helps in the regulation of metabolism, or builds, maintains, or repairs tissues.

Nutrient Density: A relatively high proportion of nutrients for the calories provided.

Nutritious Food: A food that provides a high quantity of one or more essential nutrients, with a small quantity of calories. (See Nutrient Density.)

Obesity: Body fat weight more than 20% above ideal body weight.

Opiate: A substance that has a calming effect on the nervous system.

Oral: Pertaining to the mouth.

Organic: A substance that contains carbon.

Ovary: A glandular organ in the female reproductive system that produces the ovum (egg) and secretes the female hormones estrogen and progesterone.

Over-The-Counter Medications (OTC): Non-prescription medications.

Oxalate: Compounds in some plants, such as spinach and chard, that bind to minerals in the intestine and reduce their absorption.

Ozone: A highly reactive modification of oxygen whereby the two atoms in oxygen (O_2) are increased to three (O_3).

Palpitation: A fluttering or throbbing of the heart associated with irregular heart beat.

Pancreas: The organ responsible for the production and secretion of numerous digestive enzymes and the hormone insulin.

Parathyroid Gland: A gland in the body that secretes a hormone called parathyroid hormone that regulates calcium metabolism.

Pellagra: A disease caused by a deficiency of niacin and characterized by dermatitis, mental disorders, diarrhea, and weakness.

Periodontal Disease: Diseases of the tissues (periodontium) that surround the teeth.

Pernicious Anemia: A type of macrocytic or megaloblastic anemia caused by a deficiency of vitamin B_{12} or intrinsic factor necessary for vitamin B_{12} absorption.

Peroxide: One of a number of highly reactive free radicals.

Petechial Hemorrhages: Minute spots of hemorrhage below the skin, associated with a vitamin C deficiency.

pH: A symbol used to express the hydrogen-ion concentration and therefore the acidity or alkalinity of a substance. A pH below 7 is associated with increasing acidity and a pH above 7 is associated with increasing alkalinity.

Pharmacologic Agent: A substance with drug-like activity.

Phlegm: A thick fluid secreted by the mucous glands of the air passages. One of the four humors that caused disease described in ancient medicine.

Phospholipid: A fatty substance that has a fat-soluble end and a water-soluble end and that is an essential part of cell membranes.

Phytate: A compound in unleavened whole grains that binds to minerals in the intestine and inhibits their absorption.

Pica: The practice of eating non-food items, such as dirt or clay.

Placebo: A medicine or pill that has no pharmacologic effect, but is given to please or humor the patient.

Placebo Effect: The healing effect that faith in medicine or supplementation, even inert medicine, often has.

Plaque: An accumulation of fat, calcium, and other substances in the lining of the artery.

Platelets: Blood cell fragments that aid in blood coagulation and wound healing under normal circumstances.

Polycythemia: The presence of excessive amounts of red blood cells in the blood.

Polydipsia: Excessive thirst persisting for long periods of time.

Polyphagia: Excessive hunger persisting for long periods of time.

Polyuria: Excessive urination.

Postmenopausal: After the menopause.

Precursor: A substance used as a building block for another substance. Linoleic acid is a precursor for prostaglandins, tryptophan is the precursor for serotonin and niacin.

Premenopausal: Prior to the onset of menopause.

Primary Deficiency: A nutrient deficiency caused by inadequate dietary intake of a nutrient.

Prostaglandin: A group of hormone-like substances formed from polyunsaturated fatty acids that have a profound effect on the body, including contraction of smooth muscle and dilation or contraction of blood vessels in the regulation of blood pressure.

Protease: An enzyme that breaks down proteins to small fragments during digestion and absorption.

Prothrombin: A protein in blood necessary for normal blood clotting.

Provitamin: A substance in food that can be converted to a vitamin once it enters the body. Beta carotene is the provitamin for vitamin A.

Rectum: The lower portion of the large intestine extending to the anal canal.

Refined: The process whereby the coarse parts of plants are removed. For example, the refining of whole wheat into white wheat flour involves removing three of the four parts of the kernel: the chaff, the bran, and the germ, leaving only the endosperm or high-carbohydrate inner core.

Regional Ileitis: A chronic inflammation of the small intestine characterized by cramping, abdominal pain, diarrhea, fever, and loss of appetite.

Renal: Pertaining to the kidney.

Replication: To reproduce.

Requirement: The amount of a nutrient that will prevent clinical deficiency symptoms, in contrast the recommendation (i.e., RDAs), which contains a generous allowance.

Respiratory Tract: Pertaining to the lungs and its passageways.

Retina: The layer of light-sensitive cells lining the back of the inside of the eye.

Retinoic Acid: A form of vitamin A.

Retinol: Vitamin A.

Retinol Equivalents (RE): A unit of measurement for vitamin A; one RE is equivalent to 1 mcg or 3.33IU of vitamin A as retinol.

Retinopathy: A disease of the retina of the eye.

Riboflavin: Vitamin B_2.

Rickets: Abnormal bone development caused by a deficiency of vitamin D.

Salt: A compound composed of a positive and a negative electrical charge. For example sodium (has a positive charge) and chloride (has a negative charge) comprise table salt.

Saturated Fat: A type of fat that is solid at room temperature and is found in foods from animal sources, hydrogenated vegetable oils, and coconut or palm oil. A diet high in saturated fats is linked to the development of cardiovascular disease.

Sciatica: Pain associated with inflammation of the sciatic nerve often resulting from a damaged spinal disc and characterized by tingling, numbness, and tenderness along the nerve.

Scurvy: A diseased caused by a deficiency of vitamin C and characterized by bleeding gums, loosened teeth, small hemorrhages below the skin, and weakness.

Sebaceous Glands: Glands in the skin that secrete a greasy lubricating substance called sebum.

Sebum: An oily secretion from the sebaceous glands of the skin.

Secondary Deficiency: A nutrient deficiency caused by something other than diet, such as a disease condition that reduces absorption or excessive intake of another nutrient.

Serotonin: A neurotransmitter produced in the brain that regulates mood, sleep, and numerous other body processes.

Serum: The fluid portion of blood that is left after the clotting factors have been removed. Serum is a straw colored fluid with red blood cells.

Sinusitis: Inflammation of the sinus.

Skeletal: The bones.

Soft Water: Water with low calcium and magnesium concentrations.

Spleen: The largest lymphatic tissue in the body which is responsible for red blood formation.

Sprue: An intestinal disorder characterized by malabsorption of foods and nutrients.

Steatorrhea: Excessive amount of fat in the stool.

Sterol: A general term for compounds that resemble cholesterol, such as the sex hormones, bile acids, vitamin D, and certain adrenal hormones, such as the corticosteroids.

Strict Vegetarian Diet: A diet that contains only foods of plant origin, such as whole grain breads and cereals, cooked dried beans and peas, fruits, vegetables, and nuts and seeds. Also called a vegan diet.

Subclinical Deficiency: A nutrient deficiency that does not produce overt physical symptoms.

Sublingual: Beneath the tongue.

Superoxide Dismutase (SOD): An antioxidant enzyme.

Superoxides: A group of highly reactive compounds called free radicals.

Synthesize: The process of combining two or more substances into a new compound in the body.

Systolic Blood Pressure: The maximum pressure in the heart and arteries when the heart contracts.

Tannin: Tannic acid. A yellowish, astringent compound in tea.

Tetany: Intermittent, painful spasms of the muscles.

Therapeutics: The art of healing.

Thiamin: Vitamin B_1.

Thromboxane: A prostaglandin that causes constriction of blood vessel walls and encourages platelets to clump at the site of a damaged artery.

Thymus Gland: A gland located in the front, upper portion of the chest.

Thyroid Gland: A major endocrine gland in the body located in the front of the throat and responsible for regulation of metabolism and other endocrine glands and their hormones.

Thyroxin: The hormone of the thyroid gland.

Tocopherol: Vitamin E.

Toxemia: A disorder that sometimes develops in the later portion of pregnancy characterized by the symptoms of eclampsia, such as high blood pressure, protein in the urine, edema, salt retention, convulsions, or sometimes coma.

Toxicity: The ability of a substance to cause harmful effects. Any substance is toxic if consumed in high enough concentrations.

Trace Mineral: An essential mineral found in the body in amounts less than 0.0005% of body weight.

Triglyceride: One of the three classes of fats. Triglycerides are composed of three fatty acids (tri) and one glycerol (glyceride) molecule. They are either saturated or unsaturated.

Tyramine: A metabolite of the amino acid tyrosine which is found in foods, such as cheese and red wine.

Tryptophan: An amino acid essential for life and converted in the body to the B vitamin niacin.

Ulcer: Damage to epithelial tissues, such as the skin or lining of the stomach or small intestine, characterized by pain and inflammation.

Unsaturated Fat: A type of fat that is liquid at room temperature and is primarily found in foods of plant origin, such as vegetable oils, nuts, and seeds.

Urea: The main nitrogen-containing excretion product of metabolism, generated primarily by the breakdown of amino acids.

Ureters: The tubes that transport fluids from the kidney to the urinary bladder.

Urethra: The canal through which the urine is excreted from the body.

Urinary: Pertaining to urine.

Urticaria: An allergic skin disorder characterized by itching and reddened patches.

USRDA: The RDA figures used on labels. In most cases, the highest RDA suggested in the RDA tables for any age or gender group is used for the USRDA.

Vegan: A strict vegetarian who consumes no foods of animal origin.

Vein: A blood vessel that carries blood, carbon dioxide, and other waste products from the tissues to the heart and lungs.

Virus: Any of a large group of minute particles that are capable of infecting plants, animals, and humans.

Vitamin: An essential nutrient which must be obtained from the diet and is required by the body in minute amounts.

VLDL-cholesterol: Cholesterol carried in the blood by a type of lipoprotein that is made in the liver and is converted to LDL-cholesterol.

Wernicke-Korsakoff Syndrome: A disorder associated with excessive alcohol consumption and characterized by loss of coordination and memory.

Whole Grain: An unrefined grain that retains its edible outside layers (the bran) and the highly nutritious inner germ.

Xerophthalmia: A disease that impairs vision and is caused by a deficiency of vitamin A. This disorder is characterized by a thickening and inflammation of the outer surface of the eye.

Index

391

Index

About the Author

Elizabeth Somer, M.A., R.D. is a consulting nutritionist and author of several books, including *Cholesterol and Nutrition*; *Vitamins, Minerals, and Nutrition*; *Cancer and Nutrition*; and *Prescription Drugs and Nutrition*. She is co-author of the *Nutrition Desk Reference*, *The Lifestyle Resource Manual*, and *The Nutrition Resource Manual*. Ms. Somer is Editor-in-Chief of Health Media of America's Nutrition Book Series and the "Nutrition Report," a monthly publication that summarizes the current nutrition and health research from more than 6,000 journals.

Ms. Somer is a registered dietitian and holds a master's degree in Community Health from Ohio State University. For the past 15 years she has been active in the nutrition and health education fields, including work with the Dairy Council, public health departments, the Pritikin Program, medical centers and hospitals, and numerous universities. Ms. Somer has worked closely with cardiac, diabetic, hypertensive, cancer, and weight-management patients in the control of their disorders through lifestyle modification.